Paramedic Care: Principles & Practice

Fifth Edition

Volume 2

Patient Assessment

BRYAN E. BLEDSOE, DO, FACEP, FAAEM, EMT-P
Professor of Emergency Medicine
University of Nevada, Las Vegas School of Medicine
University of Nevada, Reno School of Medicine
Attending Emergency Physician
University Medical Center of Southern Nevada
Medical Director, MedicWest Ambulance
Las Vegas, Nevada

RICHARD A. CHERRY, MS, EMT-P
Director of Training
Northern Onondaga Volunteer Ambulance
Liverpool, New York

LEGACY AUTHOR

ROBERT S. PORTER

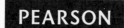

Boston   Columbus   Indianapolis   New York City   San Francisco
Amsterdam   Cape Town   Dubai   London   Madrid   Milan   Munich   Paris   Montréal   Toronto
Delhi   Mexico City   São Paulo   Sydney   Hong Kong   Seoul   Singapore   Taipei   Tokyo

Publisher: Julie Levin Alexander
Publisher's Assistant: Sarah Henrich
Editor: Sladjana Repic Bruno
Editorial Assistant: Lisa Narine
Development Editors: Sandra Breuer and
  Deborah Wenger
Director, Publishing Operations: Paul DeLuca
Team Lead, Program Management: Melissa Bashe
Team Lead, Project Management: Cynthia Zonneveld
Manufacturing Buyer: Maura Zaldivar-Garcia
Art Director: Mary Siener
Cover and Interior Designer: Mary Siener
Managing Photography Editor: Michal Heron

Vice President of Sales & Marketing: David Gesell
Vice President, Director of Marketing: Margaret Waples
Senior Field Marketing Manager: Brian Hoehl
Marketing Assistant: Amy Pfund
Senior Producer: Amy Peltier
Media Producer and Project Manager: Lisa Rinaldi
Full-Service Project Manager: Amy Kopperude/
  iEnergizer Aptara®, Ltd.
Composition: iEnergizer Aptara®, Ltd.
Printer/Binder: LSC Communications
Cover Printer: LSC Communications
Cover Image: ollo/Getty Images, Rudi Von Briel/
  Getty Images

Notice

Library of Congress Cataloging-in-Publication Data

Names: Bledsoe, Bryan E., author. | Cherry, Richard A., author. |
  Porter, Robert S., author.
Title: Paramedic care : principles & practice | Bryan E. Bledsoe,
  Richard A. Cherry, Robert S. Porter.
Description: Fifth edition. | Boston : Pearson Education, Inc., 2016- |
  Includes bibliographical references and index.
Identifiers: LCCN 2016009904 | ISBN 9780134569956 (pbk. : alk. paper) |
  ISBN 0134569954 (pbk. : alk. paper)
Subjects: | MESH: Emergencies | Emergency Medical Services | Emergency
  Medical Technicians
Classification: LCC RC86.7 | NLM WB 105 | DDC 616.02/5—dc23 LC record available
  at http://lccn.loc.gov/2016009904

Brady
is an imprint of

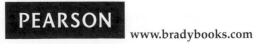

www.bradybooks.com

23 2022
ISBN 10:   0-13-456995-4
ISBN 13: 978-0-13-456995-6

This text is respectfully dedicated to all EMS personnel who have made the ultimate sacrifice. Their memory and good deeds will forever be in our thoughts and prayers.

BEB, RAC

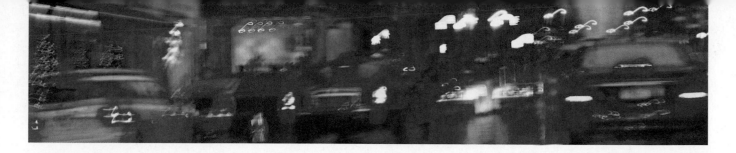

Contents

5 Secondary Assessment **70**

6 Patient Monitoring Technology **171**

7 Patient Assessment in the Field 221

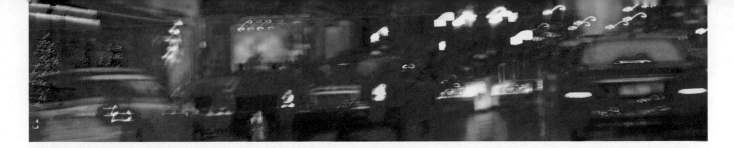

Preface to Volume 2

Today's paramedics are professional health care clinicians and practitioners of emergency field medicine. The present paramedic curriculum provides both a broad-based medical education and a specific intensive training program designed to prepare paramedics to perform their traditional role as providers of emergency field medicine. The curriculum also provides a broad foundation in anatomy and physiology, patient assessment, pathophysiology of disease, and pharmacology that allows paramedics to expand their roles in the health care industry. The five-volume *Paramedic Care: Principles & Practice* series and, in particular, *Volume 2, Patient Assessment,* reflect these broad and specific purposes.

This volume provides paramedic students with the principles of patient assessment. The first two chapters discuss scene size-up and primary assessment. The next three chapters present the techniques of conducting a comprehensive secondary assessment, along with history and physical exam, and discuss communication techniques for doing so. The sixth chapter presents an overview of patient monitoring technologies. The final chapter discusses ways to apply the techniques learned in this volume to real patient situations.

Overview of the Chapters . . . and What's New in the 5th Edition?

CHAPTER 1   Scene Size-Up discusses scene size-up in the overall context of an emergency call. On arrival at the scene, paramedics must quickly determine whether the scene is safe. They must identify indications of potential hazards, determine mechanism of injury or nature of illness, identify all patients involved, determine the need for additional resources, make decisions about Standard Precautions and personal protective equipment, and communicate their findings to the dispatcher. The chapter analyzes how to take actions that ensure the safety of both the EMS team and the patients in a variety of scenarios. **New in**

the 5th Edition: Emphasis on **ongoing scene safety assessment** throughout the call (not just on arrival).

CHAPTER 2   Primary Assessment examines how to conduct a primary assessment to identify and intervene in immediate threats to life. The first steps are identifying threats to airway, breathing, and circulation—or, in certain circumstances, circulation, airway, and breathing. The paramedic must form a general impression of the patient's condition; stabilize the cervical spine; assess baseline mental status; and assess and manage airway, breathing, and circulation. The results of the primary assessment will be used to determine the priorities of patient care and transport.

New in the 5th Edition: For significant mechanism of injury, change from recommending full immobilization to **deciding whether or not to immobilize the patient according to local protocols**. Discussion of how to use **pulse oximetry and continuous waveform capnography in evaluation of breathing adequacy**. For hemorrhage control, **updated sequence**: (1) direct pressure; and if not effective, then (2) **tourniquet** for extremity wounds or hemostatic agents for wounds to other site. **Transport triage for burns guidelines:** burns without other trauma to burn facility; burns with other trauma to trauma facility.

CHAPTER 3   Therapeutic Communications describes effective therapeutic communication strategies. This chapter provides techniques for decreasing the barriers to effective communication, building trust and rapport with patients, using nonverbal communication and responding to patients' nonverbal behaviors, and conducting patient interviews. Also discussed are ways to adapt these strategies to patients of all ages and cultures, and to patients with special challenges.

New in the 5th Edition: New emphasis on **eye contact** as the most powerful way to convey caring. Emphasis on **using language the patient can understand**, which may vary with the patient's age or other circumstances.

CHAPTER 4   History Taking discusses the components of the patient history. These components include preliminary data, the chief complaint, the present problem, the past medical history, family and social history, and the review of body systems. This constitutes a comprehensive history and is not meant to be used in its entirety in emergency field situations. Elements of the comprehensive history will be used, as appropriate, in the field.

CHAPTER 5 Secondary Assessment presents the techniques of conducting a comprehensive physical exam. Like the history, the comprehensive physical exam taught in this volume is not intended for all situations. With time and clinical experience, you will learn which components of the history and physical exam are appropriate to assess and manage each particular patient and situation. Topics in this chapter include applying the techniques of inspection, palpation, percussion, and auscultation and assessing the skin, the head, the neck, the chest (along with the respiratory and cardiovascular systems), the abdomen and digestive system, the extremities and musculoskeletal system, and the peripheral vascular system, as well as conducting a comprehensive neurologic exam. Included in each section is a review of the anatomy and physiology relevant to those areas of the exam.

CHAPTER 6 Patient Monitoring Technology covers the latest in high-tech methods for obtaining patient information. The chapter discusses continuous and 12-lead ECG monitoring, pulse and CO-oximetry, capnography, methemoglobin and total hemoglobin monitoring, glucometry, basic blood chemistries, and portable ultrasound.

New in the 5th Edition: New section on **Point of Care (POC) Testing**—performing basic blood chemistry analysis in the field with the use of portable analyzers. Completely revised and updated section on the use of **ultrasound technology** in the field to assist in assessing such factors as **internal abdominal bleeding, abdominal aortic aneurysm, impaired cardiac function, possible pneumothorax, heart failure, distinguishing cardiac from non-cardiac shock, confirming endotracheal tube placement,and obstetric factors such as early pregnancy, ectopic pregnancy, and fetal conditions**.

CHAPTER 7 Patient Assessment in the field offers a practical approach to conducting problem-oriented history and physical exams. It deals with ways to use your new skills to assess patients in the field. With time and clinical experience, you will learn which components are appropriate for different situations. Topics include scene safety, the primary assessment, the secondary assessment (for the responsive medical patient, the unresponsive medical patient, the trauma patient with significant mechanism of injury, and the trauma patient with an isolated injury), the detailed physical exam, and the reassessment.

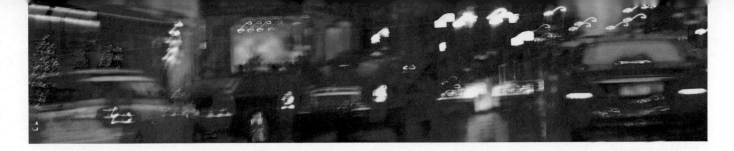

Acknowledgments

Chapter Contributors

We wish to acknowledge the remarkable talents of the following people who contributed to this five volume series. Individually, they worked with extraordinary commitment. Together, they form a team of highly dedicated professionals who have upheld the highest standards of EMS instruction.

Paul Ganss, MS, NRP (Volume 1, Chapter 2)

Michael F. O'Keefe (Volume 1, Chapter 5)

Wes Ogilvie, MPA, JD, LP (Volume 1, Chapter 7)

Kevin McGinnis, MPS, EMT-P (Volume 1, Chapter 9)

Jeff Brosious, EMT-P (Volume 1, Chapter 10)

W.E. Gandy, JD, NREMT-P (Volume 1, Chapter 15)

Darren Braude, MD, MPH, FACEP (Volume 1, Chapter 15)

Joseph R. Lauro, MD, EMT-P (Volume 2, Chapter 6)

Brad Buck, NRP, CCEMT-P (Volume 3, Chapter 10)

Bryan Bledsoe, DO, FACEP, FAAEM, EMT-P (Volume 4, Chapter 10)

Andrew Schmidt, DO, MPH (Volume 4, Chapter 10)

Justin Sempsrott, MD (Volume 4, Chapter 10)

David Nelson, MD, FAAP, FAAEM (Volume 5, Chapter 4)

Mike Abernethy, MD, FAAEM (Volume 5, Chapter 10)

Ryan J. Wubben, MD, FAAEM (Volume 5, Chapter 10)

Louis Molino, NREMT-I (Volume 5, Chapter 11)

Dale M. Carrison, DO, FACEP, FACOEP (Volume 5, Chapter 14)

Dan Limmer, AS, NRP (Volume 5, Chapter 14)

Deborah J. McCoy-Freeman, BS, RN, NREMTP (Volume 5, Chapter 15)

BEB, RAC

Instructor Reviewers

The reviewers of *Paramedic Care: Principles & Practice, Fourth Edition, Volume 2* have provided many excellent suggestions and ideas for improving the text. The quality of the reviews has been outstanding, and the reviews have been a major aid in the preparation and revision of the manuscript. The assistance provided by these EMS experts is deeply appreciated.

Fifth Edition

Michael Smith, MS, Educator, Kilgore College, Longview, TX

Edward Lee, A.A.S., BS, Ed.S., NRP, CCEMT-P, EMT Paramedic Program Coordinator, Trident Technical College, Summerville, SC

Ryan Batenhorst, BA, NRP, EMS-I, Program Director, Paramedic Program, Southeast Community College, Milford, NE

Brett Peine, BS, NRP, Director, Southern State University, Joplin, MO

Fourth Edition

John L. Beckman, AA, BS
FF/EMT-P I/C
Addison Fire Protection District
Technology Center of DuPage
Addison, IL

Bryon Bellinger, NREMT-P, BA, RN
Lead Instructor Paramedic Specialist Program
Indian Hills Community College
Ottumwa, IA

Brian Bird, AS, EMS
Firefighter/Paramedic
Santa Fe Fire Department
Santa Fe, NM

L. Kelly Kirk, III, AAS, BS, EMT-P
Director of Distance Education, Paramedic
Randolph Co. Community College/Davidson County EMS
Asheboro, NC/Lexington, NC

Gregory M. Reardon, BS, NREMT-P
Paramedic, Adjunct Faculty Cecil College/Maryland Fire and Rescue Institute
Baltimore Washington International Airport Fire and Rescue Department
Baltimore, MD

Billy Respass, NCEMT-P
EMS Programs Instructor
Beaufort County Community College
Washington, NC

Mike Smertka, EMT-P
Assistant EMS Instructor
Graduate Student of Medicine/Medical University of
  Silesia
Katowice, Poland

Kelly Weller, MA, RN, LP, EMS-C
EMS Program Director
Lone Star College-Montgomery
Conroe, TX

We also wish to express appreciation to the following EMS professionals who -reviewed the third edition of Paramedic Care: Principles & Practice. Their suggestions and perspectives helped to make this program a successful teaching tool.

Mike Dymes, NREMT-P
EMS Program Director
Durham Technical Community College
Durham, NC

Ginger K. Floyd, BA, NREMT-P
Assistant Professor
Austin Community College EMS Professions
Austin, TX

Darren P. Lacroix, AAS, EMT-P
Del Mar College
Emergency Medical Service Professions
Corpus Christi, TX

Greg Mullen, MS, NREMT-P
National EMS Academy
Lafayette, LA

Deborah L. Petty, BS, EMT-P I/C
Training Officer
St. Charles County Ambulance District
St. Peters, MO

B. Jeanine Riner, MHSA, BS, RRT, NREMT-P
GA Office of EMS and Trauma
Atlanta, GA

Aaron Weitzman, BS, NREMT-P
Lieutenant (ret.)
Faculty, Emergency Medical Services
Baltimore City Community College
Baltimore, MD

Brian J. Wilson, BA, NREMT-P
Education Director
Texas Tech School of Medicine
El Paso, TX

Photo Acknowledgments

All photographs not credited adjacent to the photograph or in the photo credit section below were photographed on assignment for Brady/Prentice Hall/Pearson Education.

Organizations

We wish to thank the following organizations for their valuable assistance in creating the photo program for this edition:

Bound Tree University
Dublin, OH. www.boundtreeuniversity.com

Canandaigua Emergency Squad
Canandaigua, NY

Flower Mound Fire Department
Flower Mound, TX

Children's Hospital St. Louis/BJC Health Care
St. Louis, MO

Christian Hospital/BJC Health Care
St. Charles, MO

Tyco Health Care/Nellcor Puritan Bennet
Pleasanton, CA

Wolfe Tory Medical
Salt Lake City, UT

Winter Park Fire-Rescue
Winter Park, FL

Chief James E. White
Deputy Chief Patrick McCabe

City of Winter Park, FL
Kenneth W. Bradley, Mayor

Technical Advisors

Thanks to the following people for providing technical support during the photo shoots in Winter Park, FL, for this edition:

Andrew Isaacs, EMS Captain
Tod Meadors, EMS Captain
Dr. Tod Husty, Medical Director
Richard Rodriguez, EMS Captain
Jeff Spinelli, Engineer-Paramedic

Models

Thanks to the following people from the Flower Mound Fire Department, Flower Mound, Texas, and from Winter Park Fire-Rescue, Winter Park, Florida, who provided locations and/or portrayed patients and EMS providers in our photographs.

FAO/Paramedic Wade Woody
FF/Paramedic Tim Mackling

FF/Paramedic Matthew Daniel
FF/Paramedic Jon Rea
FF/Paramedic Waylon Palmer
FF/EMT Jesse Palmer
Captain/EMT Billy McWhorter
Linda Kirk, Director, Winter Park Towers, Winter Park, FL

Andrew Isaacs
Richard Rodriguez
Tod Meadors
Jeff Spinelli
Mark Vaughn
Victoria Devereaux
Teresa George

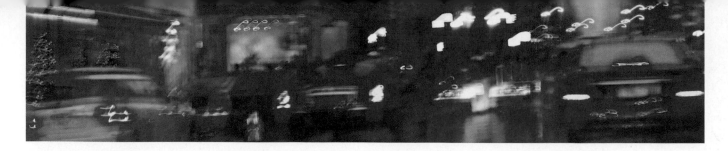

About the Authors

BRYAN E. BLEDSOE, DO, FACEP, FAAEM, EMT-P

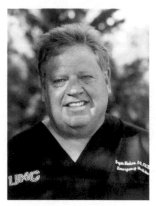

Dr. Bryan Bledsoe is an emergency physician, researcher, and EMS author. Presently he is Professor of Emergency Medicine at the University of Nevada School of Medicine and an Attending Emergency Physician at the University Medical Center of Southern Nevada in Las Vegas. He is board-certified in emergency medicine and emergency medical services. Prior to attending medical school, Dr. Bledsoe worked as an EMT, a paramedic, and a paramedic instructor. He completed EMT training in 1974 and paramedic training in 1976 and worked for six years as a field paramedic in Fort Worth, Texas. In 1979, he joined the faculty of the University of North Texas Health Sciences Center and served as coordinator of EMT and paramedic education programs at the university.

Dr. Bledsoe is active in emergency medicine and EMS research. He is a popular speaker at state, national, and international seminars and writes regularly for numerous EMS journals. He is active in educational endeavors with the United States Special Operations Command (USSOCOM) and the University of Nevada at Las Vegas. Dr. Bledsoe is the author of numerous EMS textbooks and has in excess of 1 million books in print. Dr. Bledsoe was named a "Hero of Emergency Medicine" in 2008 by the American College of Emergency Physicians as a part of their 40th anniversary celebration and was named a "Hero of Health and Fitness" by *Men's Health* magazine as part of their 20th anniversary edition in November of 2008. He is frequently interviewed in the national media. Dr. Bledsoe is married and divides his time between his residences in Midlothian, TX, and Las Vegas, NV.

RICHARD A. CHERRY, MS, EMT-P

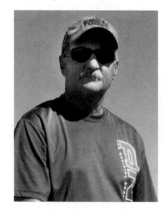

Richard Cherry is the Director of Training for Northern Onondaga Volunteer Ambulance (NOVA) in Liverpool, New York, a suburb of Syracuse. He recently retired from the Department of Emergency Medicine at Upstate Medical University where he held the positions of Director of Paramedic Training, Assistant Emergency Medicine Residency Director, Clinical Assistant Professor of Emergency Medicine, and Technical Director for Medical Simulation. His experience includes years of classroom teaching and emergency fieldwork. A native of Buffalo, Mr. Cherry earned his bachelor's degree at nearby St. Bonaventure University in 1972. He taught high school for the next ten years while he earned his master's degree in education from Oswego State -Univer-sity in 1977. He holds a permanent teaching license in New York State.

Mr. Cherry entered the emergency medical services field in 1974 with the DeWitt Volunteer Fire Department, where he served his community as a firefighter and EMS provider for more than 15 years. He took his first EMT course in 1977 and became an ALS provider two years later. He earned his paramedic certificate in 1985 as a member of the area's first paramedic class.

Mr. Cherry has authored several books for Brady. Most notable are *Paramedic Care: Principles & Practice, Essentials of Paramedic Care, Intermediate Emergency Care: Principles & Practice*, and *EMT Teaching: A Common Sense Approach*. He has made presentations at many state, national, and international EMS conferences on a variety of teaching topics. He and his wife, Sue, run a summer horse-riding camp for children with special needs on their property in West Monroe, New York. He also plays guitar in a Christian band.

A GUIDE TO KEY FEATURES

Emphasizing Principles

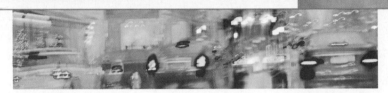

Chapter 1

Introduction to Paramedicine

Bryan Bledsoe, DO, FACEP, FAAEM

LEARNING OBJECTIVES

Terminal Performance Objectives and a separate set of Enabling Objectives are provided for each chapter.

STANDARD
Preparatory (EMS Systems)

COMPETENCY
Integrates comprehensive knowledge of EMS systems, the safety and well-being of the paramedic, and medical–legal and ethical issues, which is intended to improve the health of EMS personnel, patients, and the community.

 Learning Objectives

Terminal Performance Objective: After reading this chapter your should be able to discuss the characteristics of the profession of paramedicine.

Enabling Objectives: To accomplish the terminal performance objective, you should be able to:

1. Define key terms introduced in this chapter.
2. Compare and contrast the four nationally recognized levels of EMS providers in the United States.
3. Describe the requirements that must be met for EMS professionals to function at the paramedic level.
4. Discuss the traditional and emerging roles of the paramedic in health care, public health, and public safety.
5. List and describe the various health care settings paramedics may practice in with an expanded scope of practice.

KEY TERMS

Page numbers identify where each key term first appears, boldfaced, in the chapter.

KEY TERMS

Advanced Emergency Medical Technician (AEMT), p. 3

community paramedicine, p. 4

critical care transport, p. 7

Emergency Medical Responder (EMR), p. 3

Emergency Medical Services (EMS) system, p. 2

Emergency Medical Technician (EMT), p. 3

mobile integrated health care, p. 4

National Emergency Medical Services Education Standards: Paramedic Instructional Guidelines, p. 5

Paramedic, p. 3

paramedicine, p. 4

more rapid are the pulse and respiratory rates. | 3.0 and 3.5 kg. Because of the excretion of extracellular | As newborns make the transition from fetal to pulmonary circulation in the first few days of life, several important

1

Table 11-1 Normal Vital Signs

	Pulse (Beats per Minute)	Respiration (Breaths per Minute)	Blood Pressure (Average mmHg)	Temperature	
Infancy:					
At birth:	100–180	30–60	60–90 systolic	98–100°F	36.7–37.8°C
At 1 year:	100–160	30–60	87–105 systolic	98–100°F	36.7–37.8°C
Toddler (12 to 36 months)	80–110	24–40	95–105 systolic	96.8–99.6°F	36.0–37.5°C
Preschool age (3 to 5 years)	70–110	22–34	95–110 systolic	96.8–99.6°F	36.0–37.5°C
School-age (6 to 12 years)	65–110	18–30	97–112 systolic	98.6°F	37°C
Adolescence (13 to 18 years)	60–90	12–26	112–128 systolic	98.6°F	37°C
Early adulthood (19 to 40 years)	60–100	12–20	120/80	98.6°F	37°C
Middle adulthood (41 to 60 years)	60–100	12–20	120/80	98.6°F	37°C
Late adulthood (61 years and older)	*	*	*	98.6°F	37°C

*Depends on the individual's physical health status.

TABLES

A wealth of tables offers the opportunity to highlight, summarize, and compare information.

components of the rule of threes. Whenever BVM ventilation is difficult, however, the rule of threes should be employed.

- *Three providers.* One provider on the mask, one on the bag, and one for cricoid pressure.

- *Three inches.* A reminder to place the patient in the sniffing position (elevate the head three inches) if not contraindicated.

- *Three fingers.* Three fingers on the cricoid cartilage to perform cricoid pressure.

- *Three airways.* In a worst-case scenario, the airway can be maintained, if necessary, with an oropharyngeal airway and two nasopharyngeal airways (one in each nostril).

CONTENT REVIEW

Content review boxes set off from the text are interspersed throughout the chapter. They summarize key points and serve as a helpful study guide—in an easy format for quick review.

PHOTOS AND ILLUSTRATIONS

Carefully selected photos and a unique art program reinforce content coverage and add to text explanations.

index, and middle finger of one hand. If a lesser-trained provider is performing the maneuver, you should confirm that they are in the correct position (Figure 15-47).

Use caution not to apply so much pressure as to deform and possibly obstruct the trachea; this is a particular danger in infants. The necessary pressure has been estimated as the amount of force that will compress a capped 50-mL syringe from 50 mL to the 30 mL marking. In the event that the patient actively vomits, it is imperative to release the pressure to avoid esophageal rupture. Similarly, if cricoid pressure is being performed during intubation, reduce or release the pressure if the intubator is having difficulty visualizing the vocal cords.

Optimal BVM Ventilation Using the Rule of Threes

The *rule of threes* was developed to help providers recall the components of optimal BVM ventilation. Many patients can be easily oxygenated and ventilated without using all

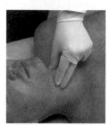

FIGURE 15-47 Cricoid pressure.

Thyroid cartilage (Adam's apple)
Cricothyroid membrane
Trachea
Esophagus
Cricoid cartilage occluding esophagus

- *Three PSI.* A gentle reminder to use the lowest pressure necessary to see the chest rise.

- *Three seconds.* A reminder to ventilate slowly and allow time for adequate exhalation.

- *Three PEEP.* Or up to 15 cm/H_2O positive-end expiratory pressure (PEEP) as needed to improve oxygen saturations.

Bag-Valve Ventilation of the Pediatric Patient

The differences in the pediatric patient's anatomy require some variation in ventilation technique. First, the child's relatively flat nasal bridge makes achieving a mask seal more difficult. Pressing the mask against the child's face to improve the seal can actually obstruct the airway, which is more compressible than an adult's. You can best achieve the mask seal with the two-person BVM technique, using a jaw-thrust to maintain an open airway.

For BVM ventilation, the bag size depends on the child's age. Full-term neonates and infants will require a pediatric BVM with a capacity of at least 450 mL. For children up to 8 years of age, the pediatric BVM is preferred, although for patients in the upper portion of that age range you can use an adult BVM with a capacity of 1,500 mL if you do not maximally inflate it. Children older than 8 years require an adult BVM to achieve adequate tidal volumes. Additionally, be

Summary

The scene size-up is the initial step in the patient care process. Sizing up the scene and situation begins at your initial dispatch and does not end until you are clear of the call. As the call unfolds, you should be making constant observations and adjustments to your plan of action. Remember that your safety and the safety of your partner are paramount—it is hard to effectively treat both yourself and others.

Scene size-up should be practiced so much that it becomes second nature to you. It is like noticing veins on people in public after you begin starting IVs. (You have all done it—looked across the room at the back of someone's hand and noticed what nice veins they had.) Sizing up a scene is no different. After a while, you begin to notice mechanisms of injury and other important details almost subconsciously. But be careful and do not get complacent! Always make it a point to pause for just a few seconds and consciously look around the scene before proceeding into any situation.

Scene size-up is not a step-by-step process, but a series of decisions you make when confronted with a variety of circumstances that are often beyond your control. It is a way to make order out of chaos, keep yourself and your crew safe, and ensure that all necessary resources are focused on patient care and outcomes. With time and experience, you will learn to perform a scene size-up quickly and focus on important issues. Your careful size-up lays the foundation for an organized and timely approach toward patient care and scene management. And always remember that scene size-up is not a one-time occurrence. It is an ongoing process.

SUMMARY

This end-of-chapter feature provides a concise review of chapter information.

airway management in every patient, you should learn and use advanced skills such as intubation, RSI, and cricothyrotomy. You must maintain proficiency in all airway skills, especially the more advanced techniques, through ongoing continuing education, physician medical direction, and testing with each EMS service. If you cannot do this, it is in the patient's best interest to focus on less sophisticated airway skills. If you anticipate that every airway will be complicated, apply basic airway skills before using advanced procedures, and perform frequent reassessments, you will give the patient his best chance for meaningful survival.

You Make the Call

You and your paramedic partner, Preston Connelly, are assigned to District 4, a quiet suburban neighborhood, on a warm Saturday in June. At 2:00 P.M., you are dispatched to care for a choking child at the Happy Hotdog Restaurant on Main Street. On your way to the location, the dispatcher advises you that they are currently giving prearrival choking instructions to the bystanders at the scene. On arrival, you find a frantic mother who tells you that her 6-year-old son was eating a hot dog and drinking a soda when he started coughing and gasping for air. She keeps yelling for you to do something. Bystanders surround the child and are attempting to perform the Heimlich maneuver without success. On your primary assessment, you find a 6-year-old boy lying on the floor, unconscious and apneic, with a pulse rate of 130. There is cyanosis surrounding his lips and fingernail beds, with a moderate amount of secretions coming from his mouth. There are no signs of trauma. You and Preston immediately start management of this child.

1. What is your primary assessment and management of this child?
2. What are your first actions?
3. What are your options for managing the airway after the obstruction is relieved?
4. What are the major anatomic differences between pediatric and adult patients in terms of airway management?

See Suggested Responses at the back of this book.

YOU MAKE THE CALL

A scenario at the end of each chapter promotes critical thinking by requiring students to apply principles to actual practice.

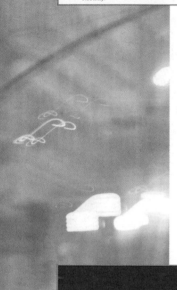

REVIEW QUESTIONS

These questions ask students to review and recall key information they have just learned.

Review Questions

1. When you couple the physical assessment findings with the patient's medical history, you are able to derive a list of _____
   - a. clinical diagnostics.
   - b. field prognoses
   - c. chief complaints
   - d. differential field diagnoses.

2. The pain, discomfort, or dysfunction that caused your patient to request help is known as the
   _____
   - a. primary problem.
   - b. nature of the illness.
   - c. differential diagnosis.
   - d. chief complaint.

3. You are assessing a patient who complains of cardiac-type chest pain that is felt in the jaw and down the left arm. This pattern of pain is known as
   _____
   - a. sympathetic pain.
   - b. tenderness.
   - c. referred pain.
   - d. associated pain.

4. Your patient has smoked 2 packs of cigarettes each day for the past 35 years. He is a _____ pack/year smoker.
   - a. 35
   - c. 730
   - b. 70
   - d. 25,550

5. The CAGE questionnaire is used as an evaluation tool to assess a patient with what type of history?
   - a. Alcoholism
   - c. Allergies
   - b. Lung disease
   - d. Pregnancy

6. What interviewing mnemonic should be used for each presenting problem a patient has?
   - a. SAMPLE
   - b. DCAP–BTLS
   - c. OPQRST–ASPN
   - d. AEIOU–TIPS

7. The mnemonic GPAL is used to evaluate a patient's
   _____
   - a. alcoholism.
   - b. allergies.
   - c. pregnancy history.
   - d. endocrine dysfunction.

Match the following elements of the present illness of the patient with a chief complaint of chest pain with their respective examples:

1.	O	a.	Pain is 6 on a scale of 1–10
2.	P	b.	Patient also complains of shortness of breath and nausea
3.	Q	c.	Pain had a sudden onset
4.	R	d.	Pain began 2 hours ago
5.	S	e.	Pain worsens while lying down
6.	T	f.	Patient denies dizziness
7.	AS	g.	Pain goes through to the back
8.	PN	h.	Pain is heavy and vise-like

See Answers to Review Questions at the back of this book.

6. Which radio frequencies may be used by cities and municipalities for their ability to better transmit through concrete and steel?
   - a. UHF
   - c. 800-mHz
   - b. VHF
   - d. none of the above

7. Which frequency band is typically used by county and suburban agencies due to its ability to transmit over various terrains and longer distances?
   - a. UHF
   - c. 800-mHz
   - b. VHF
   - d. none of the above

8. What is the name of the basic communications system that uses the same frequency to both transmit and receive?
   - a. Multiplex
   - c. Simplex
   - b. Duplex
   - d. Complex

9. A communications system that uses a different transmit and receive frequency allowing for simultaneous communications between two parties is called _____
   - a. multiplex.
   - b. duplex.
   - c. simplex.
   - d. complex.

10. _____ communications systems are capable of transmitting both voice and electronic patient data simultaneously.
    - a. Multiplex
    - c. Simplex
    - b. Duplex
    - d. Complex

See answers to Review Questions at the back of this book.

REFERENCES

This listing is a compilation of source material providing the basis of updated data and research used in the preparation of each chapter.

References

1. Department of Homeland Security. SAFECOM. (Available at http://www.dhs.gov/safecom/)
2. National EMS Information System (NEMSIS). The NEMESIS Technical Assistance Center (TAC). (Available at http://www.nemsis.org//.)
3. American College of Emergency Physicians (ACEP). "Automatic Crash Notification and Intelligent Transportation Systems." *Ann Emerg Med* 55 (2010): 397.
4. National Emergency Number Association (NENA). National Emergency Number Association. (Available at: http://www.nena.org)
5. Association of Public-Safety Communications Officials (APCO). [Available at: http://www.its.apco911.org/]
6. Department of Transportation, Research and Innovative Technology Administration. Next Generation 911. (Available at: http://www.its.dot.gov/ng911/.)
7. Centers for Disease Control and Prevention. Recommendations from the Expert Panel: Advanced Automatic Collision Notification and Triage of the Injured Patient. (See NHTSA summary at http://www.nhtsa.gov/Research/Biomechanics+&+Trauma/Advanced+Automatic+Collision+Notification+-+AACN)

8. Wilson, S., M. Cooke, R. Morrell et al. "A Systematic Review of the Evidence Supporting the Use of Priority Dispatch of Emergency Ambulances." *Prehosp Emerg Care* 6 (2002): 42–29.
9. Billittier, A. J., 4th, E. B. Lerner, W. Tucker, and J. Lee. "The Lay Public's Expectations of Prearrival Instructions When Dialing 911." *Prehosp Emerg Care* 4 (2000): 234–237.
10. Munk, M. D., S. D. White, M. L. Perry, et al. "Physician Medical Direction and Clinical Performance at an Established Emergency Medical Services System." *Prehosp Emerg Care* 13 (2009): 185–192.
11. Cheung, D. S., J. J. Kelly, C. Beach, et al. "Improving Handoffs in the Emergency Department." *Ann Emerg Med* 55 (2010): 171–180.
12. Chan, T. C., J. Killeen, W. Griswold, and L. Lenert. "Information Technology and Emergency Medical Care during Disasters." *Acad Emerg Med* 11 (2004): 1229–1236.
13. DREAMS Ambulance Project. (See article at: https://www.ems1.com/ems-products/technology/articles/1183110-DREAMS-revolutionizes-communication-between-ER-and-ambulance/.)
14. Haskins, P. A., D. G. Ellis, and J. Mayrose. "Predicted Utilization of Emergency Medical Services Telemedicine in Decreasing Ambulance Transports." *Prehosp Emerg Care* 6 (2002): 445–448.

FURTHER READING

This list features recommendations for books and journal articles that go beyond chapter coverage.

Further Reading

Bass, R., J. Potter, K. McGinnis, and T. Miyahara. "Surveying Emerging Trends in Emergency-related Information Delivery for the EMS Profession." *Topics in Emergency Medicine* 26 (April–June 2004): 2, 93–102.

Fitch, J. "Benchmarking Your Comm Center." *JEMS* 2006: 98–112.

McGinnis, K. K. "The Future of Emergency Medical Services Communications Systems: Time for a Change." *N C Med J* 68 (2007): 283–285.

McGinnis, K. K. *Future EMS Technologies: Predicting Communications Implications.* National Public Safety Telecommunications Council, National Association of State EMS Officials, National Association of EMS Physicians, June, 2010.

McGinnis, K. K. "The Future Is Now: Emergency Medical Services (EMS) Communications Advances Can Be as Important as Medical Treatment Advances When It Comes to Saving Lives." *Interoperability Today* (SafeCom, U.S. Department of Homeland Security), Volume 3, 2005.

McGinnis, K. K. *Rural and Frontier Emergency Medical Services Agenda for the Future.* National Rural Health Association Press: October 2004.

cleaning, p. 70	isotonic exercise, p. 61	sterilization, p. 70
Code Green Campaign, p. 78	pathogens, p. 65	stress, p. 74
disinfection, p. 70	personal protective equipment	stressor, p. 74
exposure, p. 70	(PPE), p. 66	Tema Conter Memorial Trust, p. 78

CASE STUDY

This feature at the start of each chapter draws students into the reading and creates a link between text content and real-life situations.

Case Study

Howard is a 15-year veteran of a high-volume, inner-city EMS service. When he first started his career, Howard thought he knew what he was getting into, but the years have taught him differently.

Right now, Howard is in the spotlight for saving the life of a police officer who was shot in a hostage situation. "That call forced me to reflect on a few important things," he says. "Two years ago, I had a minor heart problem, and it was a good wake-up call. Since then I've been lifting weights and running, so I was able to get to the officer with enough strength to carry him to safety.

"Another thing is that I always use personal protective equipment. I never go to work without steel-toed boots and I never leave the ambulance without a pair of disposable gloves. Can you believe there are still paramedics who knock the concept of infection control? If any one of my partners sticks a needle into the squad bench in my ambulance, they know I'll speak up."

Howard, a mild-mannered, nondescript man, doesn't realize that his young colleagues regard him as a role model. They've seen him handle himself at chaotic scenes as well as when a situation demands sensitivity, patience, and gentleness. "Howard is the man I'd want to tell bad news to my mother," one of his partners says. "He can handle people involved in just about any circumstance—death situations, panicked parents, lonely elderly people, and even hostile drunks. I've never seen anyone treat others with such dignity and respect. He's the best partner anyone could want, especially when we have to manage patients who are thrashing around. But that was not always so, was it, Howard?"

"No, it wasn't," Howard replies. "There was a time when no one wanted to work with me. I was a rebel, and I figured there was only one way to do things: my way. But an incident that occurred a few years ago changed all that. It's a long story. But the upshot is that when I recovered from the stress, my outlook had been altered. I realized that though I couldn't save the world, I could save myself. That's when I learned how to deal with the effects of a stressful job. I started eating right, lost a lot of weight, and adopted a new attitude. Anyway, if I can maintain my own well-being, I can do a lot more to help others. Right? Isn't that what we're about?"

Introduction

The safety and well-being of the workforce is a fundamental aspect of top-notch performance in EMS.[1] As a paramedic, it includes your physical well-being as well as your mental and emotional well-being. If your body is fed well and kept fit, if you use the principles of safe lifting, observe safe driving practices, and avoid potentially addictive and and insidious infections. If you let your spirit appreciate the fear and sadness on other faces, you will find ways to combat your prejudices and treat people with dignity and respect. By doing all these things, you will also be able to promote the benefits of well-being to your EMS colleagues.

Death, dying, stress, injury, infection, fear—all these threaten your wellness and conspire to interfere with your good intentions. However, you can do something about

PROCEDURE SCANS

Visual skill summaries provide step-by-step support in skill instruction.

Procedure 7-4 Reassessment

7-4a Reevaluate the ABCs.

7-4b Take all vital signs again.

7-4c Perform your focused assessment again.

7-4d Evaluate your interventions' effects.

laryngospasm may be occurring. Airway and breathing management requires constant reevaluation.

oxygenation. Lip cyanosis indicates central hypoxia (overall oxygen status), whereas peripheral cyanosis indicates decreased oxygen to the tissues. Pallor and coolness sug-

---

Special Features

PATHO PEARLS

Offer a snapshot of pathological considerations students will encounter in the field.

the present illness. Common sense and clinical experience will determine how much of the following history to use.

Preliminary Data

For documentation, always record the date and time of the physical exam. Determine your patient's age, sex, race, birthplace, and occupation. This provides a starting point for the interview and establishes you as the interviewer. Who is the source of the information you receive about your patient? Is it the competent patient himself, his spouse, a friend, or a bystander? Are you receiving a report from a first responder, the police, or another health care worker? Do you have the medical record from a transferring facility?

After you have gathered the information, you should establish its reliability, which will vary according to the source's knowledge, memory, trust, and motivation. Again, reconfirm the information with the patient, if possible. This is a judgment call based on your experience. For example, if the patient information you received from a particular EMT first responder has been accurate in the past, you probably will trust it again. On the other hand, if the nurse at a physician's office has repeatedly provided you with erroneous information, you probably will doubt its accuracy.

scious patient, the chief complaint becomes what someone else identifies or what you observe as the primary problem. In some trauma situations, for instance, the chief complaint might be the mechanism of injury, such as "a penetrating wound to the chest" or "a fall from 25 feet."

Patho Pearls

The renowned Canadian physician Sir William Osler said, "Listen to the patient, and he will tell you what is wrong." This advice is as true today as it was 100 years ago. A great deal of information can be determined from a skillful history taking. As you listen to a patient's medical history, try to understand the underlying pathophysiologic processes that might cause the symptoms the patient describes. This will help you to fully comprehend the disease process or processes affecting the patient.

For example, consider the following case. Mrs. J. Franklin is a 72-year-old pensioner, twice widowed, who lives in an older section of town. She summons EMS with what initially seem like vague complaints. She reports to the dispatcher, when queried, that she is "just sick." You arrive and begin an assessment, starting with a pertinent history. The patient reports that her symptoms began about two weeks ago after several family members came to her house with dinner, which included a baked ham. Since that time, she has developed some fatigue, progressive dyspnea, and occasional chest pain. She now reports that she often wakes up at 3:00 A.M. with breathing trouble that resolves when she walks around the room or

---

LEGAL CONSIDERATIONS

Offer a snapshot of pathological considerations students will encounter in the field.

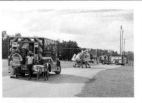

FIGURE 2-11 Patients may be transported by ground or air. Medical helicopter transport was introduced in the 1950s during the Korean War. (© Ed Effron)

Vietnam, and success of military evacuation procedures led to their use in civilian ambulance systems. In 1970, the Military Assistance to Safety and Traffic (MAST) program was established. This demonstration project set up 35 helicopter transportation programs nationwide to test the feasibility of using military helicopters and paramedics in

Legal Considerations

Emergency Department Closures. Numerous factors have resulted in emergency department closures and ambulance diversions. This can have a significant impact on the EMS system. All systems must address this situation so that patient care does not suffer.

In 1974, in response to a request from the DOT, the General Services Administration (GSA) developed the "KKK-A-1822 Federal Specifications for Ambulances." This was the first attempt at standardizing ambulance design to permit intensive life support for patients en route to a definitive care facility. The act defined the following basic types of ambulance:

- **Type I (Figure 2-13).** This is a conventional cab and chassis on which a module ambulance body is mounted, with no passageway between the driver's and patient's compartments.
- **Type II (Figure 2-14).** A standard van, body, and cab form an integral unit. Most have a raised roof.

CULTURAL CONSIDERATIONS

Provide an awareness of beliefs that might affect patient care.

An important part of patient assessment is gathering information that is accurate, complete, and relevant to the present emergency. To begin, you must identify the patient's chief complaint. Although dispatch probably will have given you an idea of what the emergency is about, it is

Cultural Considerations

Eye contact is a major form of nonverbal communication. Short eye contact is often seen as friendly, whereas prolonged eye contact may be interpreted as threatening. Thus, timing is an important factor in how a person interprets eye contact.

One's culture also influences how eye contact is interpreted. Eye contact can mean respect in one culture and disrespect in another. Often, Asians will avoid eye contact even when they have nothing to hide. Eye contact between people of different sexes is problematic in Muslim cultures, in which a prolonged look in the face of a member of the opposite sex might be misinterpreted. Because of this, people in Middle Eastern countries might look a person of the same sex in the eye and not look into the eyes of a person of the opposite sex.

If you work in a culturally diverse community, you should learn the customs of eye contact and other forms of nonverbal communication of those you might encounter during the course of your work.

unexpected but important facts. For example, instead of asking your patient with abdominal pain, "Did you have breakfast today?" which can be answered with either a "yes" or a "no," ask: "What have you eaten today?"

- *Use direct questions when necessary.* Direct questions, or **closed questions**, ask for specific information. ("Did you take your pills today?" or "Does the abdominal pain come and go like a cramp, or is it constant?") These questions are good for three reasons: They fill in information generated by open-ended questions. They help to answer crucial questions when time is limited. And they can help to control overly talkative patients, who might want to tell you about their gallbladder surgery in 1969 when their chief complaint is a sprained ankle.
- *Ask only one question at a time, and allow the patient to complete his answers.* If you ask more than one question, the patient may not know which one to answer and may leave out portions of information or become confused. Equally important is having one person do the interview. Don't force your patient to discern questions from multiple interviewers.
- *Listen to the patient's complete response before asking the next question.* By doing so, you might find that

ASSESSMENT PEARLS

Offer tips, guidance, and information to aid in patient assessment.

Provocation/Palliation

What provokes the symptom (makes it worse)? Does anything palliate the symptom (make it better)? In many

Assessment Pearls

Chest pain is a common reason that people summon EMS. However, the causes of chest pain are numerous. In emergency medicine or EMS, we often look to exclude the most serious causes before determining whether chest pain is of a benign origin. Internal organs do not have as many pain fibers as do such structures as the skin and other areas. Pain arising from an internal organ tends to be dull and vague. This is because nerves from various spinal levels innervate the organ in question. The heart, for example, is innervated by several thoracic spinal nerve segments. Thus, cardiac pain tends to be dull and is sometimes described as pressure. It also tends to cause referred pain (i.e., pain in an area somewhat distant to the organ), such as pain in the left arm and jaw. Dull pain that is hard to localize (or to reproduce with palpation) may be due to cardiac disease. One sign often seen with patients suffering cardiac disease is Levine's sign. With Levine's sign, the patient will subconsciously clench his fist when describing the chest pain. Levine's sign is associated with pain of a cardiac origin (e.g., angina or acute coronary syndrome).

Ask about any activity, medication, or other circumstance that either alleviates or aggravates the chief complaint.

Quality

How does your patient perceive the pain or discomfort? Ask him to explain how the symptom feels, and listen carefully to his answer. Does your patient call his pain crushing, tearing, oppressive, gnawing, crampy, sharp, dull, or otherwise? Quote his exact descriptors in your report.

Region/Radiation

Where is the symptom? Does it move anywhere else? Identify the exact location and area of pain, discomfort, or dysfunction. Does your patient complain of pain "here," while holding a clenched fist over the sternum, or does he grasp the entire abdomen with both hands and moan? If your patient has not done so, ask him to point to the painful area. Identify the specific location, or the boundary of the pain if it is regional.

Determine whether the pain is truly pain (occurring independently) or **tenderness** (pain on palpation). Also determine whether the pain moves or radiates. Localized pain occurs in one specific area, whereas radiating pain

---

the result of a head injury, hypothermia, severe hypoxia, or drug overdose. Bradycardia is a common finding in the well-conditioned athlete, but it may be found in almost anyone. Treat bradycardia only if it compromises your patient's cardiac output and general circulatory status.

Tachycardia usually indicates an increase in sympathetic nervous system stimulation as the body compensates for another problem, such as blood loss, fear, pain, fever, drug overdose, or hypoxia. It is an early indicator of shock and may indicate ventricular tachycardia, a life-threatening cardiac dysrhythmia.

The pulse's quality can be weak, strong, or bounding. Weak, thready pulses indicate a decreased circulatory status, such as shock. Strong, bounding pulses may indicate high blood pressure, heat stroke, or increasing intracranial pressure. The pulse location may be another indicator of your patient's clinical status. The presence of a carotid pulse generally means that his systolic blood pressure is at least 60 mmHg. The presence of peripheral pulses indicates a higher blood pressure; their absence suggests circulatory collapse. Practice locating each of the pulse locations (Figure 5-12). As with other vital signs, take your patient's pulse frequently in the emergency setting and note any trends.

To take the pulse of a conscious adult or large child, the most accessible and commonly used location is the radial artery. With the pads of your first two or three

Pediatric Pearls

In infants and small children, use the brachial artery or auscultate for an apical pulse. Remember that auscultating an apical pulse does not provide information about your patient's hemodynamic status. To locate the brachial artery, feel just medial to the biceps tendon. Auscultate the apical pulse just below the left nipple.

fingers, compress the radial artery onto the radius, just below the wrist on the thumb side (Procedure 5-1b). In the unconscious patient, begin by checking his carotid pulse. To locate the carotid pulse, palpate medial to and just below the angle of the jaw. Locate the thyroid cartilage (Adam's apple) and slide your fingers laterally until they are between the thyroid cartilage and the large muscle in the neck (sternocleidomastoid).

First, note your patient's pulse rate by counting the number of beats in 1 minute. If his pulse is regular, you can count the beats in 15 seconds and multiply that number by 4. If his pulse is irregular, you must count it for a full minute to obtain an accurate total. Also note the pulse's rhythm and quality.

Blood Pressure

Blood pressure is the force of blood against the arteries' walls as the heart contracts and relaxes. It is equal to cardiac output times the systemic vascular resistance. Any

PEDIATRIC PEARLS

Offer tips, guidance, and information on how to deal with pediatric patients encountered in the field.

Customer Service Minute

Following Up. Last week, a man took his dog to the vet for an upper respiratory infection. The dog was pretty sick, but the vet assured the owner that she was not critical, and with antibiotics she would be better in a few days, so he brought her home. The next day, the veterinarian called to find out how the dog was doing. She called every day until the dog was back to normal. Needless to say, the man was delighted in the service he received from that vet.

Physicians' offices, dentists' offices, and veterinary offices often call their patients a few days following a visit to see how things are going. Why don't we? Before you leave your patient and the family, why not ask them for permission to call the next day or in a few days to see how they're doing? If they say no or are hesitant to give permission, drop it. If they give permission, call them and see if there is anything you can do for them.

The follow-up has many benefits. You get to reconnect with the people in your community. It is great for public relations. It is educational because you can see whether your diagnosis was accurate. It's a winner from every angle. When they hang up, they'll be thinking, "Wow!"

Introduction

Patient assessment means conducting a problem-oriented evaluation of your patient and establishing priorities of

your patient en route to the hospital to detect changes in patient condition.

Your proficiency in performing a systematic patient assessment will determine your ability to deliver the highest quality of prehospital **advanced life support** (ALS) to sick and injured people. Paramedic patient assessment is a straightforward skill, similar to the assessment you might have performed as an EMT. It differs, however, in depth and in the kind of care you will provide as a result.

Your assessment must be thorough, because many ALS procedures are potentially dangerous. Safely and appropriately performing advanced procedures such as administration of drugs, defibrillation, synchronized cardioversion, needle decompression of the chest, or endotracheal intubation will depend on your assessment and correct field diagnosis. If your assessment does not reveal your patient's true problem, the consequences can be devastating.

As always, common sense dictates how you proceed in the field. When you assess the responsive medical patient, the history reveals the most important diagnostic information and takes priority over the physical exam. For the trauma patient and the unresponsive medical patient, the reverse is true. However, trauma may cause a medical emergency, and, conversely, a medical emergency may cause trauma. Only by performing a thorough patient assessment can you discover the true cause of your patient's problems. This chapter provides problem-oriented patient assessment examples based on the information and techniques presented in the previous six chapters.

CUSTOMER SERVICE MINUTE

Shows how extending extra kindness and compassion can make an important difference to patients and families coping with an emergency.

In the Field

The Tools of Your Trade. The Ophthalmoscope
An **ophthalmoscope** (Figure 5-27) is a medical instrument used to examine the internal eye structures, especially the retina, located at the back of the eye. Although it is most often used to diagnose eye conditions, you can discover information that may be relevant to other medical and traumatic events.

The ophthalmoscope is basically a light source with lenses and mirrors. It has a handle, which houses the batteries, and a head, which includes a window through which you visualize the internal eye; an aperture dial, which changes the width of the light beam; a lens dial to bring the eye into focus, and a lens indicator, which identifies the lens magnification used (i.e., 0 to +40 or 0 to −20). You examine the eye by looking through a monocular eyepiece into the eye of your patient. You can view different depths of the eye at different magnifications by rotating a disk of varying lenses within the instrument itself.

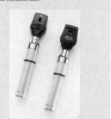

FIGURE 5-27 An ophthalmoscope is used to visualize the interior of your patient's eyes.

eye while the patient continues to fix his gaze on an object in the distance. Adjust the lens disk as needed to focus on the retina. Farsighted patients will require more "plus" diopters (black or green numbers), whereas nearsighted patients will require more "minus" diopters (red numbers) to keep the retina in focus.

Try to keep both your eyes open and relaxed. The optic disk should come into view when you are about 1.5 to 2 inches from the eye while you are still aiming your light 15 to 25 degrees nasally. If you are having difficulty finding the disk, look for a branching (bifurcation) in a retinal blood vessel. Usually the bifurcation will point toward the disk.

Follow the vessel in the direction of the bifurcation and you should arrive at the optic disk. The disk should appear as a yellowish-orange to pink round structure. Within the center of the disk there should be a central physiologic cup, which normally appears as a smaller, paler circle. The cup should be less than half the diameter of the disk. An enlarged cup may indicate chronic open-angle glaucoma. Indistinct borders or elevation of the optic disk may indicate papilledema, which is a marker of increased intracranial pressure.

Next, look at the arteries and veins of the retina. The arteries are usually brighter and smaller than the veins. Spontaneous venous pulsations are normal. Abnormalities of the retina such as hemorrhages, arteriovenous (AV) nicking, and cotton wool spots may indicate local or systemic disease such as retinal vein occlusion, hypertension, or many other conditions.

Finally, look at the fovea and surrounding macula. This area is where vision is most acute. It is located about two disk diameters temporal to the optic disk. You may also find the macula by asking the patient to look directly into the light of your ophthalmoscope. Prepare for a fleeting glimpse as this area is very sensitive to light and may be uncomfortable for your patient to maintain. A "cherry red" macula with surrounding pallor of tissue in the setting of acute painless monocular visual loss indicates a central retinal artery occlusion. Irreversible damage occurs

IN THE FIELD

Provides extra tips that can help ensure success in real-life emergency situations.

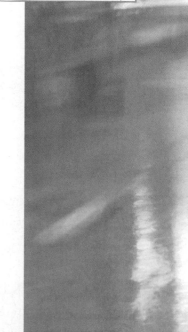

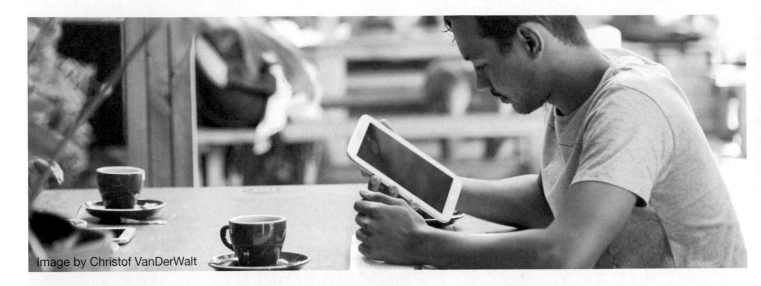
Image by Christof VanDerWalt

MyBRADYLab®

Our goal is to help every student succeed.
We're working with educators and institutions to improve results for students everywhere.

MyLab & Mastering is the world's leading collection of online homework, tutorial, and assessment products designed with a single purpose in mind: to improve the results of higher education students, one student at a time. Used by more than 11 million students each year, Pearson's MyLab & Mastering programs deliver consistent, measurable gains in student learning outcomes, retention, and subsequent course success.

Highlights of this Fully Integrated Learning Program

- **Gradebook:** A robust gradebook allows you to see multiple views of your classes' progress. Completely customizable and exportable, the gradebook can be adapted to meet your specific needs.

- **Multimedia Library:** allows students and instructors to quickly search through resources and find supporting media.

- **Pearson eText:** Rich media options let students watch lecture and example videos as they read or do their homework. Instructors can share their comments or highlights, and students can add their own, creating a tight community of learners in your class.

- **Decision-Making Cases:** take Paramedic students through real-life scenarios that they typically face in the field. These cases give students the opportunity to gather patient data and make decisions that would affect their patient's health.

**For more information,
please contact your BRADY sales representative at 1-800-638-0220,
or visit us at www.bradybooks.com**

ALWAYS LEARNING   PEARSON

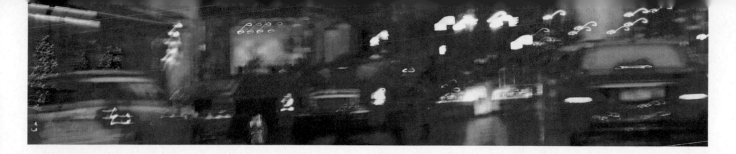

Chapter 1
Scene Size-Up

Richard A. Cherry, MS, EMT-P

STANDARD
Assessment

COMPETENCY
Integrate scene and patient assessment findings with knowledge of epidemiology and pathophysiology to form a field impression. This includes developing a list of differential diagnoses through clinical reasoning to modify the assessment and formulate a treatment plan.

 ## Learning Objectives

Terminal Performance Objective After reading this chapter, you should be able to apply findings obtained through a scene size-up to decision making about the scene and patient.

Enabling Objectives: To accomplish the terminal performance objective, you should be able to:

1. Define key terms introduced in this chapter.

2. Discuss how the scene size-up integrates into the overall context of an emergency call.

3. Identify the individual components that compose the scene size-up.

4. Define Standard Precautions and discuss how they integrate into the scene size-up.

5. Define scene safety and discuss how it integrates into the scene size-up.

6. Define resource determination and discuss how this and the number of patients integrate into the scene size-up.

7. Define mechanism of injury/nature of illness and discuss how these integrate into the scene size-up.

8. Given a scenario, discuss how you would integrate these components into a comprehensive scene size-up.

KEY TERMS

hazardous materials, p. 9

index of suspicion, p. 15

mechanism of injury, p. 15

personal protective equipment (PPE), p. 4

scene safety, p. 6

Standard Precautions, p. 4

Case Study

On a quiet afternoon, paramedic Dean Barker hears the tones for a person slumped over the steering wheel of his car. He and his partner, Sarah Santorini, a new EMT, respond immediately. En route, Dean emphasizes to his rookie partner the need to put safety first and not to rush in without a quick evaluation of the scene. His partner nods agreeably but is obviously both excited and nervous about her first real emergency call.

When they arrive, Dean notices a very unusual and troubling scene. Dean grabs his partner and stops her from jumping out of the vehicle. He asks her to stop and look around. "Tell me what you see," he says. His partner nervously answers, "Right, OK, I see one car parked alongside a cemetery and it looks like someone might be inside. There seems to be a white cloud inside the car and I smell a strong odor of sulfur or rotten eggs. I also see a sign on the driver's side window with what looks like a hazard emblem on it."

"So, is there anything we should do before jumping out and entering this scene? What is our first priority? asks Dean. "Patient care." answers his partner. "No, safety first. We'll park our vehicle upwind from the car and I'll make a quick report to dispatch and call for more help. We already know this is more than we can handle by ourselves."

Dean assumes the role of incident commander; he calls for the fire department's hazmat team, cordons off the area, and alerts all responding personnel that the potential for fire and explosion exists. There also may be a need to evacuate the area. Waiting for the fire department to arrive seems like hours to his energetic partner. Dean asks her what they can do until they arrive. Sarah responds that they can shut down the road and secure the scene from bystanders.

When the hazmat team arrives, they read the signs that someone left on three of the four windows. They appear to be suicide notes and a warning to rescuers of the toxic atmosphere inside the car. The hazmat team begins the arduous process of identifying the toxic substance, containing the exposure, and decontaminating the victim and all rescuers. Dean and his partner are released and head back to the station.

Sarah asks Dean what the substance was inside that car and asks why they didn't try to extricate and resuscitate the driver. Dean calmly explains that the white cloud and rotten-egg odor strongly suggested a deadly asphyxiant, hydrogen sulfide, and if they had opened the door to extricate him, they would have been just as dead as their victim. This day a rookie learned a crucial lesson—on an EMS call, nothing is more important than her safety. Nothing.

Customer Service Minute

Exceeding Expectations. A suburban fire department was fighting a fire in a residence where one elderly woman lived with her 11 cats. The house was totally destroyed but, miraculously, she got out in time. Unfortunately her cats didn't—except for one. This lucky cat was found by one of the rescue teams alive, but barely breathing. They took the cat into the rescue truck and evaluated it. They provided oxygen and eventually inserted an endotracheal tube and transported it to an emergency animal clinic a few miles away. The cat survived. The woman was absolutely thrilled to have at least one family member survive the fire. She was overwhelmed that the firefighters would do something like that.

People call 911 because they're having a day that's worse than bad. Like all customers, they want two things: They want their problem solved and they want to be treated well. Like all customers, they have expectations and they will evaluate your agency based on whether you met those expectations. In the end, they will be either dissatisfied, satisfied, or delighted.

Some occupations don't require good customer service skills. In others, it is a necessity. In EMS you are delivering your service to people on their worst days. Your ability to delight them during these times with competent, compassionate care can make all the difference in the world.

Customer service is a mindset. Train yourself to be open to new ways of thinking. Look for opportunities to go beyond what is expected. Take that extra step. Perform one unexpected, random act of kindness to someone on your next shift. Just one. It's something they probably will never forget. You can't change the world, but you can make a world of difference in someone's life by a simple act of kindness. And you'll want to do it again.

Introduction

Scene size-up is the essential first stage of every emergency call. Sizing up an emergency scene is not a step-by-step process, but a series of timely decisions you will make to ensure that you and your crew remain safe and to begin to secure the necessary resources to manage the scene and care for your patient. These informed, critical decisions will be based on judgment and instinct—the sum total of your education and experience. They will be some of the most important decisions you will ever make as a paramedic. The size-up components presented in this chapter can be done in order, but most likely you will perform your scene size-up as the situation dictates. In other words, you will make critical decisions about the scene as it reveals itself to you. Although you must consider all the elements of scene size-up important, circumstances will determine the priority you give to each one. And always remember—just because the scene appears safe right now doesn't mean it will stay that way. You don't just perform a scene size-up when you arrive at the scene. You repeatedly assess your scene all throughout the call.

Before you enter a scene, take the necessary time to assess the situation. The term *size-up* originated in the fire service, in which fire officers drive just past a burning house so they can see three of its sides before they make strategic decisions. Follow their lead. Never rush into any scene; first stop and look around (Figure 1-1).

On arrival, quickly determine whether the scene is safe. Are there any obvious hazards that could impede your efforts and threaten your lives? Does the situation require special personal protective clothing or equipment? Is the mechanism of injury or the nature of illness obvious? Are there multiple patients? Do you need immediate additional resources? After an initial scene assessment, if necessary, report to your dispatcher what you have, what you need, and what you are doing. This way, you keep every-

one informed and your dispatcher can send any necessary additional support.

Although size-up is your initial responsibility, remember that it is an ongoing process. Emergency scenes are dynamic and can change suddenly. A call for an injury to a child can erupt into a violent domestic dispute if one parent blames the other. A patient, a bystander, a family member, and even a family pet can turn on you in an instant. A hazardous material spill can ignite. An improperly stabilized car can shift. Any scene involving a large number of inebriated people can be extremely unpredictable and dangerous. Always be alert for subtle signs of danger, and avoid becoming a patient yourself. There is a little voice inside everyone that alerts us to an impending catastrophe. It is our subconscious mind trying to warn us through a sudden uneasy feeling, as when the hairs at the back of your neck stand up and you don't really know why. If there ever was a time to listen to that little voice, it is during an emergency call, especially when sizing up a scene.

Scene size-up actually begins when you first receive the call. The emergency medical dispatcher will provide the address of the incident, the nature of the call, and any other pertinent information. From this information, you should begin to formulate a basic plan. For example, what immediately comes to mind when you hear the following dispatch? "Ambulance 6, respond priority one to Elm Street and James Avenue on a possible head-on collision involving a school bus and a tractor-trailer." A flood of possibilities should assault your conscious mind at this time:

- The possibility for a serious situation involving many underage patients

- The need to establish command and triage until help arrives

- The need to make an initial radio report and secure additional resources

- The need for safety precautions to protect you, your partner, and other responders from harm's way

- The possibility that the truck might be carrying hazardous materials

Imagining these possibilities en route can save you precious time when you arrive. You may be familiar with the address from previous incidents—a frequent patient, a nightclub known for violent activity, a vacant house in a run-down crime-infested neighborhood, traffic jams during rush hour, a strip mall with limited access and egress. Your experience with the location may alert you to possible hazards prior to arrival. Determine the need to stage away from a potentially unsafe scene until it is secured.

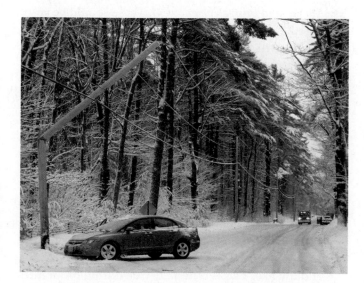

FIGURE 1-1 Always stop to size up the scene before approaching.

(© Daniel Limmer)

The nature of the incident also allows you to formulate an initial differential diagnosis prior to arrival. Take the following example:

EXAMPLE

"Unit 1, respond to 1337 Washington Boulevard, apartment 4B on a person with stridor."

You begin to think about some common causes for stridor (such as foreign body obstruction, infection, anaphylaxis, or respiratory burns) and the treatment strategies for each. The dispatcher usually provides you with enough important information to begin your scene size-up en route to the call.

An effective and efficient scene size-up will guide your actions. In trauma, the accident scene reveals the mechanism of injury. From this, you can estimate the degree of energy transfer and possible seriousness of injuries. In a medical emergency, you can sometimes determine the nature of your patient's illness from clues at the scene. The smell of a lower gastrointestinal bleed, the sound of a hissing oxygen tank, or the sight of drug paraphernalia provides clues and an initial insight into your patient's situation.

Learn to use all your senses when sizing up the scene. The components of a scene size-up include the following critical decisions:

- Is the scene safe for us to enter? Later on: Is it safe to stay?
- Which standard infection control precautions will be appropriate?
- What additional resources will be necessary?
- Have we located all the patients?
- What does the mechanism of injury or nature of the illness suggest?

You will revisit these critical decisions throughout the call, because conditions can change at any time. Always be aware of your surroundings and be prepared to change strategies and tactics on a moment's notice. Never allow complacency to lure you into a false sense of security.

Now, let us take an in-depth look at the five components of sizing up an emergency scene.

CONTENT REVIEW

➤ Components of Scene Size-Up
- Standard Precautions
- Scene safety
- Resource determination
- Location of patients
- Mechanism of injury/ nature of illness

Standard Precautions

An integral component of scene safety is using a **Standard Precautions** strategy that matches your circumstances.

You certainly do not want to wear a hazmat suit to assess a patient with an ankle injury from playing soccer. Likewise, do not approach a coughing or sneezing sick-looking patient without respiratory protection. When you list scene hazards, you must include the vast array of infectious diseases that your patient's body fluids may transmit to you and your crew. The most common risks for health care workers include HIV, hepatitis B and C, tuberculosis, and any bacterial or viral infection that your body may be susceptible to.

Standard Precautions is a strategy designed to reduce the risk of transmission of microorganisms from both recognized and unrecognized sources of infection.[1] You should assume that every person is potentially infected with an organism that he could transmit, and routinely apply the following infection control practices. Standard Precautions dictate that all EMS personnel take the same (standard) precautions with every patient. To achieve this, make sure that the appropriate **personal protective equipment (PPE)** is available in every emergency vehicle (Figure 1-2). The minimum recommended PPE includes the following:

- *Hand hygiene.* Have a waterless antimicrobial handwashing dispenser or alcohol-based towelettes available in each emergency vehicle and encourage proper handwashing whenever you have had contact with your patient's body substances. Perform a more thorough handwashing at the receiving facility after transferring your patient.

- *Protective gloves.* Wear disposable protective gloves before initiating any emergency care. When an emergency involves more than one patient, change gloves between patients. When gloves have been contaminated or torn, remove and dispose of them properly as soon as possible.

- *Masks and protective eyewear.* These should be worn together whenever blood spatter is likely to occur, such as with arterial bleeding, childbirth, endotracheal intubation and other invasive procedures, oral suctioning, and cleanup of equipment that requires heavy scrubbing or brushing. Both you and your patient should wear masks whenever the potential for airborne transmission of disease exists.

- *HEPA and N-95 respirators* (Figure 1-3). Because of the resurgence of tuberculosis (TB), you must protect yourself from infection through the use of a high-efficiency particulate air (HEPA) or N-95 respirator. Wear one whenever you care for a patient with confirmed or suspected TB or any other airborne communicable disease, such as meningitis, swine flu, H1N1, avian flu, and the like. This is especially true during procedures that involve the airway, such as the administration of nebulized medications, endotracheal intubation, or suctioning.

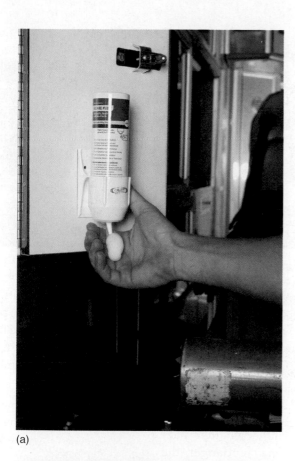

(a)

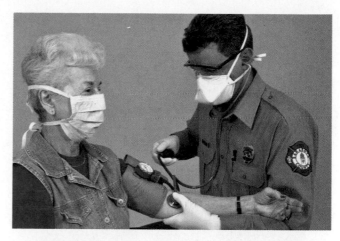

FIGURE 1-3 With a suspected tuberculosis patient, you may place a surgical-type mask on the patient while you wear a NIOSH-approved respirator. Monitor the patient's airway and breathing carefully.

- *Gowns.* Disposable gowns protect your clothing from splashes. If large splashes of blood are expected, such as with childbirth or major wounds with severe hemorrhage, wear an impervious gown.
- *Disposable resuscitation equipment.* Use disposable resuscitation equipment as your primary means of artificial ventilation in emergency care. Such items should be used once, then disposed of properly.[2]

The garments and equipment described here are intended to protect against infection through contact with potentially contaminated body substances, such as blood, vomit, and urine, as well as other agents, such as airborne droplets. When you are finished with them, place all contaminated items in the appropriate biohazard bag (Figure 1-4).

Infectious diseases also are minimized through the use of appropriate work practices and equipment especially engineered to minimize risk. For example, most invasive equipment is now used on a one-time, disposable basis. Of course, it is important to launder reusable clothing with infection control in mind.

General cleanliness and appropriate personal hygiene will do much to prevent infection. Probably the most important infection control practice is handwashing (Figure 1-5). As soon as possible after every patient contact and decontamination procedure, thoroughly wash your hands. To do so, first remove any rings or jewelry from your hands and arms. Then use soap and water. Lather your hands vigorously front and back for at least 15 seconds up to 2 or 3 inches above the wrist. Be sure to lather and rub between your fingers and in the creases and cracks of your knuckles. Scrub under and around the fingernails with a brush. Rinse your hands well under running water, holding your hands downward so that the water drains off your fingertips. Dry your hands on a clean towel. Plain soap works perfectly well for handwashing. As stated earlier, at times when soap is not available, you might use an antimicrobial

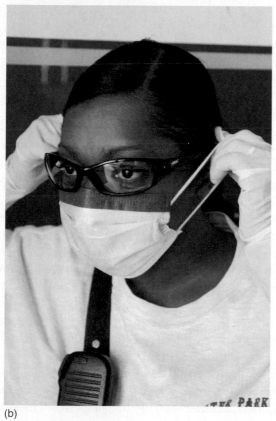

(b)

FIGURE 1-2 Always have personal protective supplies, including (a) a waterless handwashing dispenser and (b) eyewear and masks, available in the ambulance.

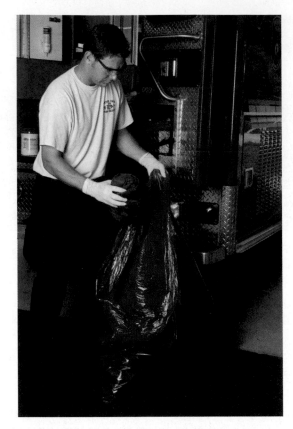

FIGURE 1-4 Place all contaminated items in the appropriate biohazard bag.

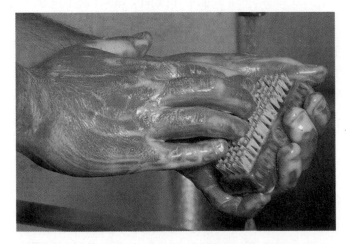

FIGURE 1-5 Careful, methodical handwashing helps reduce exposure to contagious disease.

handwashing solution or an alcohol-based foam or towelette. Finally, be sure to wash rings and other jewelry before putting them back on.

Scene Safety

Scene safety means doing everything possible to ensure a safe environment for yourself, your crew, other responding personnel, your patient, and any bystanders. Your personal safety is the top priority at any emergency scene. Make

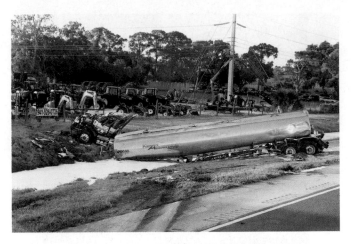

FIGURE 1-6 Look for potential hazards during scene size-up. (© *Ed Effron*)

sure you do not become injured while attempting to provide care. If you become a patient yourself, you will do your own patient little good. Quickly determine whether hazards may endanger the lives of people on the scene. If your scene is unsafe, either make it safe or wait until someone else does (Figure 1-6). You have no obligation to enter an unsafe scene unless you are trained and equipped to manage it. In these cases your responsibility is to establish a safe perimeter, evaluate the hazard, and call for help.

> **CONTENT REVIEW**
> ➤ Order of Priorities for
>   Scene Safety
>   1. You
>   2. Your crew
>   3. Other responding
>   personnel
>   4. Your patient
>   5. Bystanders

Many factors can make an emergency scene unsafe. Through experience, you will learn to identify them quickly. Although there are specific dangers inherent in responding to a trauma, especially those involving violence, you can encounter the majority of hazards discussed in this chapter on any scene. Do not become complacent en route to a medical emergency on a quiet street in a small village. Sometimes even the most harmless-looking scene can turn into a disaster (Figure 1-7). If you are not sure the scene is safe, do not enter.

As you approach the scene, immediately evaluate the surrounding area. Is it as your dispatcher's information has led you to expect, or does something just not look right? Is the house completely dark? Do bystanders look angry, scared, or panicked? Be alert for situations that look or feel suspicious. If necessary, wait until law enforcement, the fire department, or other specially trained personnel secure the scene. Use all your senses to evaluate a scene, and learn to trust your intuition. If your instincts tell you not to enter or to get out, follow them. They are the subconscious sum of all your experiences. Listen to them; they are probably correct. Carefully look for and identify on-scene hazards before

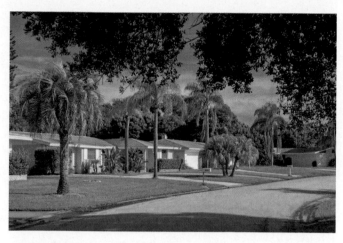

FIGURE 1-7 Even the most peaceful-looking scene can pose potential dangers.

even attempting to reach your patient. To do otherwise places you, other rescuers, and your patient at risk.

If the scene is unsafe, do not enter unless you have the necessary training and equipment. Entering an unsafe scene is unacceptable unless there is an immediate life-threatening situation you are reasonably sure you can mitigate or avert to save your patient's life. If you are injured entering an unsecured scene, you only add to the problem: More resources will be needed to assist you and take care of the original problem.

Unsafe scene hazards come in a variety of forms. Let us look at some common types of hazards encountered in emergency services: environmental hazards, hazardous materials, roadway operations, and violence.

Environmental Hazards

Nature, and its environment, can provide a variety of obstacles that inhibit your ability to reach your patient, deliver care, and transport him to the appropriate facility. This section focuses on some common types of environmental hazards that may complicate your scene and threaten your well-being—weather, terrain, water, electricity, and confined spaces.

Weather

The most common obstacle, depending on where you practice your craft, may be extreme weather conditions. These everyday phenomena can make even the most basic emergency situations a challenge. For example, carrying a patient down an icy flight of stairs, trying to navigate your stretcher through a snow-covered driveway, or accessing your patient in a blinding rainstorm are just a few of the everyday hazards you can encounter (Figure 1-8). Working outdoors on extremely hot and humid days can result in serious heat-related injuries, such as heat exhaustion or heat stroke.

Even wind gusts can make simple tasks much more difficult. Extended operations on cold and windy days can

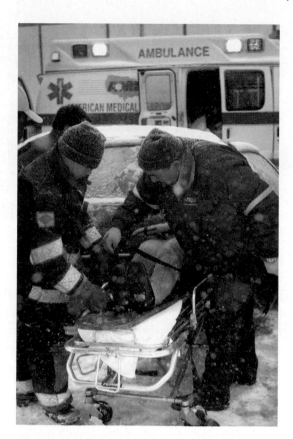

FIGURE 1-8 Inclement weather can pose a variety of challenges at any emergency scene.
(© Mark C. Ide/Science Source)

produce cold injuries, such as frostbite and hypothermia. More treacherous natural phenomena, such as tornados, hurricanes, lightning strikes, hailstorms, and dust storms, can create life-threatening conditions for emergency responders. Unfortunately, there is nothing anyone can do to mitigate nasty weather conditions. But when you are up against nature's powerful and sometimes destructive forces, you are wise to be overly cautious and not take unnecessary chances with your crew.

Terrain

Unstable terrain can severely hinder your efforts to reach your patient. Mudslides, avalanches, rock slides, high-angle cliffs, earthquake crevices, and steep slopes challenge even the most skilled and experienced rescuer (Figure 1-9). Hikers, mountain climbers, and other outdoor enthusiasts will continue to find new ways of becoming trapped in the very terrain they love to navigate. Remember that in any case involving moving earth, such as rock or mud slides, avalanches, and cave-ins, there can be a second and third movement. Do not become complacent thinking that the event has "happened." Make sure things have been secured or stabilized prior to entering the scene. In every case, it is your responsibility to recognize the need for specialized rescue teams and control the scene until they arrive. Refer to the hazardous terrain rescue section in the chapter

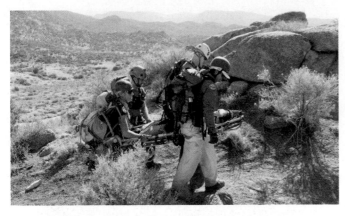

FIGURE 1-9 Uneven and hazardous terrain that compromises your footing can create an extremely difficult situation.

"Rescue Awareness and Operations" for more information on this topic.

Hazardous terrain can also exist inside a building such as a house or an apartment. Poorly lit entranceways and hallways, broken stairs, slippery floors, loose floorboards, and rooms cluttered with trash all pose a significant risk of injury to responders. Uneven sidewalks and potholes can make navigating to and from your patient's location treacherous. Carry a flashlight and always be aware of your footing.

Water

Rescue scenarios can occur in standing water, such as a lake or swimming pool, or in rushing water, such as a raging river or the open sea. The potential for serious injury or death is real for the victims and their rescuers in these situations (Figure 1-10). Like their hiking counterparts, water-sport enthusiasts also seem to find new and ingenious ways of getting into trouble. When sizing up your scene, you must decide whether you can safely perform a water rescue or whether you need specialized resources. As always, do not place yourself in harm's way unless you believe you can mitigate the circumstance effectively.

One simple water rescue method is the Reach (with a long pole)–Throw (a flotation device)–Row (boat)–Go

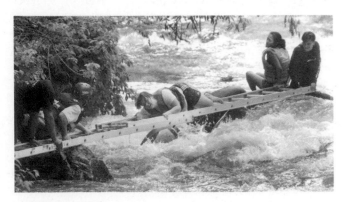

FIGURE 1-10 Never enter a specialized rescue situation without proper training and equipment.

(© AP Photo/Standard Examiner, Brian Nicholson)

(water entry) technique. However, consider "Go" as a last-ditch effort and be aware of the life dangers inherent in that type of rescue attempt. In addition, anyone participating in a water rescue should wear a personal flotation device. Swift water rescues involve a number of underwater terrain situations that pose a unique and dangerous challenge to rescuers. Becoming trapped in recirculating currents, strainers, foot and extremity pins, and dam intakes can be lethal for the rescuer. These types of rescues should only be attempted by specialized personnel. Refer to the water rescue section in the chapter "Rescue Awareness and Operations" for more information on this topic.

Electricity

Always approach a scene with downed power lines with extreme caution. Assume that the lines are energized and potentially dangerous until the power company removes the power lines or isolates them. Do not make the potentially fatal mistake of thinking you have the proper equipment to move a charged power line. You don't. Secure a safe perimeter and do not allow responders to enter. Use your public address system to warn car occupants to stay in the car and everyone else to stay outside the established perimeter.

Lightning strikes pose a significant hazard. Even though the chance of being hit by lightning is extremely remote, it still remains in the top three causes of environmental deaths.[3] A person can be hit directly, hit by an arc from a nearby object that was hit, or hit by ground current as much as 50 yards away from the original strike. Injuries can include respiratory and cardiac arrest, skin and vascular disruption, and blunt force trauma. The only real safe action is to seek shelter indoors. If you have to access or move a patient during a thunderstorm, do it quickly.

Confined Space

Confined space situations pose a number of fatal possibilities. These include oxygen deficiency, toxic or explosive chemicals, cave-ins, machinery entrapment, electricity, and structural collapse (Figure 1-11). Again, unless you are properly trained and equipped, your role includes recognition, assuming incident command, securing the scene, and calling for the help of a specialized rescue team. Confined spaces include, but are not limited to, underground vaults, tanks, storage bins, manholes, pits, silos, process vessels, and pipelines. OSHA defines a *confined space* as having one or more of the following characteristics:

- Contains or has the potential to contain a hazardous atmosphere
- Contains a material that has the potential to engulf an entrant
- Has walls that converge inward or floors that slope downward and taper into a smaller area that could trap or asphyxiate an entrant

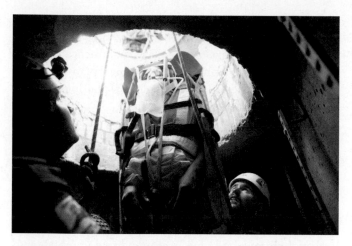

FIGURE 1-11 Confined space rescues pose a special threat for victims and rescuers. Never enter confined spaces without adequate training, equipment, and experience.

- Contains any other recognized safety or health hazard, such as unguarded machinery, exposed live wires, or heat stress[4]

Because you may encounter a confined space in virtually any industry, recognition is the first step in preventing fatalities. The majority of deaths associated with confined spaces or hazardous atmospheres are rescuers rushing in for the patient and failing to recognize the hazard. These atmospheres often are toxic, oxygen deficient, or combustible. Because every industry has standards and references that aid in recognizing and evaluating hazards and possible solutions related to their confined spaces, you should simply secure the scene and wait for assistance from the appropriate personnel. Refer to the hazardous atmosphere rescue section in the chapter "Rescue Awareness and Operations" for more information on this topic.

Hazardous Materials

Hazardous materials are found everywhere. You may encounter them at any scene involving fires, automobile accidents, medical emergencies, transportation containers, or industrial or mercantile facilities (Figure 1-12). The pri-

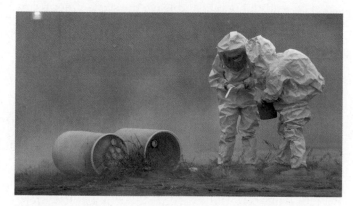

FIGURE 1-12 Toxic chemical spills can ignite or explode at any time.

(© AP Photo/Topeka Capital Journal, Chris Landsberger)

Table 1-1 Hazardous Materials

Agent	Examples
Chemical	Liquids, gases, solids, corrosives, poisons, nerve agents, and toxic industrial materials
Biological	Viruses (e.g., smallpox, swine flu, hemorrhagic fever), bacteria (e.g., plague, anthrax), and biotoxins (e.g., ricin, botulism)
Radiological	Nuclear weapons, "dirty bombs," nuclear waste products
Explosive	Low order (e.g., gunpowder), high order (e.g., TNT, dynamite), or improvised (e.g., pipe bombs, backpacks)

mary hazards include chemical, biological, radiological, nuclear, and explosive agents (Table 1–1). These agents can cause thermal injuries, asphyxiation, neuromuscular paralysis, coma, and even death depending on the exposure and potency of the agent.

Hazards can occur during production, storage, transportation, use, or disposal of any of these agents. You and your crew are at risk if you arrive on a scene at which a chemical was used unsafely or released in harmful amounts into the environment. Hazardous materials in various forms can cause death, serious injury, and long-lasting health effects. Many products containing hazardous chemicals are used and stored in homes routinely, though usually not in quantities that cause major hazards. These products are also shipped daily on the nation's highways, railroads, waterways, and pipelines. Unfortunately these come in quantities large enough to cause a major environmental disaster.

Coming into contact with a hazardous material while performing your job is inevitable. These substances are most often released as a result of transportation accidents or chemical accidents in plants. Incidents involving hazardous material exposure can pose life-threatening problems for all responding personnel. A devastating chain of explosions can be set off by a simple spark near chemical spills or gas leaks.

Several training levels exist for managing a hazardous materials incident. As a paramedic student, you are most likely trained to the awareness level. This means that your main responsibilities are to recognize that the incident involves a hazardous material, establish incident command, and control the scene until help arrives.

A good pair of binoculars may be your best tool in assessing a possible hazmat scene (Figure 1-13). Stage your vehicle uphill, upwind, and far enough away from the site to need binoculars. If you don't have a set of binoculars, use the rule of thumb: Stick your thumb in front of you and in the direction of the scene. If you can still see the scene, you are too close.

Keep people away from the scene and avoid any contact with the material. *Do not enter* the scene unless you are properly trained and equipped. If possible, establish

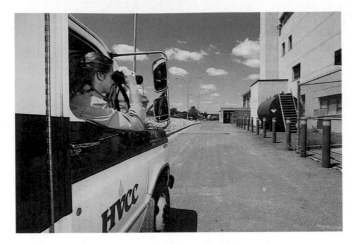

FIGURE 1-13 Don't take any chances. Use binoculars to make a visual inspection of a potentially hazardous situation from a safe distance.

danger and safe (upwind, same level as danger zone) zones. Assume that all patients are contaminated. Call for help immediately and use an incident management system. Refer to the *North American Emergency Response Guidebook*, a common item in any ambulance or rescue vehicle, for help in identifying hazardous materials, managing the scene, and treating exposed patients (Figure 1-14). Adhere to the four "don'ts" when you approach a hazardous scene:

1. Don't rush in.
2. Don't assume anything.
3. Don't become a victim.
4. Don't test (smell, taste, touch) a foreign substance.

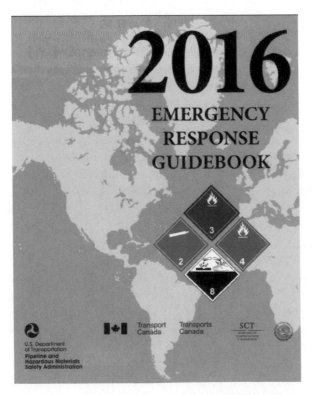

FIGURE 1-14 Carry a copy of the *Emergency Response Guidebook* in your vehicle at all times.

The ideal time for size-up is before the incident occurs. Survey your district and identify any sites of potential hazmat incidents. Develop preplans and practice the plan. Visit any industrial plants and work out a plan with their response teams. Refer to the chapter "Hazardous Materials" for more information on this topic.

Violence

Violence, especially violence aimed at emergency responders, can happen suddenly anywhere, anytime. It is not limited to a dark alley in the bad parts of town. You may encounter violence in the form of domestic abuse between husband and wife at home. You may drive up on a gang-related fight or a school shooting involving semiautomatic weapons. You may even arrive on scene of a terrorist bomb explosion in a crowded restaurant. Inner cities, suburbs, and rural areas are all affected by this recent surge in violent activity. You cannot escape it. You must be on high alert whenever responding to an emergency. As always, staying safe is your primary responsibility in these cases.

You may learn of a potentially violent situation on dispatch. In these cases, do not approach the scene until law enforcement personnel have secured it. In fact, do not even enter the neighborhood, because sitting in your ambulance on the scene may undermine an already unstable environment. If possible, turn off your lights and siren and stage your vehicle a few blocks away, where it cannot be seen from the scene. Do not assume that because police are on the scene, it is safe. You may come on a situation in which police are struggling to secure a weapon from a perpetrator. This unfortunate mistake in judgment could cost you and your partner your lives. Always keep your level of awareness up even if law enforcement personnel arrive before you do.

You may not know of the potential for violence until you arrive. Look for signs of trouble during your size-up. Is a crowd gathering? Is there an unusual silence or escalating noise? Does the scene match the dispatch information, or does your instinct tell you something is wrong? In these cases, be ready to retreat and leave the scene if necessary. Violence may erupt during the course of the call. Bystanders may become agitated and violent at any point, and you may opt to remove your patient to a safe location or transport him from the scene. Your personal safety should come before patient abandonment considerations. The law does not expect you to place yourself in grave danger while providing care. Always have a way out. Never allow yourself to be trapped inside a room or on a scene.

When responding to a crime scene, remember that dangerous weapons probably were used and that the perpetrator may still be on the scene, or could return. If your patient is the perpetrator, he may attack you in an attempt to flee the scene and escape prosecution. Gang activity occurs in the cities, the suburbs, and rural areas. No one is immune. Be alert for classic signs of gang activity in your district: clothing colors, graffiti, tattoos, and hand signals. When responding to an area of known gang activity, be overly cautious, especially if you wear a uniform that closely resembles that of law enforcement.

Domestic violence is an ever-rising situation that can turn from bad to worse in a matter of seconds. Things may escalate once the police attempt to arrest the violent offender. These types of scenes can become very ugly very quickly. Always be aware of your positioning in the room and have your emergency egress in sight.

Methamphetamine (meth) labs pose a double threat. The volatile chemicals used to manufacture illicit drugs may be present and provide a high possibility for explosion. In addition, the people who participate in this illicit, highly profitable criminal activity will be extremely uncooperative with your efforts to manage the scene and probably disrupt their lucrative livelihood. If you suspect a meth lab, wait for help.

Sometimes even a family pet can become a safety hazard to responders if the pet believes it is protecting its master from intruders. The loyalty of a dog, in these cases, is amazing. If you respond to an automobile collision involving a police canine unit and the dog is loose in the car, for example, do not attempt to reach the injured officer. That officer and his dog are as close as any two partners can be, and the dog will sacrifice its own life to protect him. Call for someone who works with these dogs, preferably another canine unit officer, to mitigate the situation before accessing your patient.

Maintain a vigilant awareness of your surroundings. If you find yourself in the middle of a potentially violent situation, try to back away to a safe location. Use the equipment you brought with you as cover, if necessary. Make sure you always have a way out if things escalate. Try to de-escalate the situation by using a calm tone and being empathetic. If possible, try to understand the other person's point of view. Avoid phrases such as "calm down, relax, settle down." Never use threats and continue to try to reason with the agitated person. If none of these tactics works, and law enforcement has not yet arrived, make every effort to retreat to a safe location. If you cannot, and things are still escalating, you may be forced to defend yourself. Use whatever force is necessary, but no more.

Patho Pearls

Here are a dozen tips to help keep you safe:

1. Park so you can make a fast exit from a potentially lethal situation.

2. Always make sure the dispatchers know your exact location. If you move from your original location, notify them.

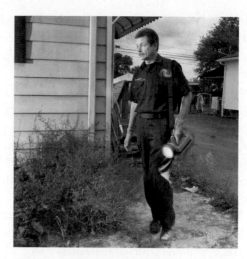

FIGURE 1-15 Hold a flashlight to the side of your body, not in front of it. Armed assailants usually aim at the light.

3. At night carry your flashlight to the side, never in front of your body, while you and your partner approach a building separately. Do not present a large, lit, easy target for some shooter (Figure 1-15).

4. When knocking on a door, always stand off to the side. You never know what awaits you on the other side of the door (Figure 1-16). Have someone lead you to the patient, but do not let this person follow. Always know who and what are behind you.

5. When talking with agitated people, speak calmly, maintain a monotone voice, watch your posture, and make sure they can see that you are there to help and not be an intrusion.

6. Watch your tone with crowds of people; identify yourself as a paramedic so there is no confusion if you are dressed like law enforcement.

7. Keep your hair tied up so it cannot be grabbed. Avoid wearing anything around your neck, including your stethoscope, for the same reason.

8. Look for traditional (e.g., knives, guns) and nontraditional (e.g., bats, broken bottles, sharp objects) weapons when you survey the scene. Be especially wary of patients' bulging pockets. They may be concealing weapons.

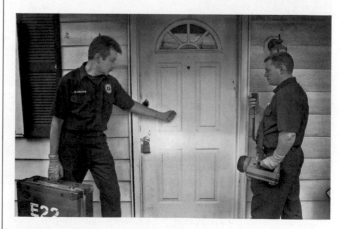

FIGURE 1-16 Always stand to the side of a door when knocking.

9. If possible, never get between people who are fighting. This is not your job.

10. Crews that work together should have a "code of trouble" if something happens.

11. If the police tell you to get out, listen to them.

12. If your gut tells you something is wrong, listen to it.

Refer to the chapter "Crime Scene Awareness" for more information on this topic. It is worth repeating that when you are on the scene of a potentially unstable situation always be aware of your exit route. Never allow yourself to be blocked from exiting a room. Under no circumstances should you ever allow yourself to be placed in grave danger.

Roadway Rescue Operations

You will encounter a number of rescue scenarios as a paramedic. By far the most common rescue situation is the motor vehicle collision on a major roadway. The greatest hazard to any emergency worker during a roadside rescue operation is traffic flow. The obvious danger of passing motorists gazing at the scene often results in secondary responder injuries and, often, death.

Never work at a roadside incident, even during the day, without wearing a safety vest that readily identifies you as an emergency worker (Figure 1-17). Position your ambulance to protect the scene but do not allow the patient load-ing area to be exposed to traffic. Place traffic cones and flares strategically to reroute traffic a safe distance from where you will be working. Always assess your scene with a special eye for circumstances that may cause harm to you, your crew, other responders, and bystanders. Look for fuel leaking and the potential for fire and explosion, downed electrical wires, unstable vehicles, and automobile systems intended to prevent harm, such as energy-absorbing bumpers, air bags, and other supplemental restraint systems. Do not overlook the obvious. Sometimes it is just the potential for injuries from working around broken glass or jagged metal.

How involved you become in any rescue is determined by your training and equipment. Match the rescue scenario and conditions with the gear you will use. Refer to the chapter "Rescue Awareness and Operations" for more information on this topic.

Resource Determination

If you need additional resources to manage your scene, request them as early as possible. Crash scenes requiring heavy-duty rescue procedures, scenes at which toxic substances are present, crime scenes with a potential for violence, or scenes with unstable surfaces, such as slippery slopes, ice, or rushing water, all call for specialized crews, additional medical supplies, and sophisticated equipment. As stated earlier, do not even consider entering such situations unless you have the proper clothing, equipment, and training to work in them. Because getting backup requires extra time, this phase is critical. A prompt call to your dispatch center can save critical minutes in a life-threatening situation.

As the first unit on the scene, you may overestimate your capability to manage a particular rescue situation. Individual acts of courage are sometimes necessary, but modern rescue operations emphasize safety first, not heroics. Foolish heroics often end in tragedy. If in doubt, it is better to err on the side of caution than to risk personal harm.

Without the appropriate protective gear, you will jeopardize your safety and that of your patient. To participate in a rescue operation, you should have at least the following equipment immediately available: four-point suspension helmets, eye goggles or industrial safety glasses, high-quality hearing protection, leather work gloves, high-top steel-toed boots, insulated coveralls, and turnout gear

> **CONTENT REVIEW**
>
> ➤ Minimum Rescue Operation Equipment
> - Four-point suspension helmets
> - Eye goggles or industrial safety glasses
> - High-quality hearing protection
> - Leather work gloves
> - High-top steel-toed boots
> - Insulated coveralls
> - Turnout gear

> **CONTENT REVIEW**
>
> ➤ Minimum Patient Safety Equipment
> - Construction-type hard hats
> - Eye goggles
> - Hearing and respiratory protection
> - Protective blankets
> - Protective shielding

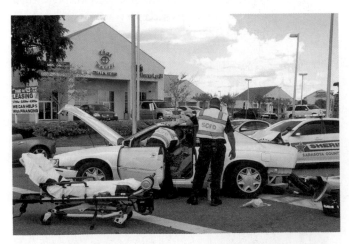

FIGURE 1-17 Always wear reflective clothing whenever working at a roadside incident. Make sure oncoming traffic can easily see you.

(© Ed Effron)

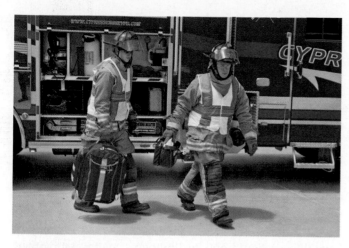

FIGURE 1-18 Full protective gear, including eye protection, helmet, turnout gear, and gloves.

(Figure 1-18). Only personnel thoroughly trained in hazardous material suits or self-contained breathing apparatus (SCBA) should use them (Figure 1-19). These items are often supplied on specialty support vehicles such as hazmat response units and heavy-rescue trucks (Figure 1-20).

After you ensure that responding personnel have adequate safety equipment to manage the rescue scene, con-

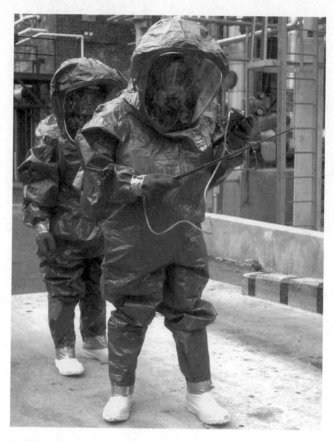

FIGURE 1-20 Hazardous materials responses require special training and equipment.

sider patient safety. Many considerations for rescuer safety also apply to patients. Additionally, patient safety equipment should at least include construction-type hard hats, eye goggles, hearing and respiratory protection, protective blankets, and protective shielding. You will need these to protect your patient during rescue operations (Figure 1-21). Patient safety also includes simple measures such as removing patients from unstable environments such as temperature extremes, smoky rooms, or hostile crowds. For example, the simplest way to begin managing

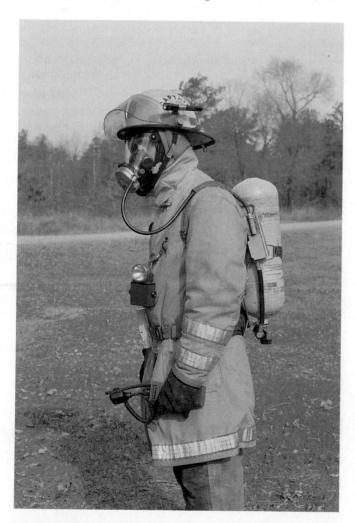

FIGURE 1-19 Self-contained breathing apparatus (SCBA).

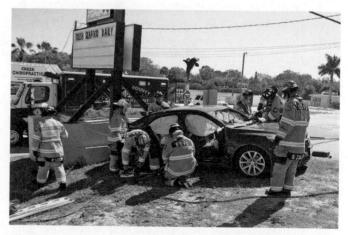

FIGURE 1-21 Protect the patient from hazards at the scene.

(© Ed Effron)

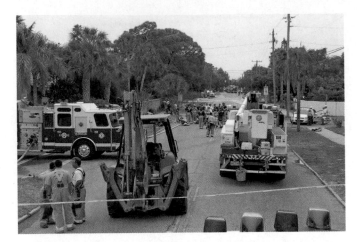

FIGURE 1-22 A tape line can help to keep bystanders out of hazardous scenes.

(© Ed Effron)

a patient suffering from hypothermia is to move him into a warm environment. In every case, let common sense dictate scene management.

Safe, orderly, and controlled incident management is essential for everyone's safety. Call for specialty personnel to stabilize wreckage or turn off electrical power. Make sure someone routes traffic safely around a vehicle collision. Control bystanders and spot potential human hazards. Be certain that a hostile crowd or someone who assaulted your patient is not ready to attack you. Scenes involving toxic exposures, environmental hazards, and violent patients are especially worrisome. When possible, have law enforcement personnel establish a tape line to cordon off the hazard zone or use other measures to protect bystanders who do not realize the potential dangers of watching operations (Figure 1-22).

Location of Patients

Scene size-up also includes a search of the area to locate all the patients. Ask yourself whether other persons could be involved in the crash or affected by the medical problem. Determine where you are most likely to find the most seriously injured patients and how many will need transport. The mechanism of injury or the nature of the illness can help you determine the number of patients. For example, a two-car crash must include at least two drivers. Clues such as diaper bags, child auto seats, toys, coloring books, clothing, or twin spider-web impact marks in the windshield should lead you to search for more patients, especially children, than those who may be readily apparent. Some medical situations such as carbon monoxide poisoning can affect an entire household. A hazardous liquid spill in the chemistry lab can affect students and staff in an entire wing of a school.

If you find more patients than you can manage safely and effectively, call for assistance early. If possible, you should do this before you make contact with any patients, because you are less likely to call for help once you become involved with patient care. Often, as you proceed into a scene, more patients become apparent. It is wise to overestimate when asking for help at the scene.

Multiple-casualty incidents can range from two to hundreds of patients. For example, you respond to an imminent delivery at a residence in the suburbs. You deliver a normal, healthy baby but the mother still complains of labor pains. You suddenly realize that a second baby is coming. It is born pulseless and apneic. Now you have three patients: one healthy baby, one frantic mother, and one clinically dead baby. It is not necessarily how many patients you have but how many patients will overtax your resources. A simple motor vehicle collision with three or four patients can overwhelm a rural EMS system or a large system already taxed beyond its capacity.

For any multiple-patient incident, it is wise to implement an incident management system according to local protocols. If the first unit to arrive establishes incident command and begins the triage process, it will save time and energy playing catch-up later on. Initiate the incident management system according to local protocols (Figure 1-23). Again, try not to become immediately involved in patient care, because two important functions must occur in the initial stages of any multiple-casualty incident: command and triage.

If you and your partner find yourselves in a situation that overwhelms your resources, one of you should establish command while the other begins triaging patients. The command person performs a scene size-up, determines the needs of the incident, makes a radio report requesting the necessary additional help, and directs oncoming crews to their duties until he transfers command duties to an

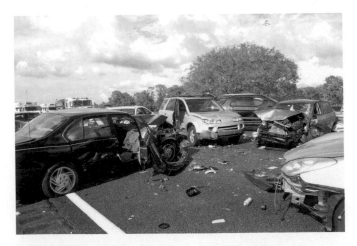

FIGURE 1-23 Follow local protocols when you respond to a multiple-casualty incident.

(© Ed Effron)

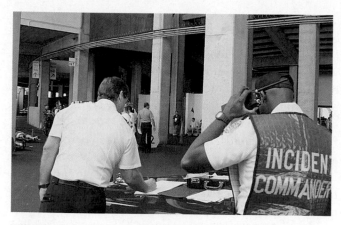

FIGURE 1-24 The incident commander directs the response and coordinates resources at a multiple-casualty incident.

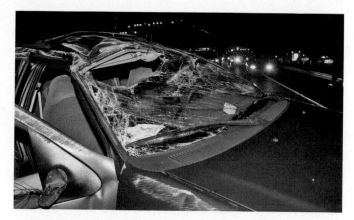

FIGURE 1-26 With trauma, try to determine the mechanism of injury during scene size-up.

(© Daniel Limmer)

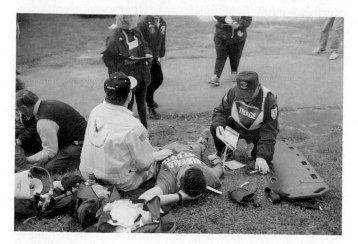

FIGURE 1-25 The triage person examines and prioritizes patients.

arriving officer (Figure 1-24). The triage person performs a triage exam on every patient and prioritizes them for immediate or delayed transport (Figure 1-25). He may perform simple lifesaving procedures such as opening the airway or controlling bleeding, but as a rule he should not stop to provide intensive care for any one patient. Refer to the chapter "Multiple Casualty Incidents and Incident Management" for more information on this topic.

Mechanism of Injury / Nature of Illness

The **mechanism of injury** is the combined strength, direction, and nature of forces that injured your patient. It is usually apparent through careful evaluation of the trauma scene and can help you anticipate both the location and the seriousness of injuries. Identify the forces involved, the direction from which they came, and the bodily locations potentially affected (Figure 1-26). For example, in a fall injury, how high was the patient, what did he land on, and

what part of his body hit first? If your patient jumped from a significant height and landed on his feet, for example, expect lower extremity, pelvis, and lumbar spine injuries.

Although trauma poses a serious threat to life, its appearance often masks your patient's true condition. Extremity injuries, for example, are frequently obvious and grotesque, yet they rarely cause death. Conversely, life-threatening problems such as internal bleeding and rising intracranial pressure often occur with only subtle signs and symptoms. Your assessment of trauma patients must look beyond obvious injuries to significant mechanisms of injury for evidence that suggests life-threatening situations. Although now downplayed, certain significant mechanisms predictably cause serious internal injury.

In an automobile crash, the mechanism of injury is the process by which forces are exchanged between the automobile and what it struck, between your patient and the automobile's interior, and among the various tissues and organs as they collide with one another within the patient. Close inspection of the automobile and the forces, or various collisions, can lead to an **index of suspicion** (a prediction of injuries based on the mechanism of injury) for possible injuries. What does the car look like? If the windshield is cracked, expect head and neck injuries. If the steering wheel is bent, expect chest and abdominal injuries. With a major intrusion into the passenger compartment, expect major multisystem trauma.

Other significant mechanisms of injury can result from seat belts, air bags, and child safety seats. Do not rule out serious injury just because your patient wore a seat belt. Seat belts can actually cause injuries, even when worn properly. Always ask your patient whether he wore a seat belt and look for bruises across the chest or around the waist. If these are present, expect hidden internal injuries.

In general, air bags have been effective devices in preventing serious injury by protecting passengers from hitting the windshield, steering wheel, and dashboard. Originally, they deployed only when the front of the car hit another object. Many automakers currently have installed side air bags that deploy when the car is struck from the side. Air bags are not without complication, however. For example, they are designed to cushion the chests of large adults. If the passenger is a child or a short adult, the air bag will hit him in the face, possibly causing injury. In addition, air bags are designed to deflate automatically within seconds after inflation, which may allow passengers to be propelled into the steering wheel or dashboard. For this reason, they may not be effective without the seat belt. Always lift the deployed bag and inspect the steering wheel for deformity. Suspect serious internal injuries if you discover a bent steering wheel (Figure 1-27). There is also danger of the bag not deploying in the crash. It may deploy during the rescue operation, putting rescuers in danger of serious injury.

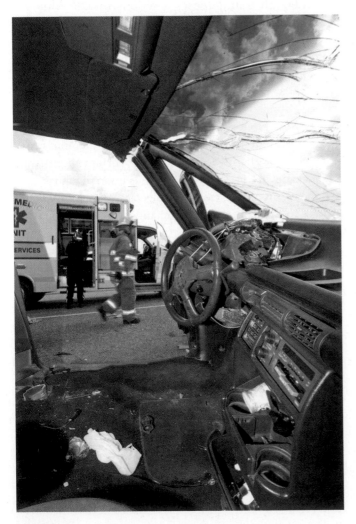

FIGURE 1-27 A bent steering wheel signals potentially serious injuries.

(© Kevin Link)

A child safety seat, when used appropriately, also can save a life. If the safety seat is not securely fastened to the car seat, though, it can come loose and be thrown when the collision occurs, causing severe head, neck, and body cavity trauma to its occupant. If the harness straps are not tight on the child, the child may come out of the seat during the crash. If the safety seat is used in the car's front seat, the child can suffer a serious injury when the air bag deploys.

Expect a pedestrian struck by a car to have fractures of the lower extremities. If the auto was moving at 20 miles per hour, expect less-severe fractures than if it had been moving at 55 miles per hour. Internal injuries are also less likely at lower speeds than at higher speeds. By evaluating the strength and nature of impact, you can anticipate which organs are injured and the degree of their damage.

For a gunshot patient, determine the type of gun used, the range of the shot, and whether an exit wound exists. This information will enable you to estimate the damage along the bullet's path and to formulate an index of suspicion for your patient's possible injuries. Expect the internal injuries from serious blunt trauma to be more extensive and severe than those you see externally. Often, the mechanism of injury is the only clue to the possibility of serious internal injury. The chapters "Blunt Trauma" and "Penetrating Trauma" describe the mechanisms of these injuries in depth.

Determine the nature of the illness from bystanders, family members, or your patient himself. If the patient is alert and oriented, he is usually the best source of information about his problem. If he is unresponsive, disoriented, or otherwise unable to provide information, rely on family members, bystanders, or visual cues for this information.

The scene can give additional clues to your patient's condition. How is your patient positioned? Does he sit bolt upright, gasping to breathe? Are pill bottles or drug paraphernalia nearby? Is medical care equipment, such as an oxygen tank, a nebulizer, or a glucometer, in the room? For example, if you respond to a "difficulty breathing" call and your patient is using his nebulizer when you arrive, suspect a history of pulmonary disease such as asthma, emphysema, or chronic bronchitis. If your patient is an agitated 17-year-old with a rapid pulse and you notice crack cocaine ampules on the floor, suspect a substance abuse problem.

Sometimes the nature of the illness is not readily apparent. Your patient with severe difficulty breathing, for instance, may be suffering from respiratory disease, a cardiac problem, an allergic reaction, or a toxic exposure. Remember that the nature of your patient's illness may be very different from his chief complaint.

Summary

The scene size-up is the initial step in the patient care process. Sizing up the scene and situation begins at your initial dispatch and does not end until you are clear of the call. As the call unfolds, you should be making constant observations and adjustments to your plan of action. Remember that your safety and the safety of your partner are paramount—it is hard to effectively treat both yourself and others.

Scene size-up should be practiced so much that it becomes second nature to you. It is like noticing veins on people in public after you begin starting IVs. (You have all done it—looked across the room at the back of someone's hand and noticed what nice veins they had.) Sizing up a scene is no different. After a while, you begin to notice mechanisms of injury and other important details almost subconsciously. But be careful and do not get complacent! Always make it a point to pause for just a few seconds and consciously look around the scene before proceeding into any situation.

Scene size-up is not a step-by-step process, but a series of decisions you make when confronted with a variety of circumstances that are often beyond your control. It is a way to make order out of chaos, keep yourself and your crew safe, and ensure that all necessary resources are focused on patient care and outcomes. With time and experience, you will learn to perform a scene size-up quickly and focus on important issues. Your careful size-up lays the foundation for an organized and timely approach toward patient care and scene management. And always remember that scene size-up is not a one-time occurrence. It is an ongoing process.

You Make the Call

It is a cold evening, and your county has experienced record rainfall in the last few days. You and your EMT partner are dispatched to the scene of "vehicle off the roadway", along with a BLS engine company. As you approach the reported location of the accident, you see a minivan that appears to be on its side approximately 20 feet down the roadside embankment. The van sits in a depression that is flooded with standing water reaching about halfway up the vehicle. As you pass the accident you see an adult female who appears to be attempting to climb out a passenger side window.

Describe how you would size up this scene. Make sure you cover the following areas:

- Vehicle placement
- Initial radio report
- Assuming incident command
- Safety
- Hazard control
- Standard Precautions
- Location and triaging of patients
- Mechanism of injury
- Resource determination

See Suggested Responses at the back of this book.

Review Questions

1. Which of the following statements bests describes the scene size-up phase of assessment?

   a. The purpose of the scene size-up is to find and treat life threats.

   b. The scene size-up should be performed by the senior crew member.

   c. The scene size-up is an ongoing process.

   d. The scene size-up determines whether the patient is a high or low priority.

2. For which of the following situations should the HEPA mask be used by the paramedic?

   a. In an extended care facility where multiple residents have similar respiratory diseases

   b. In a child care facility where one child has bitten another on the arm for taking a crayon

   c. At a multiple-casualty incident where a commercial airliner has crashed at a regional airport

   d. When entering a home in which there is a suspicion of high levels of carbon monoxide

3. You are at the scene of a car crash where the car has been found overturned in a small river parallel to the road. You can still see the wheels and undercarriage of the car, but the patient compartment is submerged. A witness to the incident states that no one has emerged from the vehicle. In this situation, what is most important?

   a. Containing the fuel cell to prevent an environmental hazard

   b. Extricating the patient from the car if you think you can

   c. Ensuring that the witness is kept safe

   d. Your personal safety at the scene

4. As you approach a dark home at night, something just does not seem right. It is not anything you can put your finger on, just a sense that something is wrong or is about to happen. What should you do?

   a. Wait until law enforcement arrives before entering.

   b. Have your partner enter the scene while you wait outside in case an emergency occurs.

   c. Enter the scene with something with which to protect yourself.

   d. Call out for the patient to come outside so you can initiate care.

5. You are dispatched for a shooting at a local drinking establishment. You ask dispatch if law enforcement is en route also; dispatch confirms that they are, but does not know whether they are on scene yet. Given this information, what should your EMS crew do?

   a. Park the ambulance outside the bar but do not exit the ambulance until law enforcement arrives.

   b. After you arrive on the scene, send one EMS provider inside to ensure scene safety.

   c. Tell dispatch you will not respond until you are assured by the police that the scene is safe and the perpetrator is in custody.

   d. Stage your ambulance a few blocks away until law enforcement clears the scene.

6. You arrive on the scene and see that a power line lies close to your pediatric patient. You are fairly certain the line is live and decide to move it with a dry piece of equipment. Which of the following should you use?

   a. A wooden-handled ax

   b. A fallen tree branch

   c. A nylon rope

   d. None of the above

7. Early one morning, near the end of your 12-hour shift, you are dispatched to a school bus-versus-truck crash. You are the first to arrive and you notice that the bus is lying on its side. Numerous children are crawling out of the bus, others are walking around, and some are lying on the ground nearby. What should be the first task(s) completed by your EMS unit?

   a. Begin treating the first patients you encounter.

   b. Establish incident command and begin the triage process.

   c. While you start triaging patients, your partner should begin loading the minimally wounded into the ambulance.

   d. Start at opposite ends of the scene and begin assessing patients.

8. The most important infection control measure you can employ to prevent contracting or spreading disease is _____

   a. handwashing

   b. wearing gloves

   c. donning eyewear

   d. wearing a full body gown

9. Most paramedics are trained to what level concerning a hazardous material spill?

   a. Awareness level

   b. Action level

c. Coordination level

d. Technician level

10. The "Reach–Throw–Row–Go" technique is used to
    _____

    a. remove power lines from a car with entrapped people.

    b. isolate a hazardous material that endangers civilians.

    c. conduct a search in a confined space.

    d. rescue a drowning victim.

See Answers to Review Questions at the back of this book.

References

1. Centers for Disease Control and Prevention. *Standard Precautions III, 2009.* (Available at http://www.cdc.gov/ncidod/dhqp/gl_isolation_standard.html. Accessed July 26, 2015.)

2. Centers for Disease Control and Prevention. *Standard Precautions IV, 2011.* (Available at http://www.cdc.gov/ncidod/dhqp/gl_isolation_standard.html. Accessed July 27, 2015.)

3. Usatch, B. "When Lightning Strikes, Bolting Down the Facts and Fiction." *JEMS* 34(4) (2009): 36–39.

4. U.S. Department of Labor Occupational Safety and Health Administration. *Confined Spaces: 2009.* (Available at http://www.osha.gov/SLTC/confinedspaces/index.html. Accessed June 14, 2015.)

Further Reading

Federal Emergency Management Administration: NIMS Resource Center. 2009. (Available at http://www.fema.gov/emergency/nims/. Accessed July 20, 2015.)

Friese, G. The Methamphetamine Crisis. 2006. (Available at www.emsworld.com/article/10323126/the-methamphetamine-crisis. Accessed July 25, 2015.)

International Fire Service Training Association (IFSTA). *Principles of Vehicle Extrication,* 3rd ed. Upper Saddle River, NJ: Pearson/Prentice Hall, 2010.

Meyer, M. *Chemistry of Hazardous Materials with MyFireKit,* 5th ed. Upper Saddle River, NJ: Pearson/Prentice Hall, 2009.

Tompkins, S. Emergency Services Control of Aggressive Patients Education. 2009. (Available at http://escapeprogram.net/. Accessed July 11, 2015.)

U.S. Department of Homeland Security. National Incident Management System. 2009. (Available at http://www.dhs.gov/xlibrary/assets/NIMS-90-web.pdf. Accessed July 11, 2015.)

U.S. Department of Labor Occupational Safety and Health Administration. Hazardous Waste Operations and Emergency Response. 2009. (Available at http://www.osha.gov/pls/oshaweb/owadisp.show_document?p_table5standards&p_id59765. Accessed July 19, 2015.)

U.S. Department of Transportation, Pipeline and Hazardous Materials Safety Administration. Emergency Response Guidebook. 2012. (Available at http://www.phmsa.dot.gov/hazmat/library/erg. Accessed July 11, 2015.)

Weber, C. H. *Pocket Reference for Hazardous Materials Response.* Upper Saddle River, NJ: Pearson/Prentice Hall, 2008.

Wilder, S. S. and C. Sorensen. *Essentials of Aggression Management in Health Care.* Upper Saddle River, NJ: Pearson/Prentice Hall, 2000.

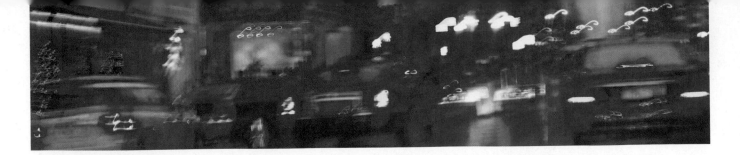

Chapter 2
Primary Assessment

Richard A. Cherry, MS, EMT-P

STANDARD
Assessment

COMPETENCY
Integrate scene and patient assessment findings with knowledge of epidemiology and pathophysiology to form a field impression. This includes developing a list of differential diagnoses through clinical reasoning to modify the assessment and formulate a treatment plan.

 Learning Objectives

Terminal Performance Objective: After reading this chapter, you should be able to perform a primary assessment in which you identify and intervene in all immediate threats to life.

Enabling Objectives: To accomplish the terminal performance objective, you should be able to:

1. Define key terms introduced in this chapter.

2. Discuss how the primary assessment integrates into the overall context of an emergency call.

3. Identify the individual components that comprise the primary assessment.

4. Discuss the forming of a general impression and integrate this into the primary assessment.

5. Identify the clinical need to stabilize the cervical spine during the primary assessment.

6. Discuss how to assess baseline mental status and integrate this into the primary assessment.

7. Discuss how to assess and manage the airway as it integrates into the primary assessment.

8. Discuss how to assess and manage breathing as it integrates into the primary assessment.

9. Discuss how to assess and manage circulation as it integrates into the primary assessment.

10. Discuss how to establish patient priorities as it relates to the primary assessment findings.

11. Given a scenario, discuss how you would integrate these components into a comprehensive primary assessment.

KEY TERMS

circulation assessment, p. 29

decerebrate, p. 25

decorticate, p. 25

general impression, p. 22

primary assessment, p. 22

Case Study

En route to the scene, paramedic Andy Illingston and EMT Diane Tomlinson prepare for the worst. The initial report from bystanders at the scene says that a woman jumped from a fourth-floor balcony at the downtown shopping mall. She reportedly landed four stories below on the marble floor and lies bleeding with multiple injuries. If this is true, Andy thinks, he and Diane will find a critical patient with serious injuries.

On arrival, Andy's worst fears come true. A woman in her mid-30s is lying on the floor in a pool of blood with signs of obvious multiple trauma. Immediately, Andy directs Diane to stabilize the woman's head and neck and manually open her airway with a jaw thrust. Andy begins the primary assessment by evaluating their patient's level of response. He quickly notes that the patient is unresponsive to all stimuli. He then assesses the airway, which is noisy with gurgling blood, and immediately suctions the oropharynx and listens for air movement. The patient has shallow respirations at a rate of 38 per minute. Andy instructs Diane to insert an oropharyngeal airway and begin ventilations with a bag-valve mask and supplemental oxygen while he continues his assessment.

Because the patient exhibits signs of severe respiratory distress, Andy decides to assess her neck and chest before proceeding with the primary assessment. He quickly exposes the patient's chest and notices deformity to the right side with probable multiple rib fractures. He auscultates the chest and, noticing decreased breath sounds on the right side, suspects a flail chest and a pneumothorax. Andy feels for radial and carotid pulses. He notes the absence of a radial pulse and the cool, pale look of the patient's skin. The carotid pulse is weak at a rate of approximately 130 beats per minute. Diane comments that the patient is in shock. Andy designates her as a priority 1 patient, indicating rapid transport to the appropriate medical facility.

While Diane continues to maintain manual stabilization of the patient's neck, Andy begins a rapid secondary assessment. He starts at the head and quickly palpates a depressed skull fracture. Andy notes that the patient's trachea is midline and jugular veins are flat, temporarily ruling out a tension pneumothorax. He notices a rigid, distended abdomen and suspects an intraabdominal bleed, which is most likely causing the profound shock. Next, he palpates the pelvis and notes an unstable pelvic ring, indicating fracture. He also notes severe deformity and angulation to both femurs, suggesting bilateral fractures. As additional help from the fire department arrives, he instructs them to quickly immobilize the patient on a vacuum mattress while he prepares the back of the ambulance for transport.

Once in the ambulance, Andy reassesses his patient's mental status and ABCs during the 4-minute ride to Memorial Hospital. At this time, he takes a full set of vital signs and notes the following: heart rate, 130 and weak; blood pressure, 76/40 mmHg; respirations, 38 and shallow. Andy decides to administer a rapid fluid bolus. Advanced EMT Joe Calloway, one of the firefighters, performs the procedure and runs both lines "wide open." Andy contacts the hospital and gives a quick report to Dr. Prasad, the attending physician. On arrival, they transfer their patient to the emergency department staff and watch as an experienced team of trauma specialists prepares the patient for a quick ride to surgery.

Customer Service Minute

The Human Touch A paramedic field preceptor was working with a student one afternoon when they responded to a call for an unknown illness. The patient was an elderly woman who drifted in and out of consciousness. The paramedic student provided first-class medical care. He conducted an efficient and relevant assessment, provided advanced life support, and did everything right. By the end of this call, he was exhausted. The only thing the preceptor did was sit by the patient's head en route to the hospital and talk with her. He put a hand on her shoulder and provided some reassurance during her lucid moments. When they arrived at the emergency department and prepared to get out of the ambulance, she suddenly gave the preceptor a big hug and thanked him. The student was dumbfounded. Afterward he asked his mentor, "Why did she hug you? I did all the work!" But he eventually understood.

What do our patients expect from us? First, they want us to respond quickly. If it's not quick, it's not emergency service. They expect us to solve their problem by being smart (book smart and street smart), by being skillful, and by using good, sound clinical judgment.

Mostly, they expect us to be nice. Treat your patients just as you would your mother. Focus on them, explain things, and say good-bye before you leave the hospital. They will remember how you treated them long after they've forgotten that you missed the IV three times. Patient care is about human contact. Let your patients know that they've been taken care of by an EMS professional.

Customer service is always human being to human being. This is especially true in EMS. We bring with us thousands of dollars in patient care monitoring technology, but what patients remember most was how we treated them. When we make a connection with our patients, we remind patients that we, in EMS, care about people.

Introduction

The **primary assessment** is the basis of all prehospital emergency medical care. Its goal is to identify and correct immediately life-threatening conditions of the patient's airway, breathing, or circulation (ABCs). If you find these conditions during this part of your assessment, treat them at once. For example, open a closed airway, provide ventilation, or control hemorrhage before moving on.

Immediately following the primary assessment, decide whether to provide immediate transport or to perform further on-scene assessment and care. As with the scene size-up, think of the primary assessment not as a step-by-step process, but as a series of critical decisions based on what you find. In most cases, you will proceed systematically through the ABCs, but sometimes the situation may determine how much priority you give to any one component. For example, if you suspect that your patient is in cardiac arrest, begin your assessment with a circulation check, followed by airway and breathing. In another situation, if you find your patient bleeding profusely from an arterial wound, it would be a waste of time to secure his airway first if, by the time it was secured, he would have exsanguinated. Think

---

CONTENT REVIEW

➤ Steps of Primary Assessment
   • Form a general impression.
   • Stabilize cervical spine as needed.
   • Assess baseline mental status.
   • Assess and manage airway.
   • Assess and manage breathing.
   • Assess and manage circulation.
   • Determine priorities.

---

of the primary assessment as a solid framework from which to begin but always allow common sense to dictate the best way to proceed.

The primary assessment consists of the following components:

• Forming a general impression
• Stabilizing the cervical spine as needed
• Assessing a baseline mental status
• Assessing and managing the airway
• Assessing and managing breathing
• Assessing and managing circulation
• Determining priorities of care and transport

The primary assessment should take less than 1 minute, unless you have to intervene with lifesaving measures. Perform the primary assessment again as part of your reassessment throughout the patient contact, especially after any major intervention or whenever your patient's condition changes.

Let's now take an in-depth look at the components of a primary assessment.

Forming a General Impression

The **general impression** is your first, intuitive evaluation of your patient. It is also known as your "view from the door." It will help you determine his general clinical status (stable versus unstable) and priority for immediate transport. Base your first impression on the information you gather from the environment, the mechanism of injury, the nature of the illness, your patient's posture and overall look, the chief complaint, and your instincts.

One of the first determinations you will make is whether your patient "looks dead or doesn't look dead." Because this is a critical step in the management of a patient in cardiac arrest, it must be determined as soon as possible. If your patient looks dead, make a quick evaluation of responsiveness and breathing. If he is unresponsive and is apneic or has agonal respirations, quickly feel for a pulse and, if the pulse is absent, begin chest compressions immediately. Continue the standard CPR sequence of 30 compressions and 2 quick breaths. If your patient shows any signs of life, such as moaning, groaning, or moving, or if he shows a significant breathing effort, conduct the standard primary assessment (ABC) as outlined in this chapter.

Your patient's age, gender, and race often influence your index of suspicion. Very old and very young patients are more apt to have severe complications from injury or illness. This is because their compensation mechanisms are either not yet fully formed or have deteriorated with age. Suspect a woman of childbearing age with lower abdominal pain and vaginal bleeding to have a life-threatening gynecologic emergency known as ruptured ectopic pregnancy. Black Americans have a higher incidence of hypertension and cardiovascular disease than members of other races.

Determine whether your patient's problem results from trauma or from a medical problem. Sometimes this will not be readily apparent. For example, did your patient slip and fall or get dizzy and fall? Note your patient's face and his posture and decide whether rapid intervention or a more deliberate approach is warranted. With experience, you will be able to recognize even the most subtle clues of a patient in critical condition. Generally, the more serious the condition, the quieter your patient will be. Look at, listen to, and smell the environment. Gather as many clues as possible as you enter the scene.

Take the necessary Standard Precautions with every patient. Then, if your patient is alert, identify yourself and begin to establish a rapport. For example, "Hello, I'm Marko Johnson, a paramedic with AVON Ambulance Service. I'm here to help you." This establishes your level of training, authority, and reason for being at your patient's side. It also allows your patient to refuse care. As discussed in the chapter, "Medical–Legal Aspects of Prehospital Care," you cannot provide care without either implied or informed consent.

Reassure your patient. Listen to him and do not trivialize his complaints. Frequently, we forget how significant an injury or illness, even a minor one, seems to a patient. With your experience, his problem may seem insignificant to you, but for your patient it is a real concern. There is a fine line between reassuring your patient and minimizing his condition. Remain calm and reassure him while you take his situation seriously. The ill or injured patient may worry about the long-term consequences for work, child care, and finances. Understand these fears and support your patient psychologically as well as physiologically.

If the mechanism of injury is significant or if your patient is unresponsive, have your partner manually stabilize your patient's head and neck (Figure 2-1). Approximately 2 percent of victims with blunt trauma have a spinal injury; this risk is tripled if the victim has a craniofacial injury.[1] Do this before establishing his mental status and continue manual stabilization until you make the decision whether or not full spinal motion restriction is indicated as directed by local protocols. If your patient is awake, explain what you are doing and ask him not to move his neck. You do not want him to turn his head when you try to assess mental status. Ask your partner to maintain your patient's head in a neutral position as you begin your assessment. If your patient is a small child, place a small towel or pad

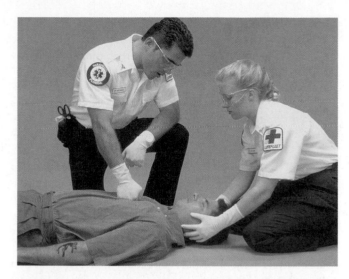

FIGURE 2-1 Manually stabilize the head and neck on first patient contact.

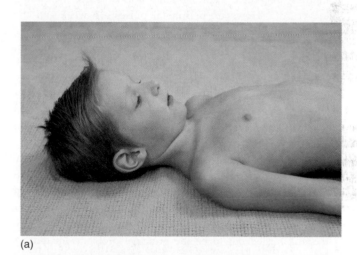

(a)

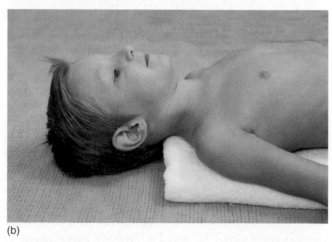

(b)

FIGURE 2-2 Place a folded towel under your young patient's shoulders to keep the airway aligned. (a) Airway not aligned. (b) Airway aligned after using a towel.

beneath the shoulders to maintain proper alignment of the cervical spine (Figure 2-2). This will compensate for the large occiput of the child's head, which normally would flex his neck when he is placed on a flat surface.

Patho Pearls

Patient assessment actually starts as soon as you approach the scene. Clues about the patient's underlying pathophysiology might be evident from such things as positioning of a vehicle, downed power lines, or the appearance and actions of bystanders. However, your safety, and that of your fellow rescuers, is always paramount. Never approach a scene that appears unsafe. With time, you will develop a "sixth sense" about emergency scenes and bystanders.

As you begin the patient encounter, process all that you see into your patient assessment and care. For example, consider this scenario: A car with two 16-year-old girls fails to negotiate a turn on a country road and overturns into a flowing creek adjacent to the road. Although the ambient temperature is in the 60s, you know that the temperature of the water in this area often is in the 40s. Thus, you should immediately suspect the possibility of hypothermia.

As the girls are removed from entrapment, no obvious injuries are noted. Vital signs are normal other than slight tachycardia. However, peripheral pulses are weak and the skin is pale and cool. Is it shock? Is it hypothermia? Is it both? Your index of suspicion is high for both hypothermia and blunt force trauma. You follow local protocols with regard to immobilization, fluid therapy, and monitoring. Once in the ambulance and wrapped in blankets, both girls start to show signs that blood flow to the skin is improving. By the time you reach the hospital, their skin has a normal color and their pulse rates are normal.

Following a comprehensive assessment in the emergency department, the girls are discharged to their parents with no apparent injuries. Thus, your instincts were right. The potential for shock was a greater risk to the girls than the potential for hypothermia, and you had to treat based on this risk. But hypothermia turned out to be the principal problem. Integrating information from the scene size-up, patient history, and patient examination gave you a clear picture of the patients' underlying pathophysiologic process.

Mental Status Assessment

Your assessment of baseline mental status is crucial for all patients.[2] For example, when you deliver your head injury patient to the emergency department, the neurosurgeon will want a chronological report of your patient's mental status from the time you arrived on the scene. This vital information helps the surgical team diagnose a deteriorating brain injury. For example, if the patient was alert and oriented when you arrived, then became sleepy en route, and within 30 minutes was responsive only to deep pain stimuli, the suspicion for epidural hematoma with subsequent rising intracranial pressure is high. Rapid surgical intervention in these and many other cases can save lives if the diagnosis is made quickly. Your baseline mental status documentation is critical to these patients' emergency care.

Establishing a baseline mental status is also crucial in assessing the variety of medical situations that cause altered levels of response. Drug overdoses, poisonings, diabetic emergencies, sepsis, hypoxia, and hypovolemia are just a few of the many conditions that result in altered mentation. For the stroke patient, identifying the time of the symptoms' onset is critical for the emergency physician to consider administering clot-dissolving drugs. This is possible only with your accurate assessment of your patient's change in mental status.

AVPU Levels

To record your patient's mental status, use the acronym AVPU. Your patient is either **A**lert, responds to **V**erbal stimuli, responds only to **P**ainful stimuli, or is **U**nresponsive. Perform this exam by starting with verbal stimuli, then moving to painful stimuli only if he fails to respond to your verbal cues.

Alert

An alert patient is awake, as evidenced by open eyes. He may be oriented to person (who he is), place (where he is), time (day, month, and year), and situation (what is going on) and give organized, coherent answers to your questions. In contrast, an alert patient also may be disoriented and confused. For example, a patient with a suspected concussion will often present as dazed and confused. A hypoxic or hypoglycemic patient may present as combative. A shock patient may be restless and anxious. If his eyes are open and he appears awake, however, he is categorized as alert.

Children's responses to your questions will vary with their age-related physical and emotional development. Infants and young children usually will be curious but cautious when a stranger approaches. Their level of response may not indicate the gravity of their condition. In fact, the quiet child is usually the seriously injured or ill child.

Verbal

If your patient appears to be sleeping but responds when you talk to him, he is responsive to verbal stimuli. He can respond by speaking, opening his eyes, moaning, or just moving. Note the level of his verbal response. Does he speak clearly, mumble inappropriate words, or make incomprehensible sounds? Children may respond to your verbal commands by turning their heads or stopping activity. For infants, you may have to shout to elicit a response.

Pain

If your child or adult patient does not respond to verbal stimuli, try to elicit a response with painful stimuli. Pinch his fingernails or perform a "horsebite" (pinching tender areas such as under the arms, flanks, inner thigh, or back of the knee) and watch for a response. Again, the patient may respond by waking up, speaking, moaning, opening his eyes, or moving. Note the type of motor response to the painful stimuli. Is his response purposeful or nonpurposeful? If he tries to move your hand away or to move himself away from the pain, it is purposeful.[3] **Decorticate** (arms flexed, legs extended) or **decerebrate** (arms and legs extended) posturing is nonpurposeful and suggests a serious brain injury. For the infant, flick the soles of the feet and expect crying as the appropriate response.

Unresponsive

The unresponsive patient is comatose and fails to respond to any noxious stimuli.

The AVPU scale describes your patient's general mental status. Avoid using terms such as "semiconscious," "lethargic," or "stuporous" because they are interpreted broadly and you have not had a chance to conduct a comprehensive neurologic exam at this point.

Your patient's response to stimulation will tell you a great deal about his condition. Any alteration or deterioration in mental status may indicate an emergent or already serious problem. A patient with an impaired mental status may have lost, or be in danger of losing, the ability to protect his airway. Take immediate steps to protect your patient's airway by proper positioning and the use of basic and advanced airway adjuncts as appropriate. Provide oxygen if your patient exhibits a pulse oximetry reading below 95 percent and provide only enough until your reading is in the normal range (95 to 100 percent).

Airway Assessment

If your patient is responsive and can speak clearly, you can assume that his airway is patent. If your patient is unconscious, however, his airway may be obstructed. The supine unconscious patient's tongue often obstructs his upper airway. Because the mandible, tongue, and epiglottis are all connected, gravity allows these structures to block the patient's upper airway as his facial muscles relax. Assume that the unconscious patient has no gag reflex and cannot protect his airway. Because of this, secretions probably have settled in the hypopharynx even if you do not hear a gurgling sound. Routine oropharyngeal suctioning will clear these secretions effectively.

You can open your patient's airway with one of two simple manual maneuvers: the jaw-thrust maneuver or the

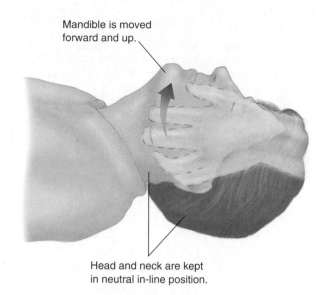

Mandible is moved forward and up.

Head and neck are kept in neutral in-line position.

FIGURE 2-3 Use the jaw-thrust maneuver to open your patient's airway if you suspect a cervical spine injury.

head-tilt/chin-lift maneuver. If you suspect a cervical spine injury, open the airway using a jaw thrust without head extension.[4] Place your thumbs on your patient's cheeks and lift up on the angle of the jaw with your fingers (Figure 2-3). For all other patients, use the head-tilt/chin-lift maneuver. Place one hand on your patient's forehead and lift up under the chin with the fingers of your other hand (Figure 2-4). Because maintaining a patent airway and providing adequate oxygenation and ventilation are priorities in managing critical patients, use a head-tilt/chin-lift maneuver if the jaw thrust does not open the airway.

To open the airways of infants and young children, apply a gentle and conservative extension of the head and neck (Figure 2-5). These patients' upper airway structures are very flexible and are easily kinked when their necks are flexed or hyperextended. It may be necessary to move the child's head through a range of positions to obtain optimal airway patency and effective rescue breathing.[5]

To assess your patient's airway, look for chest rise while you listen and feel for air movement. If the airway is clear, you should hear quiet airflow and feel free air movement. A noisy airway is a partially obstructed airway. Snoring occurs when the tongue partially blocks the upper airway. In this case, reposition the head and neck and reevaluate. Gurgling indicates that fluid, such as blood, secretions, or gastric contents, is blocking the upper airway. Gently open and examine the mouth for foreign bodies you can remove easily and quickly. Use aggressive suctioning to remove blood, vomit, secretions, and other fluids.

The high-pitched inspiratory screech of stridor is caused by a life-threatening upper airway obstruction that may be caused by a foreign body, severe swelling, allergic reaction, or infection. If you suspect a foreign body obstruction and your patient exhibits poor air movement,

ADULT

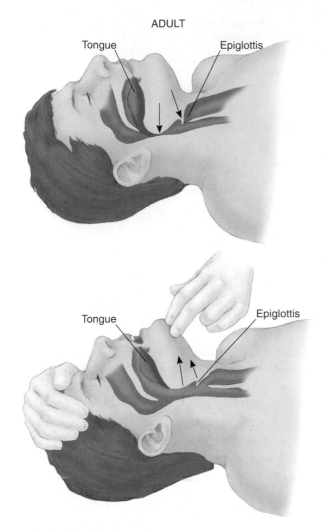

FIGURE 2-4 The head-tilt/chin-lift maneuver in an adult.

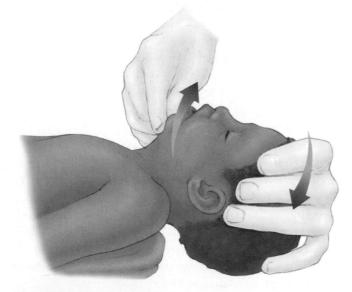

FIGURE 2-5 The head-tilt/chin-lift maneuver in an infant. Do not overextend the head and neck.

a weak cough, or a diminishing mental status, immediately deliver abdominal thrusts to dislodge the object. If your patient is less than 1 year old, use back blows and

chest thrusts instead of abdominal thrusts. If these maneuvers are ineffective, remove the object under direct laryngoscopy with Magill forceps. If these attempts fail, try inserting an endotracheal tube in the hope of passing it past or through the object or pushing it down into the right mainstem bronchus, thereby clearing the way for left lung ventilation.

Other causes of stridor require vastly different approaches. Upper respiratory infections such as croup or epiglottitis call for oxygen administration (if your patient's pulse oximetry is below 95 percent) and a quiet ride to the hospital. In croup cases, vaporized epinephrine is helpful, and minimally invasive, in opening the upper airway. More invasive maneuvers, such as positive pressure ventilation, continuous positive airway pressure (CPAP), bilevel positive airway pressure (BiPAP), intubation, and cricothyrotomy, are indicated only if the airway becomes totally obstructed.

Respiratory burns can cause rapid massive swelling of the upper airway and require rapid endotracheal intubation. Anaphylaxis necessitates vasoconstrictor medications to decrease upper airway swelling. Because these vastly different management techniques are potentially life threatening when applied inappropriately, your correct field diagnosis is critical. If your patient presents with stridor, take time to evaluate the history and clinical signs and symptoms for the common causes of stridor: foreign body obstruction (sudden onset while eating), epiglottitis (fever, illness, drooling, inability to swallow), respiratory burns (history of facial burns, hoarseness), and anaphylaxis (hives, history of allergies).

The softer, expiratory whistle of wheezing is caused by constricted bronchioles, the smaller, lower airways. You may hear it audibly (without a stethoscope) in cases such as asthma, bronchitis, emphysema, acute pulmonary edema, or other causes of bronchospasm. Bronchiolitis, a lower respiratory infection, often causes these sounds in infants and young children. If you do hear wheezing, use a stethoscope to better hear and identify the sounds before you proceed with treatment. Wheezing patients require a bronchodilator medication to dilate the bronchioles and reduce airway resistance. Use aerosolized medications, such as albuterol and ipratroprium, for this purpose.

If your patient is not moving air, quickly feel for a pulse. If he is pulseless, begin CPR immediately. If he has a pulse, he is in respiratory arrest. Immediately provide ventilation with a bag-valve mask and high-concentration oxygen (Figure 2-6). Give two rescue breaths, each over 1 second, with enough volume to produce visible chest rise. Be careful not to overventilate (by breathing either too fast or too deeply). Ventilate adult patients at a rate of 10 to 12 breaths per minute and all children at a rate of 12 to 20 breaths per minute.[5, 6] If you cannot ventilate the lungs,

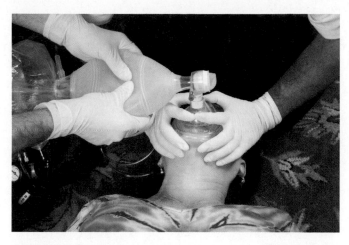

FIGURE 2-6 Immediately use a bag-valve mask to ventilate patients who are not moving air.

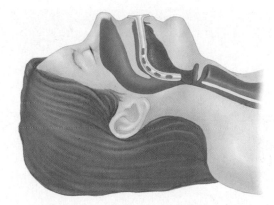

FIGURE 2-7 Use an oropharyngeal airway for unconscious patients without a gag reflex.

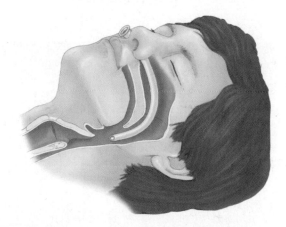

FIGURE 2-8 The nasopharyngeal airway rests between the tongue and the posterior pharyngeal wall.

reposition the head and neck and try again. If there is still no air movement, assume a complete obstruction and apply the measures explained earlier.

In an infant, if you have difficulty making an effective seal over the mouth and nose, try either mouth-to-mouth or mouth-to-nose ventilation.[6] If you use the mouth-to-mouth technique, pinch the nose closed. If you use the mouth-to-nose technique, close the mouth. In either case, make sure the chest rises when you give a breath.

Sometimes, in cases of massive face and neck trauma, you may have to use unorthodox methods to find and secure the airway. For example, a patient with facial trauma and a massive open neck wound may require you to look for the presence of bubbles in the neck wound and trace them to an opening in the larynx or trachea. Then insert an endotracheal tube or other tracheal device into the opening and ventilate your patient. These types of situations are extremely challenging, but managing the difficult airway is certainly part of a paramedic's scope of practice.

Once you have cleared the airway, keeping it open may require constant attention. In these cases, insert a basic airway adjunct to help keep the tongue from blocking the upper airway. If your patient is unconscious and lacks a gag reflex, insert an oropharyngeal airway (Figure 2-7). If he has a gag reflex or significant orofacial trauma, insert a nasopharyngeal airway (Figure 2-8). Be cautious when using a nasopharyngeal airway if you suspect a basilar skull fracture because these airways have been passed through the skull fracture and into the brain. If the patient has no gag reflex and cannot protect his airway, you will need to use advanced techniques to maintain airway patency.[5, 6] These include the many forms of endotracheal intubation (Figure 2-9), the many multilumen airways (Figure 2-10), and transtracheal techniques such as needle or surgical cricothyroidotomy (Figure 2-11). The multilumen airways are not appropriate for use in

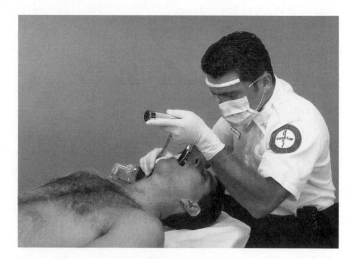

FIGURE 2-9 Endotracheal intubation.

children. If your patient has an airway problem and shows signs of hypoxia (pulse oximetry below 95 percent), administer oxygen by nonrebreather mask. All these devices for maintaining upper airway patency are described in detail in the chapter "Airway Management and Ventilation."

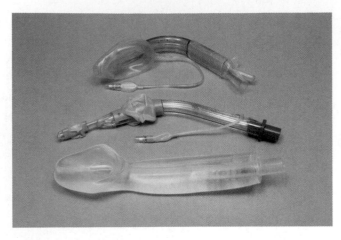

FIGURE 2-10 A variety of multilumen airways are becoming more popular in managing the airway of critical patients.

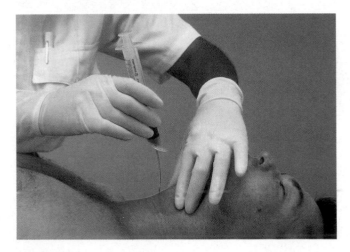

FIGURE 2-11 QuickTrach® device.

Breathing Assessment

Assess your patient for adequate breathing. Immediately note any signs of inadequate breathing:

- Altered mental status, confusion, apprehension, or agitation
- Shortness of breath while speaking
- Retractions (supraclavicular, suprasternal, intercostal)
- Asymmetric chest wall movement
- Accessory muscle use (neck, abdominal)
- Cyanosis
- Audible sounds
- Abnormally rapid, slow, or shallow breathing
- Nasal flaring

Assess the respiratory rate and quality. Normal respiratory rates vary according to your patient's age. Abnormally fast or slow rates (Table 2–1) actually decrease the

Table 2-1 Respiratory Rates

Age	Low Rate	High Rate
Newborn	30	60
Infant (<1 year)	30	60
Toddler (1–2 years)	24	40
Preschooler (3–5 years)	22	34
School age (6–12 years)	18	30
Adolescent (13–18 years)	12	26
Adult (>18 years)	12	20

amount of air that reaches the alveoli for gas exchange. For patients with abnormally fast or slow respiratory rates and decreased tidal volumes, provide positive-pressure ventilation with, for example, a bag-valve mask and supplemental oxygen, to ensure full lung expansion and maximum oxygenation.

Note the respiratory pattern. Rapid (tachypneic), deep (hyperpneic) respirations are a compensatory mechanism and suggest that the body is attempting to rid itself of excess acids. They may indicate a diabetic problem, severe acidosis, or head injury. They also may result from hyperventilation syndrome or from simple exertion. Kussmaul's respirations (deep, rapid breathing) accompanied by a fruity breath odor are a classic sign of a patient in diabetic ketoacidosis. In either case, always ensure an adequate inspiratory volume and administer only enough oxygen to correct hypoxia.

Cheyne-Stokes respirations, a series of increasing and decreasing breaths followed by a period of apnea, most likely result from a brainstem injury or increasing intracranial pressure. Biot's respirations, identified by short, gasping, irregular breaths, may signify severe brain injury. Again, ensure adequate inspiratory volume and provide ventilation with supplemental oxygen as needed. Some patients with acute pulmonary edema can benefit from a CPAP unit (Figure 2-12). These devices provide a constant back pressure that keeps the airways open, especially during exhalation, when they tend to collapse. They can also help drive oxygen across the alveolar–capillary membrane and prevent the need for endotracheal intubation.

If your patient's breathing appears inadequate, immediately assess the neck and chest before moving on to circulation. Quickly inspect and palpate the rib cage for rigidity and wounds. Auscultate bilaterally high and low for adequate and equal breath sounds. Identify and correct any life-threatening conditions before moving on. If you find a sucking chest wound, cover it immediately at

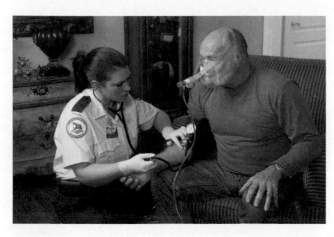

FIGURE 2-12 CPAP can provide positive airway pressure, which will maintain lower airway patency.

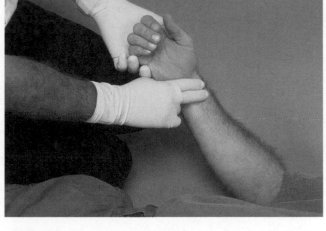

FIGURE 2-13 To assess an adult's circulation, feel for a radial pulse.

CONTENT REVIEW

➤ Signs of Inadequate Breathing
  - Altered mental status, confusion, apprehension, or agitation
  - Shortness of breath while speaking
  - Retractions
  - Asymmetric chest wall movement
  - Accessory muscle use
  - Cyanosis
  - Audible sounds
  - Abnormally rapid, slow, or shallow breathing
  - Nasal flaring

the end of exhalation (to prevent trapping air in the pleural space) with an occlusive dressing taped on three sides. This will act as a relief valve, allowing air to escape but not enter.

If you find signs of a tension pneumothorax (absent breath sounds on one side, diminished breath sounds on the other side, distended neck veins, unequal chest expansion), immediately decompress the affected side with a large IV catheter at the second intercostal space, midclavicular line. If you find a flail segment and resultant hypoventilation, immediately perform positive pressure ventilation. If you visualize or feel paradoxical movement of the segment, apply a large dressing to stabilize it. If your patient exhibits adequate breathing, or if you have successfully corrected his breathing problem move directly to circulation.

Two noninvasive devices can be extremely helpful in objectively assessing the adequacy of your patient's breathing: the pulse oximeter and the continuous waveform capnography monitor. Pulse oximetry is a useful tool in quantifying the oxygen saturation of the red blood cells and, ultimately, the tissues. Continuous waveform capnography can be invaluable in assessing not only your patient's ventilatory status, but also his general circulation. Whether these simple procedures should be routinely used during the primary assessment is debatable and situation dependent. Refer to the chapter "Patient

Monitoring Technology" for more information on these two devices.

Circulation Assessment

The **circulation assessment** consists of evaluating the pulse and skin and controlling hemorrhage. Go directly to the wrist and feel for a radial pulse (Figure 2-13). Its presence suggests adequate peripheral perfusion. If the radial pulse is absent, check for a carotid pulse (Figure 2-14). The carotid pulse's presence along with the absence of a peripheral pulse suggests a low flow state. In the infant, palpate the brachial pulse (Figure 2-15) or, if necessary, auscultate the apical pulse. If your patient is pulseless, begin chest compressions immediately, evaluate the cardiac rhythm, and provide prompt defibrillation as needed.

Assess your patient's pulse for rate and quality. The normal heart rate varies with your patient's age (Table 2–2). Very fast rates (tachycardia) and very slow rates

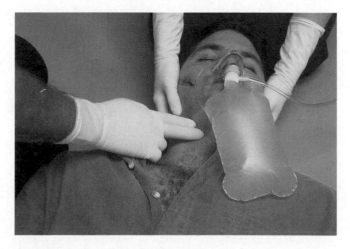

FIGURE 2-14 If you cannot feel a radial pulse, palpate for a carotid pulse.

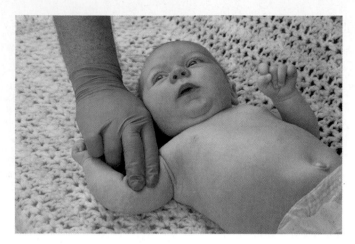

FIGURE 2-15 To assess an infant's circulation, palpate the brachial pulse.

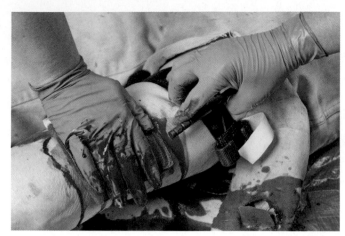

FIGURE 2-16 Combat application tourniquet.

(bradycardia) may indicate a life-threatening cardiac dysrhythmia. Abnormally fast or slow rates may result in decreased cardiac output. If your patient is hemodynamically unstable (i.e., altered mental status, hypotension, cool ashen skin) with an abnormally fast rate, quickly attach your monitor and prepare to perform synchronized cardioversion as appropriate. If the rate is abnormally slow, prepare to administer atropine and/or perform external cardiac pacing. For more information on this topic, refer to the chapter "Cardiology."

Note the quality of the pulse. The normal pulse should be regular and strong. An irregular pulse may indicate a cardiac arrhythmia requiring advanced cardiac life support procedures. In head injury, heat stroke, or hypertension, you will often find a strong, bounding pulse. A weak, thready pulse usually indicates poor perfusion due to fluid loss, pump failure, or massive vasodilation.

Stop your patient's bleeding if you have not already done so (Figure 2-16). Major bleeding usually originates with trauma, but it also can result from a medical emergency. For example, vaginal bleeding, rectal bleeding, and

even a nosebleed associated with hypertension can result in life-threatening blood loss. For external bleeding, employ any appropriate measures for hemorrhage control. First try direct pressure with elevation for an extremity wound followed quickly by a tourniquet (Figure 2-16) if the bleeding isn't controllable. For places not suitable for applying a tourniquet, for example the head or abdomen, use hemostatic agents (Figure 2-17) such as HemCon®,[7] QuikClot®,[8] and Celox™. Internal bleeding is not easily controlled in the prehospital setting and demands initiating transport as soon as possible.

Assess the skin for temperature, moisture, and color (Figure 2-18). Peripheral vasoconstriction decreases peripheral perfusion to the skin early in shock. The skin may appear mottled (blotchy), cyanotic (bluish), pale, or ashen. It may also feel cool and moist (clammy). This often indicates that warm, circulating blood has been shunted away from the skin to the core of the body to maintain perfusion of vital organs. If you find any of these signs, suspect conditions related to or caused by poor perfusion. In infants and young children, capillary refill is a reliable indicator of

Table 2-2 Normal Pulse Rate Ranges

Age	Low Rate	High Rate
Newborn	100	180
Infant (<1 year)	100	160
Toddler (1–2 years)	80	110
Preschooler (3–5 years)	70	110
School age (6–12 years)	65	110
Adolescent (13–18 years)	60	90
Adult (>18 years)	60	100

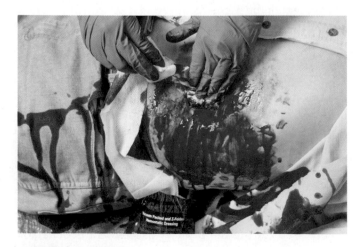

FIGURE 2-17 Hemostatic agent.

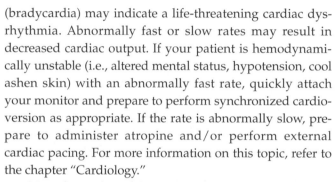

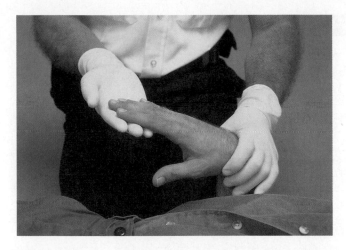

FIGURE 2-18 Assess the skin for color, temperature, and moisture.

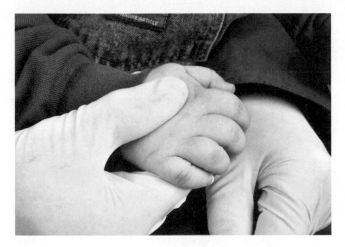

FIGURE 2-19 Capillary refill time provides important information about the circulatory status of infants and young children.

circulatory function (Figure 2-19). In adults, smoking, medications, cold weather, or chronic conditions of the elderly may affect capillary refill, so you should always consider the other indicators of circulatory function.

Priority Determination

Once you have conducted a primary assessment, determine your patient's priority. If the primary assessment suggests a serious illness or injury, conduct a rapid head-to-toe assessment to identify other life threats and transport the patient immediately to the nearest appropriate facility that can deliver definitive care. Do not delay transport for detailed assessments and procedures that you can provide en route to the hospital.

In 2011, the Centers for Disease Control and Prevention published a revised set of guidelines for field-triaging injured patients (Figure 2-20).[9] Its recommendations include a four-step process designed to decrease morbidity and mortality from trauma. Let's look at this process.

Step 1 is aimed at vital signs and level of consciousness. If your patient's Glasgow Coma Scale score is less than 14, his systolic blood pressure is less than 90 mmHg, or the respiratory rate is less than 10 or greater than 29 (less than 20 in infants <1 year), transport him to the highest-level trauma center in your community.

Step 2 is aimed at the anatomy of injury. If your patient has any of the following injuries, transport him to the highest-level trauma center in your community: penetrating injuries to the head, neck, torso, or extremities proximal to the elbow or knee; chest wall instability or deformity; two or more proximal long bone fractures; crushed, degloved, mangled, or pulseless extremity; amputation proximal to the wrist or ankle; pelvic fracture; open or depressed skull fracture; paralysis.

Step 3 is aimed at mechanism of injury and evidence of high-energy impact. If your patient suffered from one of the following mechanisms, transport him to the closest appropriate trauma facility (it need not be the highest level of trauma center): a fall of more than 20 feet for an adult, more than 10 feet for a child or two to three times the height of the child; high-risk auto crash (more than 12 inches intrusion into occupant site or more than 18 inches into any site; partial or complete ejection, death in same passenger compartment, vehicle telemetry data consistent with high risk of injury); auto-versus-pedestrian/bicyclist thrown, run over, or with significant (>20 mph) impact; and/or motorcycle crash >20 mph.

Step 4 is aimed at miscellaneous findings. If any of the following conditions exist, contact medical control and consider transport to a trauma center or specific resource hospital: age greater than 55; children; anticoagulants or bleeding disorders; burns without other trauma mechanism: triage to burn facility; burns with other trauma mechanism triage to trauma center; pregnancy greater than 20 weeks; EMS provider judgment.

In these cases, decide whether to stabilize your patient on the scene or expedite transport and initiate advanced life support procedures en route. On the way to the hospital you can conduct a general secondary assessment and provide additional care as time allows. If your patient is stable, before transport you can conduct a problem-oriented secondary assessment, followed by reassessment during transport as the situation requires, if time allows.

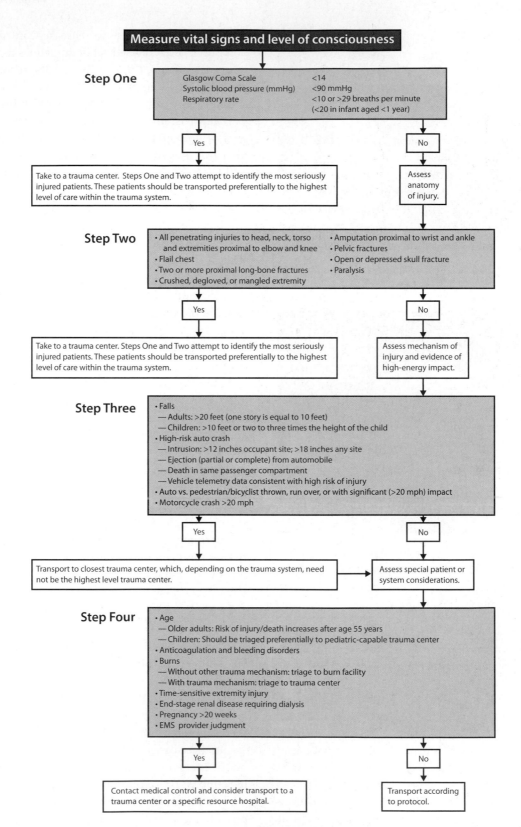

When in doubt, transport to a trauma center.

FIGURE 2-20 The 2011 Centers for Disease Control and Prevention Field Triage Guidelines.

(Centers for Disease Control and Prevention, http://www.cdc.gov/mmwr/pdf/rr/rr6101.pdf)

Summary

The primary assessment is the crucial first stage in providing lifesaving measures to seriously ill or injured patients—with the key term being "lifesaving" measures. The primary assessment is used to identify and correct immediate life threats to your patient. You will generally save more lives during the primary assessment than anywhere else in your patient care. It is here that you will reopen an obstructed airway, decompress a tension pneumothorax, seal an open pneumothorax, provide emergency ventilation and oxygenation, stop a major hemorrhage, or defibrillate a cardiac arrest. The list could go on. There is no more important element of your patient assessment than conducting a systematic primary assessment. It is time well spent.

After securing the scene and ensuring your personal safety, your goal is to identify and correct, if possible, any life threats in airway, breathing, circulation, and mental status. If you are systematic and have practiced, it should take you less than 1 minute to perform the primary assessment, yet it will provide you with enough vital information to begin correcting any life threats and confirm your priority determination for the patient and for transport.

Along with the obvious life threats, the primary assessment includes a "gut check" component that takes the patient's general appearance into account. What does your gut say when you first encounter the patient? If you walk in the room and your gut says "Oh crap!" you can mark that patient as a higher priority. If you walk into the room and your gut is saying "hmm," you need a little more information before you can make a decision. Either way, the primary assessment is a quick assessment of potentially life-threatening injuries, including cervical spine injuries, airway or breathing problems, circulatory issues, or any other situation that would cause an immediate threat to life.

In the next few chapters we will discuss continuing assessments for patients, including obtaining a thorough history, performing detailed physical exams, communicating effectively, and making clinical decisions based on your assessments.

You Make the Call

You respond to a residence for a report of a patient having difficulty breathing. You enter the living room and see a young man sitting on the couch. You notice he is slumped forward, resting his elbows on his knees, and that he does not look up at you as you enter. As you perform your primary assessment, you identify that his airway is patent and a rapid and strong radial pulse is present. While assessing his breathing, you see his head bobbing with each breath and identify a respiratory rate of about 10 breaths per minute with accessory muscle use. A family member states "He has asthma and has been working hard to breathe for several hours now."

1. How would you describe this patient's respiratory status? What factors influence this determination? What immediate interventions, if any, would you provide at this time?

See Suggested Responses at the back of this book.

Review Questions

1. Of the following components of the primary assessment, which should you normally perform first?

   a. Determine airway adequacy.

   b. Assess for breathing adequacy.

   c. Access circulatory parameters.

   d. Determine the patient's mental status.

2. During the primary assessment of an unresponsive pediatric patient who was ejected from a vehicle during a crash, you are providing manual cervical spine immobilization. To help maintain proper alignment of the child's head and neck, you should place a folded towel under which region of the body?

a. Head   c. Shoulders

b. Neck   d. Occiput

3. Your patient presents with his eyes open, and he responds to you when you speak to him. He answers your questions but is obviously disoriented as to time and place. Given this response to your stimulation, how would you grade him on the AVPU scale?

a. Alert   c. Painful

b. Verbal   d. Unresponsive

4. During your primary assessment, you determine that your trauma patient responds to loud verbal stimuli with moaning, he has a weak carotid pulse with no peripheral pulse, his breathing is labored at 32/minute, his airway displays sonorous sounds, and you note cyanosis to the face and hands. Given this information, what is your priority for treatment?

a. Apply high-flow oxygen via nonrebreather mask.

b. Suction the airway with a rigid-tip catheter.

c. Apply a manual airway technique.

d. Insert an oropharyngeal airway.

5. At what point should you initially determine that your patient has a partially occluded airway?

a. During the primary assessment

b. During the scene size-up

c. During the rapid trauma assessment

d. After making your patient priority determination

6. Your patient presents unconscious, without a gag reflex, and with decreased respirations that yield no airway sounds. During your initial management of the patient during the primary assessment, you should perform all of the following *except*

_____

a. open the airway manually.

b. perform bag-valve-mask ventilation.

c. administer oxygen.

d. provide full spinal immobilization.

7. Your trauma patient presents with cool, pale skin; a weak central pulse rate of 110/minute; absence of peripheral pulses; and a capillary refill time of 5 seconds. From this information, what can you conclude about his circulatory condition?

a. It is normal, given a history of traumatic injury.

b. It shows findings of early circulatory compromise.

c. It shows findings of severe circulatory collapse.

d. He requires immediate CPR, starting with chest compressions.

8. While caring for a trauma patient, which of the following would be the *last* finding to be managed during the primary assessment?

a. Airway compromise

b. Inadequate ventilation

c. Major hemorrhage

d. Lumbar spinal cord transection

9. Of the following assessment parameters, which would be the *least* reliable indicator of ventilatory adequacy?

e. Chest rise and fall

f. Air movement in and out of the mouth

g. Presence of bilateral breath sounds

h. Pulse oximetry

10. You are managing an unresponsive medical patient who had a large amount of blood in the airway. During oral suctioning, you noted that the patient had an intact gag reflex. Following the suctioning, the airway now displays snoring sounds, and manual airway techniques have failed. What should you do next?

a. Insert an oropharyngeal airway.

b. Insert an endotracheal tube.

c. Insert a nasopharyngeal airway.

d. Perform a surgical cricothyrotomy to secure the airway.

11. If your afebrile patient presents with a sudden onset of severe respiratory distress and an inability to speak or cough, what intervention should you perform?

a. Attempt to intubate.

b. Deliver abdominal thrusts.

c. Perform needle cricothyrotomy.

d. Administer humidified oxygen.

12. If your patient presents with a self-inflicted open chest wound to the anterior right thorax, what would be the appropriate intervention?

a. Perform needle chest decompression.

b. Intubate the trachea.

c. Apply a sterile dressing to stop the bleeding.

d. Seal the wound with an occlusive dressing.

13. Your patient presents with marked severe respiratory distress, jugular venous distention, unequal chest expansion, absent lung sounds on the left, and diminished lung sounds on the right. What should be your priority intervention?

a. Perform BVM ventilation with oxygen.

b. Decompress the chest with a large-gauge IV needle.

c. Continue with the primary assessment.

d. Splint the chest wall with a bulky dressing.

14. You are on the scene of an altercation during which a male patient was stabbed in the leg. The wound is bleeding profusely and the emergency medical responders on scene cannot control the bleeding with direct pressure. What priority treatment should you perform next?

    a. Place cold compresses over the bleeding site to promote vasoconstriction, and raise the leg.

    b. Apply more vigorous direct pressure and raise the leg higher than the heart.

    c. Apply digital pressure to the site of bleeding to tamponade the lacerated artery.

    d. Apply a tourniquet proximal to the injury.

15. Which statement best describes the types of treatment the paramedic should perform during the primary assessment?

    a. Those that can be performed only by the paramedic due to scope-of-practice issues

    b. Those that support lost function to the airway, breathing, and circulation

    c. Those that can be completed in 30 seconds or less

    d. Those that replace normal functioning to the airway, breathing, and oxygenation

See Answers to Review Questions at the back of this book.

References

1. Hackl, W., K. Hausberger, R. Sailer, H. Ulmer, and R. Gassner. "Prevalence of Cervical Spine Injuries in Patients with Facial Trauma." *Oral Surg Oral Med Oral Pathol Oral Radiol Endodontics* 92 (2001): 370–376.

2. Limmer, D. and K. Monosky. "Assessment of the Altered Mental Status Patient." *Emerg Med Serv* 31(3) (2002): 54–81.

3. Mistovich, J. J., et al. "Beyond the Basics: Patient Assessment." *Emerg Med Serv* 35(7) (2006): 72–77.

4. Elam, J. O., D. G. Greene, M. A. Schneider, et al. "Head-tilt Method of Oral Resuscitation." *JAMA* 172 (1960): 812–815.

5. 2010 American Heart Association Guidelines for Cardiopulmonary Resuscitation and Emergency Cardiovascular Care Science. (Available at http://circ.ahajournals.org/content/vol122/18_suppl_3/, accessed July 26, 2015.)

6. Krost, W. S., et al. "Beyond the Basics: Airway Assessment." *Emerg Med Serv* 35(1) (2006): 85–89.

7. Wedmore, I., J. G. McManus, A. E. Pusateri, et al. "A Special Report on the Chitosan-Based Dressing: Experience in Current Combat Operations." *J Trauma* 60(3) (2006): 655–658.

8. Arnaud, F., T. Tomori, R. Saito, et al. "Comparative Efficacy of Granular and Bagged Formulations of the Hemostatic Agent QuikClot." *J Trauma* 63(4) (2007): 775–782.

9. Department of Health and Human Services Centers for Disease Control and Prevention. 2011. Guidelines for Field Triage of Injured Patients Recommendations of the National Expert Panel on Field Triage, 2011. (Available at http://www.cdc.gov/mmwr/pdf/rr/rr6101.pdf, accessed July 26, 2015.)

Further Reading

Campbell, J. E. *International Trauma Life Support for Prehospital Care Providers.* 7th ed. Upper Saddle River, NJ: Pearson/Prentice Hall, 2007.

Dickinson, E. T. *Point of Care Hemorrhage Control.* (Available at www.jems.com/articles/2013/11/point-care-hemorrhage-control.html, accessed July 26, 2015.)

Kalish, J., et al. "The Return of Tourniquets." *JEMS* 33(8) (2008): 44–46.

Limmer, D., M. F. O'Keefe, et al. *Emergency Care.* 12th ed. Upper Saddle River, NJ: Pearson/Prentice Hall, 2011.

Mistovich, J., et al. *Prehospital Emergency Care.* 9th ed. Upper Saddle River, NJ: Pearson/Prentice Hall, 2009.

Tintinalli, J. E., et al. *Tintinalli's Emergency Medicine: A Comprehensive Guide.* 7th ed. New York: McGraw-Hill, 2010.

Zeller, J., A. Fox, and J. P. Pryor. "Beyond the Battlefield: The Use of Hemostatic Dressings in Civilian EMS." *JEMS* 33(3) (2008): 102–109.

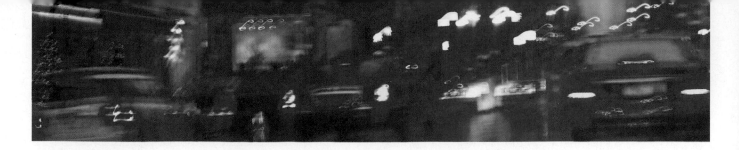

Chapter 3
Therapeutic Communications

Richard A. Cherry, MS, EMT-P

STANDARD
Assessment

COMPETENCY
Integrate scene and patient assessment findings with knowledge of epidemiology and pathophysiology to form a field impression. This includes developing a list of differential diagnoses through clinical reasoning to modify the assessment and formulate a treatment plan.

 ## Learning Objectives

Terminal Performance Objective After reading this chapter, you should be able to employ effective strategies of therapeutic communications in interactions with patients, families, and others you encounter in the course of your professional responsibilities.

Enabling Objectives: To accomplish the terminal performance objective, you should be able to:

1. Define key terms introduced in this chapter.

2. Discuss strategies that build trust and rapport with patients suffering from an emergency.

3. List and describe techniques that will foster effective communication with patients.

4. Describe strategies the paramedic can employ when interviewing a patient to improve the quality of information gained, to include nonverbal communication and feedback techniques.

5. Identify how to alter the interviewing as appropriate when communicating with a pediatric patient, geriatric patient, sensory-impaired patient, patient with sensitive needs, or otherwise challenged patient.

6. Describe communicate techniques that will allow you to effectively communicate with other health care providers, and while transferring care to them.

7. Given a scenario, discuss how you would integrate therapeutic communication into a comprehensive patient assessment.

KEY TERMS

closed questions, p. 42

closed stance, p. 41

communication, p. 38

cultural imposition, p. 48

decode, p. 38

delirium, p. 51

dementia, p. 51

depression, p. 51

empathy, p. 38

encode, p. 38

ethnocentrism, p. 48

feedback, p. 38

leading questions, p. 42

nonverbal communications, p. 47

open stance, p. 41

open-ended questions, p. 42

Case Study

Nothing illustrates the importance of good interpersonal communication better than the student in this case study. Here is his report. Read it and see what you think.

"What a study in contrasts the last two nights have been. As a paramedic student observer, I went from riding with one crew, whose members demonstrated what must be the worst possible insensitivity and callousness, to another crew, whose members showed compassion and kindness.

"Two nights ago, there was a call to an emergency for a possible heart attack. Without going into a lot of detail, I can only say that the experience was dismal. The closest Emergency Medical Responders were sent, in case CPR was needed, but when they saw the patient was awake, they quickly realized that there was little they could do while they waited for us. In the meantime, all the way there, the paramedics continued an ongoing discussion about the problems with the ambulance company's management.

"When we arrived, I noticed that the two Emergency Medical Responders were leaning disdainfully against their vehicle. I overheard one of them say to the medics, 'You got a middle-of-the-night turkey here.' I have to admit, I found their attitude shocking, and I was interested to see how the label they placed on this woman affected the paramedics. Well, they approached the patient with an obvious negative attitude, and things went from bad to worse. Concerned family and friends—about four people—were rudely pushed aside

and ignored. No one seemed to think it was important to interact with them at all. You can imagine the snide remarks that were made later when the crew found out the 'heart attack' had been abdominal gas. I'm sure the whole experience left that family feeling very unhappy with EMS.

"Then, last night, I had an entirely different experience. This paramedic crew couldn't have been more different, even though the call was very similar to the one the night before: another possible heart attack. As we arrived on scene, we saw the Emergency Medical Responders working to put the patient and the family at ease. The one in charge introduced the patient by name to the paramedics, and then told the paramedics what he had already learned. The paramedics introduced themselves to the patient, and then talked her through everything they were going to do. Their questions were polite and their manner exceptionally soothing. Everyone was efficient, kind, and calm. Someone was even assigned to help the husband get ready and into the ambulance for the ride to the hospital.

"What an amazing difference! So much about the two emergencies was the same, yet I observed absolutely opposite behaviors in the responders. The second crew's collective professionalism and excellent communication skills left me with an absolute trust that they could handle virtually anything. They restored my faith in the positive nature of EMS. They are a credit to our community, and my goal is to be like them."

Customer Service Minute

Families Are Patients, Too. I remember when my father had a cardiac arrest in the hospital like it was yesterday. It was on his birthday and one week after his quadruple cardiac bypass surgery. He was recuperating when suddenly he arrested for no apparent reason. My mother and I were rushed out of the room and the emergency code team

responded quickly. They resuscitated my dad efficiently (I peeked into the room until they rushed me out again). About 20 minutes later, my mother and I watched as the response team bounced out of the room, patting each other on the back, and one nurse said aloud, "Well that was fun, what's next?" Words cannot adequately describe how angry I was at that unprofessional, inappropriate outburst. I doubt

I will ever forget that moment or ever stop telling people about it.

Families of patients are a special group. They are overly concerned, worried storytellers. They are victims, too. Above all, they expect us to take good care of their loved one. They want to be kept informed. Tell them the truth and never give them false promises. Sometimes they need advice and direction. Remember that they are in crisis and may not be processing information normally. It's a nice touch to say goodbye to them as well. A little kindness goes a long way.

Every response involves your agency family helping a customer family. Be nice. "Nice" starts in the home—your entire organization must be committed to treating everyone with respect, kindness, and compassion. Be nice at home and your patients will be the benefactors of this home-grown attitude. Be a real family at the station and reach out to our customers. It's the right thing to do.

Introduction

Communication should be easy. After all, communication is only a matter of exchanging common symbols—written, spoken, or other kinds, such as signing and body language. Even in the best circumstances, however, communication can be a challenge. EMS providers have a particularly difficult job of it because they must communicate with strangers who are in crisis.

As a paramedic, you must use every available strategy to make sure that you understand your patients and they understand you. You also must communicate well with your patient's relatives, bystanders, and other EMS providers. In communicating, you will use verbal and nonverbal strategies such as word choices, tones of voice, facial expressions, and body language. You must minimize external and internal distractions and adjust your personal communication style to fit each new situation, especially when dealing with children, elderly people, people of different cultures, and hostile people. Helpful core traits for effective communication in EMS include a genuine liking for people, a sincere desire to be part of a helping profession, an understanding of human strengths and weaknesses, and **empathy**, or the ability to view the world through another's eyes while remaining true to yourself.

Communication consists of a sender, a message, a receiver, and feedback (Figure 3-1). First, the sender has to **encode**, or create, a message; that is, he must write, speak, or otherwise place symbols common to both parties in a format that is easy to

understand. This may include translating the message into another language, using words a child can understand, or writing the words on paper. The receiver then must **decode**, or interpret, the message, ideally getting the same meaning the sender intended to convey. Finally, the receiver gives the sender **feedback**—a response to the message. If, by way of this response, the sender believes that the message was received accurately, both parties can congratulate themselves on communicating successfully.

Unfortunately, partial or complete failure to communicate occurs often. There are abundant reasons for this. In EMS, those reasons include:

- Prejudice, or lack of empathy, particularly by the paramedic toward the patient or situation
- Lack of privacy, which inhibits a patient's responses to questions
- External distractions, such as traffic, crowds, loud music, EMS radios, smart phones, or TVs
- Internal distractions, or thinking about things other than the situation at hand

One way to minimize failure is to keep in mind that patience and flexibility are hallmarks of a good communicator. A paramedic must develop the art of effectively communicating with his patients.

Building Trust and Rapport

As a representative of EMS, you are granted a certain amount of the public's trust at each new emergency scene. You must earn the rest by putting your patient and others at ease and by letting them know you are on their side, you respect their comments, and you want to help. Little courtesies, such as asking your patient his name and thereafter pronouncing it correctly, can help to accomplish this goal.

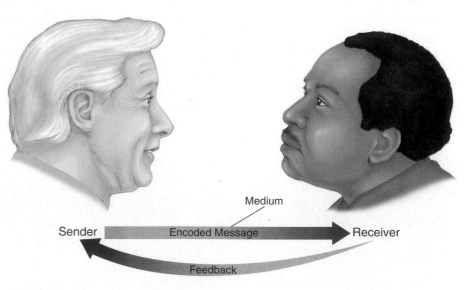

FIGURE 3-1 Communication consists of a sender, a message, a receiver, and feedback.

So can recognizing and responding with compassion to signs of discomfort or suffering. When trust is established, rapport follows.

Your patients will form an opinion about you within the first few minutes, so you must establish a positive rapport quickly. This is not always easy. The situation, your patient, and the conditions will determine your ability to establish rapport. You can do several things, however, to facilitate this task.

By asking your patients the right questions, you will discover their chief complaints and their symptoms. By responding to them with empathy, you will win their trust and encourage them to discuss freely their problems with you. Their answers will also help you decide which areas require in-depth investigation and which body systems to focus on.

With good rapport, the people you are serving will follow your lead, even if that means accepting some pain (such as with a needle stick) and tolerating inconvenience (such as canceling a trip to have a medical evaluation at the hospital). The people with whom you work also will be more motivated to do difficult, and sometimes dangerous, tasks. Remember that effective communication begins and ends with trust and rapport. Without them, your safety could be at risk.

If you expect your patient to trust you with very private information, you must establish a positive, trusting relationship. Present yourself as a caring, compassionate, competent, and confident health care professional. Because this first impression will be based largely on your appearance, your dress and grooming will play an important role in the paramedic–patient relationship. Your appearance should suggest neatness, cleanliness, pride, and professionalism. Your uniform should be clean and pressed, your shoes or boots polished, your hands and nails clean, and your hair well groomed.

Your voice, body language, gestures, and especially eye contact should communicate that you care about your patient's problems. Your questioning process should make the patient comfortable, confident in your care, and supportive of your control of the situation. Position yourself at the patient's eye level and focus your attention on him. Give his requests and concerns high priority, even if they are not medically significant. For example, if your patient complains of being cold, cover him with a blanket. Beyond making him feel warmer, it may also increase his confidence in your desire and ability to help. If you cannot care for a complaint immediately, express your concern and assure him that you will either take care of it shortly or get him to a setting where it can be cared for.

Be aware of your patient's comfort. If the setting does not lend itself to personal questions, move your patient to a more suitable location. For example, teenage girls usually will not truthfully answer questions about pregnancy with their parents nearby. Other patients may not reveal relevant items about their medical history with bystanders listening. Sometimes moving your patient to the ambulance offers the needed privacy.

If your patient is in obvious distress, try to alleviate his pain or discomfort while you interview him. For example, you may control minor bleeding and cover a wound that causes your patient distress. You might also immobilize a painful fracture site while you conduct the interview. Watch also for subtle signs of discomfort, such as squirming, grimacing, and wincing.

Other ways to help build the trust and rapport you need to conduct a patient interview include the following:

- *Introduce yourself.* Wear an identification badge. Introduce yourself by name, title, and agency. For example, "Hi, my name is Dean. I'm a paramedic with AVON Ambulance. What's your name?" Offer to shake your patient's hand or provide a comforting touch (Figure 3-2). This traditional method of greeting is a powerful tool for forming a quick bond. This short verbal and tactile exchange reveals a wealth of information about your patient's respiratory status, skin condition, level of consciousness, hearing and speech abilities, and any language barriers.

- *Use your patient's name.* A technique for remembering a name involves three steps: First, say the patient's name out loud three times in the first minute. Then "see" the patient's name in your mind in bold capital

> **CONTENT REVIEW**
>
> ➤ Ways to Build Trust and Rapport
> - Introduce yourself.
> - Use the patient's name.
> - Address the patient properly.
> - Modulate your voice.
> - Use a professional but compassionate tone.
> - Explain what you are doing, and why.
> - Keep a kind, calm expression.

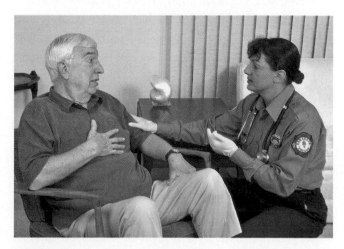

FIGURE 3-2 Introduce yourself and use an appropriate compassionate touch to show your concern and support.

letters. Finally, "feel" yourself writing the name in your imagination. Some people actually write the name on their paperwork, but this does not work as well as the mental imagery.

- *Address your patient properly.* Ask your patient how he wishes to be called—for instance, "Mr. Dobbins," "Robert," or "Bob"—and respect his wishes. Never call patients "honey," "dude," or any name other than their own. Also, be careful about shortening children's names. If a child is introduced to you as "Matthew," use that name, or ask the child if he goes by a nickname such as "Matt." It is better to be sure and not to assume.

- *Modulate your voice.* Pay attention to your volume. Speak quietly and in low tones. If the patient is hard of hearing or difficult to control, speak up. Check your pitch; some people find it hard to hear high voices. Also, check your rate of speaking. Be especially aware that people in crisis may have difficulty taking in information at a normal rate, so slow down.

- *Use a professional but compassionate tone of voice.* Avoid tones that portray sarcasm, irritation, anger, or other emotions that fail to serve the patient.

- *Explain what you are doing, and why.* This helps to ease your patient's anxiety, especially if he is in pain. For example, if you must immobilize a broken bone, explain that a splint will help to prevent movement and more pain. Also tell the patient that applying a splint may be painful but, once applied, the broken limb should be more comfortable. *Note*: Never make false promises or false assurances. They violate your patient's trust.

- *Keep a kind, calm facial expression.* Remember that facial expressions can reflect a wide variety of emotions and conditions, including relaxation, relief, pain, fear, anger, sorrow, and so on. No matter what the emergency, maintain a kind-looking poker face. It will convince others that you can handle things.

- *Use the appropriate style of communication.* A calm, reassuring voice and demeanor can put even the most apprehensive patient at ease. Remember that even though his problems may not seem extraordinary to you, they may be extremely disturbing to him. You are accustomed to handling emergency situations; he probably is not. You are not horrified by a gory scene; he probably is. You deal with life-threatening emergencies every day; he probably never does. Understanding these differences helps you to display an appropriate demeanor and begin your interview.

In general, patients will respond well to your calm demeanor, but be prepared to use a tough, authoritative approach when needed. Furthermore, if a situation requires

you to be firm, be completely firm. Do not let your facial expression, for example, kill the effect (such as one that says, "Gosh, I hope they believe me!").

At the end of a call, a final word or two can be very helpful, particularly after emotional calls. A "goodbye and good luck" can help bring the event to a close for the patient and family. It also tells everyone that you weren't just delivering "goods" to a receiving facility.

Effective Communication Techniques
General Guidelines

Patients generally respond to questioning in one of three ways: They may pour out information easily, they may reveal some things and conceal others that might be embarrassing or shameful, or they may resist, hiding information from themselves—and, therefore, from you. The patient who conceals information or resists giving it may be trying to maintain a certain image or may be fearful about how others will respond (perhaps with ridicule or rejection). Or he may simply not trust you. To get the information you need, you must be consistently professional, nonjudgmental, and willing to talk about any concern the patient may have.

Nonverbal Communication
Body Language

Body language consists of gestures, mannerisms, and postures by which a person communicates with others.[1] Your position within the environment and in relation to your patient is part of that language. Examples include the following:

- *Distance* (Table 3-1). In the United States, the socially acceptable distance between strangers is 4 to 12 feet. A "comfortable" distance may be described as twice the length of a patient's arm. In most cases, paramedics are able to break social convention and quickly enter a patient's "intimate space" (1.5 feet or less) because people intuitively understand the need for medical personnel to get "hands on" with them. However, if the patient stiffens or backs away from you, the best strategy may be to linger at a less-threatening distance until you have built more trust and rapport.

- *Relative level.* A different message is sent to the patient each time you stand at his eye level, above it, or

CONTENT REVIEW

➤ Elements of Nonverbal Communication
- Distance
- Relative level
- Stance

Table 3-1 Interpersonal Zones

Zone	Distance	Characteristics
Intimate zone	0–1.5 feet	Visual distortion occurs. Best for assessing breath and other body odors.
Personal distance, or "personal space"	1.5–4 feet	Perceived as extension of self. No visual distortion. Body odors are not apparent. Voice is moderate. Much of patient assessment, and sometimes patient interviewing, may occur at this distance.
Social distance	4–12 feet	Used for impersonal business transactions. Perceptual information is much less detailed than at personal distance. Patient interview may occur at this distance.
Public distance	12 feet or more	Allows impersonal interaction with others. Voices must be projected.

below it. Remaining at eye level indicates equality. Standing above or over the patient imparts an air of authority, but it also can be intimidating. Dropping below eye level indicates a willingness to let the patient have some control of the situation, a strategy that can be especially helpful when your patient is an elderly adult or a child (Figure 3-3).

• *Stance.* Arms extended, open hands, relaxed large muscles, and a nodding head characterize an **open stance** (Figure 3-4). A paramedic who has an open stance sends

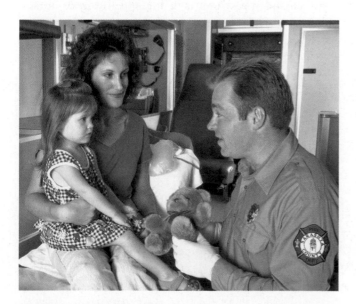

FIGURE 3-3 Getting down to a patient's level can help improve communications on a pediatric call.

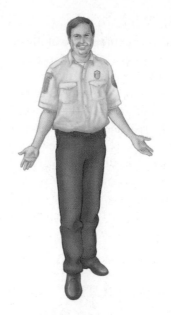

FIGURE 3-4 An open stance.

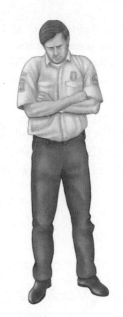

FIGURE 3-5 A closed stance.

the message that he is confident and at ease. When it is safe to do so, use this stance to communicate warmth and attentiveness. A **closed stance** is just the opposite. In this position, arms are flexed, or arms are crossed tightly over the chest (Figure 3-5). The fists are clenched or a finger may be pointing. The head may be shaking negatively. The body is square to the patient or, in some cases, may turn slightly away. This posture suggests disinterest, discomfort, disgust, fear, or anger and sends negative signals to the patient. Watch your patient's body language, too. It can tell you how well communication with him is going. If the patient has a closed stance, you may need to change your approach.

Eye Contact

A powerful source of effective communication comes with eye contact. While you are interviewing the patient, use it as much as possible. (Always remove sunglasses while working with patients.) Even when you are taking notes, look at the patient frequently. Eye contact is one way to send a message to your patient, whether it is a compassionate "I care about you" or a stern "settle down now." With eye contact, you can hold the attention of a patient so powerfully that your patient can feel that you are helping him hang on in desperate circumstances.

Of course, using eye contact means that the other person is looking at you as well. This can be unnerving if you are unfamiliar with this technique. If you feel uncomfortable, look at the bridge of the other person's nose for a bit of relief. Then try direct eye contact again. Build this skill over time, and it will serve you well. In the end, eye contact is the most powerful way to communicate with someone, because your sincerity—or lack of it—will show. "I care about you" comes across loud and clear when you make sincere eye contact with your patient.

Compassionate Touch

Another communication skill is touching. The ability to hold a hand, or even hug, in the right circumstances can yield information that would otherwise not be given. Some paramedics need to learn this skill the way they learn how to use an IV. That is, it can be awkward at first, but it is worth the effort. Nothing builds trust and rapport, or calms patients, faster than the power of touch. How effective it is depends on the patient's age, gender, cultural background, past experience, and current setting. Timing is everything. Deciding when and where to provide a compassionate touch is part of the art of medicine. Just like eye contact, it can demonstrate empathy and encourage trust.

Interviewing a Patient

From the moment of your first contact with the patient, your job is to find out all the information relevant to the present emergency. You need to identify the patient's chief complaint (the reason that 911 was called), learn the circumstances that caused the emergency, evaluate the patient's condition, and determine the best course of action to mitigate his problem. Much of this is accomplished by asking questions, observing the patient, listening effectively, and using appropriate language.

Asking Questions

An important part of patient assessment is gathering information that is accurate, complete, and relevant to the present emergency. To begin, you must identify the patient's chief complaint. Although dispatch probably will have given you an idea of what the emergency is about, it is

---

Cultural Considerations

Eye contact is a major form of nonverbal communication. Short eye contact is often seen as friendly, whereas prolonged eye contact may be interpreted as threatening. Thus, timing is an important factor in how a person interprets eye contact.

One's culture also influences how eye contact is interpreted. Eye contact can mean respect in one culture and disrespect in another. Often, Asians will avoid eye contact even when they have nothing to hide. Eye contact between people of different sexes is problematic in Muslim cultures, in which a prolonged look in the face of a member of the opposite sex might be misinterpreted. Because of this, people in Middle Eastern countries might look a person of the same sex in the eye and not look into the eyes of a person of the opposite sex.

If you work in a culturally diverse community, you should learn the customs of eye contact and other forms of nonverbal communication of those you might encounter during the course of your work.

---

important for you to let the patient state the chief complaint in his own words. If you were to ask **leading questions** (ones that guide the patient's replies), such as "Are you having difficulty breathing?" or "I see you're limping. Did you fall or hurt yourself?" you could easily miss a serious problem. So, instead, ask **open-ended questions**, such as "What happened that led you to call for an ambulance?" or "What's going on today?" Questions such as these will allow your patient to respond in an unguided, spontaneous way. They also encourage patients who are reluctant to speak to describe their complaint in a way that might not be possible otherwise.

The patient's chief complaint should then drive the evolution of all other questions to be asked. For example, if your patient's chief complaint is chest pain, you are required to obtain answers to a specific set of questions. However, instead of interviewing a patient as if you were reading a shopping list, individualize the process. For example, you would have to find out whether a patient with chest pain takes any medications. If your patient tells you that his chief complaint is "chest pain so bad even the nitroglycerin tablets aren't helping," your question about medications might be worded "What medications do you take in addition to nitroglycerin?" This tells the patient you have been listening, which can help build a greater rapport. Other questioning techniques include the following:

- *Continue to ask open-ended questions.* They do not limit the patient's responses, which can help to reveal unexpected but important facts. For example, instead of asking your patient with abdominal pain, "Did you have breakfast today?" which can be answered with either a "yes" or a "no," ask: "What have you eaten today?"

- *Use direct questions when necessary.* Direct questions, or **closed questions**, ask for specific information. ("Did you take your pills today?" or "Does the abdominal pain come and go like a cramp, or is it constant?") These questions are good for three reasons: They fill in information generated by open-ended questions. They help to answer crucial questions when time is limited. And they can help to control overly talkative patients, who might want to tell you about their gallbladder surgery in 1969 when their chief complaint is a sprained ankle.

- *Ask only one question at a time, and allow the patient to complete his answers.* If you ask more than one question, the patient may not know which one to answer and may leave out portions of information or become confused. Equally important is having one person do the interview. Don't force your patient to discern questions from multiple interviewers.

- *Listen to the patient's complete response before asking the next question.* By doing so, you might find that you need to ask a question that is different from the one you were expecting to ask. The most important skill of a great communicator is being a great listener. It's especially true when getting a medical history.

- ***Do not allow interruptions, if possible.*** Unless your partner or other EMS personnel need to give you patient care information of a critical nature, interruptions will interfere with your patient's and your trains of thought. Interruptions also can cause you to miss information that is important to the patient's medical care.

Active Listening

Few people practice the art of listening well. Usually, they think about what they are going to say next while others are still talking to them. There may be less than a half-second gap between speakers; many people cannot even wait that long, and instead finish others' sentences for them.

Listening is crucial for a skilled clinician. Listen closely to what your patients tell you and be careful not to develop tunnel vision from dispatch information. Begin your assessment without any preconceived notions about your patient's injuries or illnesses. Also watch for subtle clues that your patient may not be telling the truth. For example, your patient may tell you that his chest pain went away, but his facial expressions and body language may suggest otherwise.

Developing good communication skills takes time and practice. Listening is an active skill, not a passive one. It requires your complete attention, and it requires constant practice. To listen well, you must focus on the messenger. Stop doing other things. Discipline yourself to cease any internal dialogue that can distract or interrupt you mentally. Never finish the other person's sentences, and do not consider your response until the speaker has finished speaking. Allow some silence when the speaker has stopped.

As previously stated, avoid working your way in strict order down any prearranged list of questions (such as those in the chapter "History Taking"). Use those lists as a guide only. Listen to your patients and watch for clues to important signs, symptoms, emotions, or other factors. Then modify your questions to follow those clues. Once your patient has stopped talking, provide feedback to confirm that you have understood his message correctly. The following practices promote active listening:

CONTENT REVIEW
➤ Feedback Techniques
- Silence
- Reflection
- Facilitation
- Empathy
- Clarification
- Confrontation
- Interpretation
- Asking about feelings
- Explanation
- Summarization

- ***Silence.*** Give your patient time to gather his thoughts and add to what has been said.
- ***Reflection.*** To check your understanding and to reassure your patient, echo his message back to him using your own words. This encourages him to provide more details. Just make sure not to disturb his train of thought. For example:

Patient: My chest hurts.

You: Your chest hurts?

Patient: Yes, it hurts when I take in a full breath.

You: Are you able take in a full breath at all?

Patient: No, not since this morning when I was working in the yard and fell off my ladder.

- This simple reflection encouraged the patient to reveal facts about his recent fall. If the paramedic had merely investigated the chief complaint of chest pain, you may have focused on a cardiac issue and failed to discover his injury. Because the primary problem is not always the chief complaint, allowing your patient to take the lead is sometimes advantageous.
- ***Facilitation.*** Encourage your patient to provide more information. Maintain sincere eye contact, use concerned facial expressions, and lean forward while you listen. Cues such as "Mm-hmm," "I see," or "I'm listening" all help your patient open up. Sometimes strategic silence is also helpful.
- ***Empathy.*** Let your body language show that you understand, so your patient feels accepted and more open to talking. Your patients may be telling you very personal and sometimes embarrassing information about themselves. They may feel frightened, ashamed, and upset to have to tell a stranger these things. Show empathy by responding with "I understand" or "That must have been very scary" or "I can't imagine having not being able to breathe." Sometimes just a gesture, such as handing someone a tissue or patting him on the shoulder, conveys empathy.
- ***Clarification.*** Ask your patient to help you understand, in cases when you need to eliminate confusion about what has been said. In crisis, patients often cannot clearly describe what they feel. They will use vague, general words. Do not hesitate to ask for clarification. For example:

You: Do you have any allergies?

Patient: Yes, the last time I took penicillin I had a bad reaction.

You: Can you describe the reaction?

Patient: Well, I got itchy all over with a rash.

You: Did you have any difficulty breathing or feel like you were choking?

Patient: Oh, no, just the itching and rash.

- By asking for clarification you distinguish between a simple allergic reaction and life-threatening anaphylaxis.

- *Confrontation.* Focus the patient on one particular factor of the interview. Sometimes patients will hide the truth or mask it with other symptoms. Often you will detect inconsistencies in your patient's story. In these cases, you should confront your patient with your observations. For example, "You say you're not injured, but you keep holding your neck and it appears stiff." Confrontation may help your patient bring his hidden feelings into the open.

- *Interpretation.* State your interpretation of the information; that is, link events, make associations, identify an implied cause, or draw conclusions. Interpretation takes confrontation a step further. Here you interpret your observations and question your patient about what you believe may be the problem. For example, "You say you're not injured, but you keep holding your neck and it appears stiff. Did you hit your head or twist your neck in the crash?" Interpretation can backfire if your patient feels you are unjustly accusing him; however, if your patient trusts you and you use interpretation cautiously, it can demonstrate empathy and enhance your rapport.

- *Asking about feelings.* Your patients are people, not clinical subjects. Ask them how they feel about what they are experiencing. Let them know you are interested in them as people, not just as patients. Showing genuine interest in their problems may unlock the door to key information that they otherwise might not have shared with you.

- *Explanation.* Share factual or objective information related to the message. "If you did hurt your neck in the crash, it could be serious. Sometimes the injury doesn't start to hurt until later on. Let's not take any chances and immobilize you for the ride to the hospital."

- *Summarization.* Briefly review the interview and your interpretation of the situation. Ask open-ended questions, if needed, to allow the patient to clarify details.

Traps of interviewing, or common errors made when listening and providing feedback to patients, include the following:

- *Providing false assurances.* Never make any promises you cannot keep. For example, saying "Everything will be all right" is a terrible false reassurance. You'll make this mistake only once.

- *Giving advice.* People call 911 because they are seeking advice, but the paramedic must be careful how it is conveyed. Saying "I think we should definitely bring you to the hospital so that a doctor can take a look at your injury" is acceptable advice. Saying "You're crazy not to let us take you to the hospital. Do you want to die?" is not.

- *Abusing authority.* Remember that EMS is not a power trip. Although paramedics are entrusted with the power to do a difficult job, that power must never be used inappropriately. A paramedic provides a vital public service. Doing so correctly requires constant attention to protecting the public's trust and avoiding behaviors that might be interpreted as abuse of power.

- *Using avoidance language.* Avoidance language occurs when your patient refuses to engage in the conversation by changing the topic. For example, a person who chooses to change the conversation rather than get into a discussion about something difficult may use avoidance language. If a paramedic allows this to happen, the patient's whole story may not be revealed.

- *Improper distancing.* When the paramedic is insensitive to distancing, he may stand too close or too far from the patient to attain optimal rapport. Noticing the effects of distancing and adjusting accordingly is a hallmark of a good communicator.

- *Talking too much.* Remember that listening is also a part of communication. Don't monopolize the conversation. Allow your patient enough time to share vital, intimate information with you.

- *Interrupting.* As already discussed, good listening skills require you to wait until your patient answers you fully.

- *Using "why did you" questions.* The question "why" often steers a conversation toward blame, such as: "Why did you put your hand in the snowblower while it was running?" or "Why did you wait so long to call 911?" This type of question is counterproductive and will only serve to annoy and alienate your patient.

Demonstrating good listening and feedback skills on an emergency call is challenging. So many things are happening, it can seem like a whirlwind. For example, it may be necessary to apply monitoring equipment to the patient while you ask questions. If this happens, reassure the patient by saying something like "I know it seems overwhelming to you, but please understand that I am listening to your answers while I attach these ECG leads and prepare to start your IV."

Observing Your Patient

Observe your patient during the interview. External signs such as overall appearance, including clothing, jewelry, and other physical signs, may give you some indication of the patient's condition. Other clues you pick up may offer you a way to explore the patient's internal experiences or his mental status.

Thus, while you are interacting with the patient, observe his level of consciousness and body movements. Assess his rate and clarity of speech, his thinking, and his ability to pay attention, concentrate, and comprehend. You may be able to check the patient's orientation to person, place, and time, and his remote, recent, and immediate memory. Explore his mood and energy level, too. Watch for evidence of autonomic responses (sweating, trembling, and so on) and for unusual facial movements, such as a tic around the mouth, nose, or eyes. Note that lack of eye contact can suggest that the patient is shy, withdrawn, confused, bored, intimidated, apathetic, depressed, scared, or hiding something.

Many people do not cope well with being the center of attention. Be aware of various defense mechanisms people may use, so you can be prepared to deal with them, if necessary. For example, if your patient is self-grooming (fixing hair or straightening clothes), he may need some reassurance. If the patient keeps shifting focus away from your questions, back off for a bit and then return to the topic from a different angle.

If the patient is acting out and hostile, point out the behavior in a professional manner, ask if the behavior is intentional, let him know that such behavior defeats the purpose of calling for help, and then name behaviors you would rather see. If there is any indication that the patient's

Cultural Considerations

Communicating with Latino Families. Latinos have become the fastest-growing minority in the United States today. Mexican Americans are more than 65 percent of this community. In many first- and second-generation Latino families, Spanish remains the language of choice. In many instances, Spanish must be used to adequately convey health care information—particularly in an emergency situation.

In this culture, it is important that nonverbal communications be consistent with verbal communications. Furthermore, such communications must have an underlying tone of respect (*respeto*). The Spanish language has both informal and formal verb forms. The use of informal verb forms can be seen as a sign of disrespect and should be avoided.

In Mexican American and many Latin American cultures, the grandmother (*abuela*) is often looked to in terms of medical advice and health care decisions. Because of this, the grandmother should often be included in discussions pertaining to the patient. This is particularly true in situations in which you have a relatively young mother forced to make health care decisions about her infant. In many cases, despite what medical personnel might say, the grandmother will be sought for advice. Including the grandmother in certain situations will save time and also indicate respect.

hostility may threaten your safety or that of your crew, maintain distance and an exit path. (Additional information about hostile patients appears later in this chapter.)

Using Appropriate Language

Effective communication means connecting with your patient. They have to see you as their trusted advocate. To accomplish this effectively, it is important to use appropriate language.

Most of your patients will not understand medical terms. Nothing may distance you from your patient more quickly than sophisticated medical terminology. "Have you ever had gall bladder problems?" is better than "Have you ever had cholecystitis?" Use language the patient can understand. For example, you may need to use "pee" instead of "urine," or "breaths" instead of "respirations." Also be careful to avoid professional jargon and slang. Although it is necessary to make sure the patient knows what you are doing and why, it is unnerving for him to hear that you are going to "stick him and push some Benadryl." Also keep in mind that children are very literal and concrete-minded. Avoid telling a child, for example, that you are going to "take" his pulse. Say instead that you are going to "feel for" his pulse. In summary, watch your language and make sure you are speaking at your patient's comprehension and comfort level.

Other barriers to communication include cultural differences, language differences, deafness, speech impediments, and even blindness. When you encounter such obstacles, try to enlist someone who can communicate with your patient and act as an interpreter. An alternative is to adopt a conservative approach toward assessment, field diagnosis, and treatment, concentrating on just the crucial items.

Special Needs and Challenges

Patients generally are more than willing to answer your questions, although some will require more time and a variety of techniques. Difficult interviews stem from several sources. The patient's condition, including a developing cognitive impairment, may affect his ability to talk. The patient may be afraid to talk to you because of a psychological disorder, language or cultural difference, or even the difference between your ages. Or the patient intentionally may want to deceive you (to hide illegal drug abuse, for example).

Use the same techniques on a patient who is reluctant to talk to you as you would on any other patient, but use them in a slightly different way. For example, start your interview in the usual manner. If the patient does not respond to your questions, take time to develop rapport by reviewing the reason dispatch gave for the call. Attempt to ask open-ended questions. If unsuccessful, try direct questions, including ones that require only a yes-or-no response. Accept that you may not be able to obtain any elaboration or details about the facts. Provide positive feedback to any response the patient provides.

If the patient continues to be reluctant, be sure he understands your questions. Rule out language barriers and hearing difficulties. Once you know that the patient can understand you, continue to ask questions about the critical information you need to know to progress with treatment. If you cannot get even this much, attempt to rule out pathology (disease) by asking family members or others at the scene how long the patient has been uncommunicative.

If you determine that pathology is not the cause, you may need to continue to build trust and rapport with the patient. One way to do this is to encourage him to ask you questions about your equipment, profession, medical care, or any topic that might start a conversation. Model how you would like the patient to respond to your questions by fully answering his questions.

This next section focuses on communicating with patients who require a special effort on your part. These patients include children and their parents, elderly people, people who are blind or deaf, people of other cultures, and people who are hostile or uncooperative. No matter how long you practice as a paramedic, some patients will present with special circumstances that challenge your skills. Your ability to deal with them will improve with time and practice.

Children

Effective communication with pediatric patients (infants, children, and adolescents) depends on their age. Have a good idea of what to expect at each stage of development so your efforts to communicate can be directed appropriately (Table 3-2).

In general, you can start by talking to the caregivers, then gradually approach the patient. Remember your body language. When dealing with younger children especially, it will help to get down to their eye level. Children pick up on anxiety easily and often take cues from what they observe, so it is very important to stay calm. Introduce yourself, and use the child's name often. Be careful not to clam up and work silently.

Even if your own anxieties and the pressure of the medical requirements of the call are taxing your limits, talk! Tell the child everything: what you are looking at ("Now, let's look at your leg") and why it is important ("so we can be sure it's okay, too."). Explain your equipment; if there is time, let the child see how the equipment works. Above all, explain what you intend to do, even to very

Table 3-2 Childhood Development by Age

Common Term	Age	Characteristics and Behaviors
Infant	Birth to 1 year	Knows the voice and face of parents. Will want to be held by a parent or caregiver. Responds best to firm, gentle handling and a quiet calm voice.
Toddler	1 to 3 years old	Very curious at this age, and into everything, so be alert to the possibility of poison ingestion. May be distrustful and uncooperative. Usually does not understand what is happening, which raises level of fear. May be very concerned about being separated from parents or care caregivers.
Preschooler	3 to 5 years old	Can see the world from own perspective only. Able to talk, but may not understand what is being said. Uses simple words, short sentences, and concrete explanations. May be scared and believe what is happening is own fault.
School age	6 to 12 years old	Is more objective and realistic. Should cooperate and be willing to follow the lead of parents and EMS provider. Has active imagination and thoughts about death. May need continual reassurance.
Adolescent	13 to 18 years old	Acts like an adult. Resents being spoken to as if still a child. Considers modesty to be very important. Fears permanent scarring or deformity. May become involved in "mass hysteria."

young children. (For example, you might say, "Johnny, I am going to make your leg hurt less by putting on this splint. I will need to make the leg move first, which might hurt some. But after that, it should be a lot better. Okay?") Never tell a child that something will not hurt when, in actuality, it will. Once you have lost the trust of a child, it is very difficult to regain it.

Most important, you must build trust. Once you have that, a child will put up with a lot. Giving a child a stuffed toy may be helpful (Figure 3-6). Also, be sure to move slowly, talk gently, explain everything, and be honest. To engage children, ask questions, and when you answer their questions, be sure not to talk down to them. Use straightforward language. Never try to hide the fact that something is wrong. When something will hurt or will be at all uncomfortable, tell them. The more matter-of-fact and informative you can be, the better. If you are fair about the difficult parts and avoid springing nasty surprises, you will find greater overall cooperation. The need to be gentle whenever possible should be obvious.

If a child is especially fearful, let him play with a toy or other object and then gradually increase contact. Do not be in a hurry to touch a child unless the situation is critical. Use lots of eye contact and compassionate touch, too. Keep in mind that even if the child cannot understand you, your tone of voice is reassuring and your words and actions will be meaningful to the family and bystanders. Ask the child for feedback frequently, wait for an answer, and acknowledge that answer. Involve the child in decision making whenever possible. If he is crying, do not take it personally and do not tell him to stop. Instead, try saying, "It's ok to cry, go ahead." Lending control in this way can work wonders.

Be aware that young children are very literal. Word choice is important. As noted earlier, do not "take" a pulse, "measure" it. A blood-pressure cuff does not "squeeze," it "hugs." When one child was told that she would fly to the hospital, she started to cry. "I don't know how to fly," she wailed. Think about what you say.

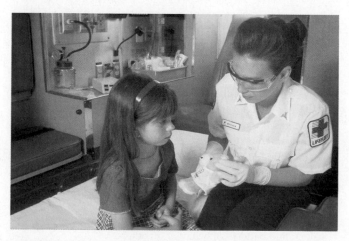

FIGURE 3-6 Use a small toy to help calm a child.

With pediatric patients, it is important to understand that caregivers, especially parents, may be very concerned and upset. Remember that you must manage them as well as your patient. Common responses include crying, emotional outbursts, anger, guilt, and confusion, which may be directed at you. Do not take it personally. You must build trust and rapport with the parents as well as with the child.

Sometimes parents interfere with emergency care and must be separated from the child. Usually, however, it is most effective to let the parents stay and, if appropriate, even hold the child. No matter how parents behave, always treat them with courtesy, respect, and understanding. Avoid raising your voice. Tell them that you know they want help for their child. They need your support and understanding, too.

With younger children (ages 1 to 6), most of your conversation will be with caregivers. Be aware that you are collecting information about the child's history from an adult's point of view, but do not put the caregiver on the defensive. Be careful to be nonjudgmental, especially if it appears that the child has not been provided with proper care or safety before your arrival. Be observant but not confrontational.

Elderly Patients

Be careful of your own prejudices with all special populations, but particularly with the elderly. Be respectful of them. Always use a formal means of address, such as "Mr." and "Mrs." or "Ms." Speak slowly and clearly. Interviews might take longer, because many elders cannot process a lot of information quickly owing to interfering physical disabilities and the fact that they can become fatigued easily. Remember that the use of compassionate touch can be a welcome and important means of nonverbal support.

Give the elderly patient choices whenever possible. Take along their "living assists," such as walkers, hearing aids, and eyeglasses, and their book of phone numbers to facilitate reaching family or friends. Many elderly people are set in their ways and can be stubborn, but if you respect their dignity and do not rush them, you usually can build enough rapport to work with them effectively.

Patients with Sensory Impairment

Blind patients, including sighted patients whose injuries may require covering the eyes, present special problems. You must identify yourself immediately, because they cannot see your uniform. Always announce yourself and explain who you are and why you are there. If possible, take your patient's hand to establish personal contact and to show him where you are. If you need to have him walk, lead him by letting him hold onto your bent arm. Remember that **nonverbal communications**, such as hand gestures, facial expressions, and body language, are useless in these cases. Your voice and touch are the only effective tools for providing reassurance and effective communication.

The challenge of communicating with a person with a hearing impairment is much like that of overcoming a language barrier. Some options, however, afford a degree of flexibility. Ask hearing-impaired and deaf patients their preferred method of communication: lip reading, signing, or writing. Writing often is necessary—and the best method of communication—in the prehospital environment. If your patient reads lips, you must modify your communication techniques accordingly. Always face him directly in a well-lit setting and speak slowly in a low-pitched voice. If he has eyeglasses, make sure he wears them. Augment your speech with hand gestures and facial expressions. Avoid covering your mouth and trailing off at the ends of your sentences. If your patient has one good ear or some hearing, use that to your advantage. Speak normally and do not exaggerate your enunciation of words or use too much volume, which can distort sound. Be aware that many hearing-impaired patients will nod "yes," even if they do not understand what was said or asked, possibly in a misguided effort to be agreeable.

Angry, Hostile, or Uncooperative Patients

You will often encounter angry patients or their families. They might be angry for many reasons. Your patient is sick, perhaps dying. Family members are anticipating their future loss. Often they will lash out at the easiest target—you. Sometimes you cannot do anything quickly enough or well enough for them. Understand that their anger is a natural part of the grieving process, and they may be merely venting their frustration. Unfortunately, you are at the receiving end of their outbursts. Try to accept their feelings without getting defensive or angry in return.

At times, you will need to build rapport with someone who cannot or does not want you to. If this is the case, be sure you are not threatening. Avoid confrontation, but keep trying until you are successful. Use the same questioning techniques you usually use. Sometimes patients open up if you clearly explain the benefits and advantages of cooperation. You also may be able to obtain the information you need from observing the scene and from questioning the patient's family, bystanders, or even law enforcement officers.

Set limits and establish boundaries with an uncooperative patient, if necessary. If the patient is sexually aggressive, for example, clarify your professional role for the patient. Tell him in a way that you are certain he understands that you are there to provide emergency medical care. Be sure to document unusual situations, and ask witnesses to document their observations as well. In extreme

Cultural Considerations

An emergency situation in which people of different cultures and languages must interact requires you to be especially compassionate. To accomplish this, you must understand that cultures vary, and **ethnocentrism**—viewing your own life as the most desirable, acceptable, or best, and acting in a superior manner—will only hinder communication. You must imagine the additional fear and frustration a patient in crisis feels when he tries to explain the emergency to a paramedic who cannot speak his language or understand his attitudes. To really empathize with him, you must be able to avoid **cultural imposition**; that is, avoid imposing on him your own beliefs, values, and patterns of behavior.

In a transcultural situation in which your patient also does not speak your language, you have the opportunity to make the experience less stressful by being caring and calm—and finding an interpreter. Some important principles when using an interpreter are the following:

- Children of immigrants may act as interpreters. If this occurs, remember to keep what you have to say at the appropriate age level.
- Recognize that the emergency may cause distressing emotions in the interpreter, especially if the interpreter is a child.
- Speak slowly.
- Phrase questions carefully and clearly.
- Address both the patient and the interpreter.
- Ask only one question at a time, and wait for a complete response.
- Understand that the information you receive may not be reliable.
- Have patience.

Cultural differences include more than just language differences. People of some cultures are more comfortable at a variety of distances when communicating; some expect health care workers to have all the answers to their illnesses; some treat ill or injured family members in different ways. Asian, Native American, Indo-Chinese, and Arab people may consider direct eye contact impolite or aggressive and may thus demonstrate respect to you by averting their eyes. The welts on a feverish Southeast Asian child may not be from abuse, but rather from a folk practice known as "coin rubbing" or "coining," which many believe will draw out fever.

Understand that both you and the patient may bring cultural stereotypes to the situation. If either of you acts as if your culture is superior, the situation could cause problems. As with any call, create an appropriate professional relationship, but keep in mind that the rules about interpersonal space, eye contact, and touching may all be very different from those you know. As you can see, it is a good idea to study the various cultures typical to your area. Be open to the different ways of people, and do not act as if your way is the only correct way to manage things. There is no reason to impose your beliefs, values, and patterns of behavior on others.

Many cultures have established and accepted folk-medicine beliefs. Even though these may seem strange, they are very important to those who believe and practice them. If you work in an area with a concentration of a particular ethnic group, try to learn about the folk-medicine beliefs and practices of that group.

cases, consider having a same-sex witness ride in the back of your ambulance or record all interactions.

If a patient is blatantly hostile, or there is any hint that your safety is jeopardized, be sure to stay far enough away from the patient. Monitor the patient closely, and never leave him alone without adequate assistance. To prevent a hostile situation from getting worse, be sure to have an appropriate show of force (enough personnel to overpower the patient), if necessary. Remember, your personal safety is paramount. Always be sure you have a clear path to the nearest exit, and always position yourself so you can observe others entering or exiting the area. Know local protocols regarding the use of restraints and psychological medications. Do not hesitate to call for law enforcement backup, if necessary.

Sensitive Topics

Paramedic students normally have difficulty questioning their patients about embarrassing, sensitive, or very personal topics such as sexual activities, death and dying, physical deformities, bodily functions, and domestic violence. Even though you may feel uneasy discussing these matters, they can help you learn important information about your patient's illness. To become more comfortable dealing with these subjects, watch experienced clinicians discuss them with their patients. Familiarize yourself with and practice some opening questions on sensitive topics that both put your patient at ease and encourage him to talk about it. If a particular area makes you most uncomfortable, attend a lecture or seminar and learn how professionals deal with this subject daily. Make the unfamiliar familiar and it will seem less imposing.

Let's look at two sensitive topics: physical violence and the sexual history. Your patient may not want to reveal a history of physical abuse. You should consider it, however, when any of the following conditions is present:

- Injuries that are inconsistent with the story given
- Injuries that embarrass your patient
- A delay between the time of the injury and seeking help
- A past history of "accidents"
- Suspicious behavior of the supposed abuser

To earn your patient's trust, try to make him or her feel that the problem is not uncommon and that you under-

stand the reasons for what has occurred. For example, you can ask your female patient, "Sometimes when husbands and wives argue a lot, it leads to physical fighting. I noticed you have some bruises on your arms and legs. Can you tell me what happened? Did someone hit you?" With active listening techniques, such questioning will help establish a rapport that encourages open communication.

Taking a sexual history can be the most embarrassing and uncomfortable topic for an inexperienced health care provider. The sexual history is normally taken later during the history, but it can be a part of the present illness or past history, depending on your patient's chief complaint. For example, if your patient complains of a genitourinary problem, the sexual history becomes important during the present illness questioning. If your patient has a history of sexually transmitted disease, then the sexual history is relevant to the past history.

Whenever you begin the sexual history, it is helpful to prepare your patient with introductory statements and questions such as "Now I need to ask you some questions about your sexual health and activity. It may help me determine the cause of your problem and provide better care for you. This information will be strictly confidential. May I begin?" If your patient consents, proceed as follows: "Are you sexually active? Have you had sex with anyone in the past six months? Do you have more than one partner? Do you have sex with men or women, or both? Do you take precautions to avoid infection or unwanted pregnancy? Do you have any problems or concerns about your sexual function?" This may seem very uncomfortable for the beginning paramedic, but with time and clinical experience you will develop a sense of where and when these questions are appropriate. It is critical that you remain calm, objective, and nonjudgmental regardless of how your patient answers.

Silence

Silence can become very uncomfortable if you are impatient. Why has your patient suddenly become silent? This question has no single answer. His silence can have many meanings and many uses. It may result from an organic brain condition that prevents him from forming thoughts.

Assessment Pearls

Remember that abuse can be physical, sexual, or emotional. The abused victim may be a husband or wife, a child or elderly parent, a boyfriend or girlfriend. If you suspect abuse, ask your patients when they feel safe or unsafe at home and watch their reaction. Are they afraid to answer? Do they act defensive and hostile? Do they seem withdrawn or show other inappropriate behaviors? If your gut tells you that your patient may have been abused, follow your local protocols about reporting your objective findings and make sure your patient remains safe while in your care.

Or it may be due to dysarthria (difficulty in speaking as a result of muscular impairment). Maybe he is just collecting his thoughts or trying to remember details. Or maybe he is deciding whether he trusts you. He might be clinically depressed or, perhaps, he simply deals with situations by being quiet.

What do you do during the silence? Stay calm and observe your patient's nonverbal clues. Is he in pain? Is he scared? Is he on the verge of becoming hysterical or combative, or is he about to cry? You can encourage him to continue speaking by confronting him with your perceptions. For example, "I see you are obviously very upset about this. Do you want to talk about it?" If you sense that your patient is not responsive to your questions, perform a brief orientation exam. Speak to him in a loud voice and call him by name. Shake him gently if he does not respond. If this does not elicit a response, assume a neurologic problem and proceed accordingly.

Sometimes your behavior might have caused the silence. Are you asking too many questions too quickly? Have you offended your patient? Have you frightened him? Have you been insensitive? Have you failed to respond to your patient's needs? If your patient suddenly becomes silent, try to determine why, what is happening, and what you should do about it.

Overly Talkative Patients

The patient who rambles on can be just as frustrating to deal with as the one who will not talk at all. Why is your patient talking so fast and so much? Some patients react to stress this way. Maybe he has a lot to say. Maybe he needs someone to talk to; some lonely patients will take any opportunity to communicate with another human being.

What can you do in the emergency setting when time is scarce? This problem has no perfect solution. You can lower your goals and accept a less comprehensive history. You can briefly give your patient free rein. You can focus on the important areas and ask closed-ended questions about them. You can interrupt him frequently and summarize what he says. Above all, try not to become impatient.

Patients with Multiple Symptoms

Patients often present with multiple complaints. For example, your elderly patient may present you with a barrage of symptoms from an extensive medical history. Your challenge is to discover the chief complaint and why the patient called for help today. If the patient complains of symptoms that suggest multiple disease states, the challenge is compounded. In these types of cases, you must sort through a multitude of information quickly and recognize patterns that lead you to a correct field diagnosis.

Some patients will answer "Yes" to every question you ask. They have every symptom you mention; although this is possible, this phenomenon is not probable. Your patient might simply misunderstand or be trying hard to cooperate; more than likely he has an emotional problem and requires a psychosocial assessment. Document your findings on your prehospital care report and request a psychological referral. Asking the patient what single complaint led him to call for help today often helps.

Anxious Patients

Anxiety is a natural reaction to stress. People who face serious illness or injury can be expected to exhibit some degree of anxiety. Sometimes this manifests itself as simple nervousness, tenseness, sweating, or trembling. Some patients will fall silent, whereas others will ramble. Still others may exhibit anxiety attacks marked by a rapid heart rate, nausea and vomiting, chest pain, and shortness of breath. When you detect signs of anxiety, encourage your patient to speak freely about it. For example, you can say, "I see you are concerned about this. Do you want to talk about it?"

Patients Needing Reassurance

Appropriate reassurance is a cornerstone of patient care. You must be careful, however, not to be overly reassuring or to prematurely reassure your anxious patient. It is natural to say, "Relax, everything is going to be all right. We are going to take care of you and get you to the hospital. Just relax and you will be all right." But your patient may have anxiety about something of which you are not aware. For instance, if your chest pain patient is anxious, you might naturally assume he is apprehensive about dying. In reality, he may be anxious about something entirely different. He may be embarrassed about his anxieties, and instead of helping him deal with them, you have helped him cover them up. Now he may decide you are not interested in what is really bothering him and block further communication. Listen carefully to your patient before offering reassurance.

Intoxicated Patients

Dealing with belligerent, intoxicated patients challenges even the most experienced paramedic.[2,3] These patients are irrational, they disrupt your control of the scene, and they rarely allow you to examine them.

First and foremost, make sure your environment is safe. If your patient acts violently, call for the police before attempting any interaction. As you approach your patient, introduce yourself and offer a handshake. Avoid any challenging body language or remarks. Appear friendly and nonjudgmental, but always stay alert for a potential violent outburst. If your patient is shouting or cursing, do not try to get him to stop or to lower his voice. Listen to what he says, not how he says it, and try to understand his situation before making a clinical judgment. Sometimes a genuine offer of a place to sit will help calm an agitated, intoxicated person. Then you can begin your assessment.

Crying Patients

Sometimes your patient will cry. This can make any paramedic uncomfortable. Crying is just another form of venting, an important clue to your patient's emotions. Accept it as a natural release and do not try to suppress it. Be patient, allow him to cry, and then offer a supportive remark. Quiet acceptance and supportive remarks will open the lines of communication once your patient composes himself.

Depressed Patients

Depression is a common problem in medicine. It is also commonly misdiagnosed or ignored. It often presents with symptoms such as insomnia, fatigue, weight loss, or mysterious aches and pains. Depression is potentially lethal, so you must recognize its signs and evaluate its severity just as you would chest pain or shortness of breath. Ask your patient whether he has ever thought about committing suicide, whether he is currently thinking about suicide, whether he has the means to commit suicide, and whether he has ever attempted it. The more exact and precise his suicide plan, the more apt he is to carry it out.

Patients with Confusing Behaviors or Histories

You may encounter a patient whose story you just cannot follow. No matter what you ask, the answers leave you confused and frustrated. You cannot seem to develop a clear picture about your patient's problems. In fact, his answers do not even seem to make any sense. For example, you ask, "When did your headache begin?" and he answers, "My head feels like a squirrel." In these cases, the problem cannot be diagnosed in the field. The list of causes could include psychotic episodes, mental illness, **dementia**, **delirium**, head injury, or other physiologic conditions, such as stroke.

Many psychotic patients live and function in their communities, with varying degrees of success. Some will provide an accurate past history; others will not. If your patient's behavior seems distant, aloof, inappropriate, or even bizarre, suspect a mental illness, such as schizophrenia. It may be helpful to focus your assessment on this patient's mental status, with special emphasis on thought, perceptions, and mood.

Delirium and dementia are disorders relating to cognitive function. Delirium is common in the acutely ill or intoxicated patient; dementia occurs more frequently in the elderly. These patients often cannot provide clear, accurate histories. Their descriptions of their symptoms and their accounts of how things happened will be vague and inconsistent. They may appear inattentive to your questions and hesitant in their answers. They may even make up stories to fill in the gaps in their memories. In these cases, do not spend too much time trying to get a detailed history, because you will only become more frustrated. Focus on the mental status exam, with special emphasis on level of response, orientation, and memory. For a more detailed discussion of these problems, see the chaper "Psychiatric and Behavioral Disorders."

Patients with Limited Intelligence

You can usually obtain an adequate history from a patient with limited intelligence. Do not assume that he will not be able to provide accurate information concerning his current or past medical status. Also, do not overlook obvious omissions because your patient appears to be giving you a good story. Try to evaluate your patient's education and mental abilities. If you suspect severe mental retardation, obtain the patient's history from family or friends. Above all, show a genuine interest in your patient and try to establish a positive relationship. Then, communication can still happen.

Talking with Families or Friends

You will often encounter patients who cannot give you any useful information. In these cases, find a third party who can augment the patient history and offer a useful adjunct to the patient's answers. The typical case is the postictal patient who cannot describe his seizure activity to you. Another example is learning from his friend that your patient's wife died in an automobile crash just three weeks ago. Now you better understand why your patient appears depressed and suicidal. Make sure that patient confidentiality is a priority when you accept personal information from a family member, friend, or bystander.

Transferring Patient Care

When you arrive at the scene of an emergency, EMS-trained first responders may already be there. Before they transfer patient care to you, be sure to listen to their report carefully. Use eye contact and say the name of the first responder, if you know it. Integrate the information the first responders give you into the questions you ask your patient; he will trust you more if he sees you have listened to your colleagues. Say something like "The first responder, John, said you felt dizzy before you fell today. Can you remember any other sensations?"

Transfer of care at the receiving medical facility can be a challenge. Remember to always interact with other emergency colleagues with respect and dignity. If the emergency department is busy, the receiving nurse or doctor may appear to be distracted. If this is true, important medical information could get lost. In noncritical circumstances, therefore, respectfully stand your ground until the nurse or doctor looks at you. Then say, "Are you the person who will be listening to my hand-off report?" If so, follow up with, "Are you ready to listen, or would you rather wait a moment?" Also, be sure to introduce the patient by name and to say goodbye to the patient before you leave.

Summary

To provide the best care for your patients, you must be able to quickly and effectively gather information about the patient and the reason he called 911. This history gathering begins when you walk through the door. The patient and bystanders quickly pick up on your body language, tone of voice, facial expressions, and how you position yourself to the patient. Within that first minute or two, you have the opportunity to set the stage for the remainder of the interview. Remember to be cognizant of the culturally acceptable communication caveats, such as eye contact and spatial relationships, as you engage in conversation. Pay particularly close attention to your body language and tone of voice as you actively listen to the patient.

As you gain experience, you will develop situational communication templates that you can draw on as scenarios unfold. Situations that require assertiveness or calm empathetic compassion call for two completely different communication styles. Each comes with its own body language, facial expressions, tone of voice, and, for your safety, personal space/distance. With practice and experience, you will be able to move quickly from compassion to assertiveness or find any necessary combination to fit the situation and obtain the maximum amount of information and trust from your patient.

Remember, much of the information you will gather from all your patients is extremely personal. (In what other line of work can a perfect stranger approach a person on the street and inquire about bowel or sexual habits?) You will need an enormous degree of sensitivity to recognize and respond to the signs of suffering to create an ideal, individualized process of communication. Showing compassion and empathy, along with demonstrating the expertise necessary to assist appropriately, will allow you to become an ally to your patients and others.

You Make the Call

You and your partner respond to a report of an attempted suicide. When you arrive at the scene, three firefighters are caring for a 17 year old boy who is sitting in a bathtub. He is conscious and alert, and appears to have cut his wrists. His airway is patent and his breathing is adequate. The bleeding has been controlled with pressure dressings and there appear to be no other life threats. The young man is sobbing and does not respond to any of your questioning, however his father appears angry and provides lengthy responses whenever you ask a question. The crying continues as you load the patient onto the gurney and move towards the ambulance, and you notice the patient pulls away from his father when he tries to take his hand. At the back of the ambulance, the father states angrily, "I'm coming with you to the hospital. You obviously can't be trusted to act like an adult without me around!"

1. Would you allow the patient's father to ride in the ambulance to the hospital? What communication techniques could you use when navigating the situation?

2. List your strategies for communicating with this patient, given that he is crying and not readily answering your questions.

See Suggested Responses at the back of this book.

Review Questions

1. Which of the following is an effective method for establishing a positive rapport with your patient when you first meet him?
   a. Stand over him when you introduce yourself.
   b. Avoid eye contact initially.
   c. Introduce yourself and offer a handshake.
   d. Use a firm voice to gain control of the situation.

2. You arrive at the nursing home of an elderly woman whose name is Helen Smith. Family members in the room refer to her as "Mom," and the nursing staff has referred to her as "Helen." Given this information how should you address her?
   a. "Dear"
   b. "Helen"
   c. "Mrs. Smith"
   d. Any of the above

3. Which of the following is an open-ended question that you might pose to an elderly patient complaining of cardiac-type chest pain?
   a. Would you please describe your chest pain?
   b. Does your chest hurt a lot?
   c. Are you having any difficulty breathing?
   d. I see you have a bottle of nitroglycerin pills. Have you taken any of these?

4. You are interviewing a patient with angina. As he tells you about his chest pain, you maintain sincere eye contact and respond with "Mm-hmm," and "Go on" when he hesitates briefly. What type of therapeutic communication is this?
   a. Clarification
   b. Reflection
   c. Confrontation
   d. Facilitation

5. Your patient denies chest pain but keeps rubbing his chest. You say to him, "You say your chest doesn't hurt but I notice you keep rubbing it." This is an example of _____
   a. facilitation.
   b. confrontation.
   c. clarification.
   d. reflection.

6. In the United States, the socially acceptable distance between strangers is _____ feet.
   a. 2 to 6   c. 4 to 12
   b. 4 to 5   d. 10 to 15

7. When a paramedic is before a patient with his arms extended, hands open, and a nodding head as the patient speaks, he is exhibiting a(n) _____.
   a. intimate zone posture.
   b. open stance.
   c. closed stance.
   d. acceptable social distance.

8. While assessing a patient with a headache, you ask him, "Since you have a bad headache, you probably feel really nauseated too, right?" What type of question is this?
   a. Direct question
   b. Leading question
   c. Inferred question
   d. Open-ended question

9. The feedback technique in which the paramedic gives the patient time to gather his thoughts and respond when ready is _____
   a. empathy.
   b. silence.
   c. facilitation.
   d. clarification.

10. You have observed your partner acting in a matter in which his words and actions are belittling to certain ethnicities on several occasions. This type of inappropriate thoughts and behaviors is known as

    _____
    a. idealism.
    b. professionalism.
    c. ethnocentrism.
    d. cultural imposition.

See Answers to Review Questions at the back of this book.

References

1. Meade, D. M. "Mixed Messages: Interpreting Body Language." *Emerg Med Serv* 28(9) (1999): 59–73.
2. Dick, T. "Stinky People. Respecting Your Limitations and Other People's Predicaments." *Emerg Med Serv* 34(11) (2005): 26.
3. Remy, J. D. "Prehospital Care of the Intoxicated Individual." *Emerg Med Serv* 33(12) (2004): 88–91.

Further Reading

Dernocoeur, K. B. *Streetsense: Communication, Safety, and Control*. 3rd ed. Redmond, WA: Laing Research Services, 1996.

DeVito, J. *Essentials of Human Communication*. 7th ed. New York: Longman, 2010.

Keeland, B. and L. Jordan. *CommuniMed: Multilingual Patient Assessment Manual*. 3rd ed. St. Louis: Mosby, 1994.

Limmer, D., M. F. O'Keefe, E. T. Dickinson, et al. *Emergency Care*. 11th ed. Upper Saddle River, NJ: Pearson/Prentice Hall, 2009.

Perez-Sabido, J. *Spanish-English Handbook for Medical Professionals*. 4th ed. Los Angeles: Practice Management Information Corp., 1994.

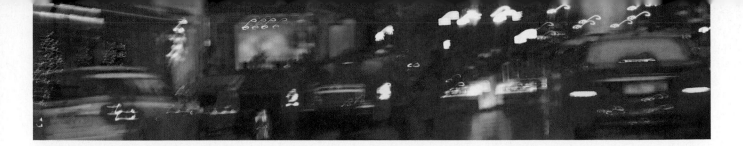

Chapter 4
History Taking

Richard A. Cherry, MS, EMT-P

STANDARD
Assessment

COMPETENCY
Integrate scene and patient assessment findings with knowledge of epidemiology and pathophysiology to form a field impression. This includes developing a list of differential diagnoses through clinical reasoning to modify the assessment and formulate a treatment plan.

 Learning Objectives

Terminal Performance Objective: After reading this chapter, you should be able to apply information obtained in a patient's history to clinical decision making.

Enabling Objectives: To accomplish the terminal performance objective, you should be able to:

1. Define key terms introduced in this chapter.

2. Explain the importance of both structure and flexibility in the approach to history taking.

3. Define and discuss what the preliminary data are, how to acquire them, and how to incorporate them into the overall history of the patient.

4. Define and discuss what the chief complaint is, how to acquire it, and how to incorporate this into the overall medical history of the patient.

5. Define and discuss what the present problem is, how to acquire it using OPQRST–ASPN, and how to incorporate this into the overall history of the patient.

6. Define and discuss what the past medical history is, how to acquire it, and how to incorporate this into the overall medical history of the patient.

7. Discuss how to use proper communication techniques while gathering the history pertinent to a review of the body systems.

8. Explain how to use clinical reasoning skills relative to the information gained in the history when developing a differential diagnosis.

9. Given a scenario, discuss communication strategies for gathering the patient's history and incorporating this information into differential diagnosis.

KEY TERMS

chief complaint, p. 58

differential field diagnosis,
   p. 57

diuretic, p. 61

dysmenorrhea, p. 64

dyspnea, p. 64

HEENT, p. 63

hematemesis, p. 64

hematuria, p. 64

hemoptysis, p. 64

intermittent claudication,
   p. 64

nocturia, p. 64

orthopnea, p. 64

paroxysmal nocturnal dyspnea,
   p. 64

polyuria, p. 64

primary problem, p. 58

referred pain, p. 60

tenderness, p. 59

tinnitus, p. 64

Case Study

En route to a call, paramedic supervisor Dan Colbert reviews the key elements of a medical interview in his head. Dan is precepting paramedic student James McConnell and wants to be a positive role model. As they approach the scene, Dan quickly sizes it up. Nothing seems unusual. To the best of his knowledge, the scene is safe.

According to the dispatch information, Dan and James are responding to evaluate an elderly man with abdominal pain. On first meeting his patient, Dan notices that the patient is in no real distress and appears stable. Dan does a primary assessment and then demonstrates taking a problem-oriented patient history for James. He introduces himself and James, and then asks for his patient's name, which he will use throughout the interview.

Dan begins with a general question. "What seems to be the problem today, Mr. O'Mara?" "My stomach hurts," Mr. O'Mara replies. Dan begins exploring the history of the present illness with questions such as "What were you doing when it started? Did it come on suddenly? Does anything make it worse or better? Can you describe how it feels? Can you point to the area that hurts? Does the pain travel anywhere else? How bad is it? On a scale of one to ten, with ten being the worst pain you have ever felt, how would you rate this pain? When did it start? Is it constant or does it come and go? Are you nauseous and have you vomited? Have you experienced a change in your bowel habits? Do you have any difficulty breathing?"

It seems that Mr. O'Mara's pain came on suddenly after he ate this afternoon. He describes it as a sharp pain in the upper right quadrant that radiates to the right shoulder area. As Mr. O'Mara answers Dan's questions, Dan leans forward, listening intently and often repeating Mr. O'Mara's words. James watches and learns.

Dan begins forming his differential field diagnosis, which includes hepatitis, acute myocardial infarction, pneumonia, aneurysm, cholecystitis, gastritis, pancreatitis, and peptic ulcer disease. He continues with the history. "Mr. O'Mara, have you ever been treated for this problem in the past? Are you being treated for any other problems right now? Do you have diabetes, heart disease, breathing problems, kidney problems, stomach problems? Have you been injured recently? Have you had any surgeries? Does this problem usually happen right after eating? Are you taking any medications for it right now? Are you allergic to any medications? Do you smoke? Do you drink? How often do you drink? Did you drink any alcohol today? Does this problem get worse when you drink? What did you eat today?"

Dan learns that Mr. O'Mara commonly has experienced pain after eating fatty foods. He then proceeds to the review of body systems, beginning with the gastrointestinal system. He learns that Mr. O'Mara often has indigestion and episodes of colicky pain. Mr. O'Mara denies vomiting blood or having blood in his stools. Hearing this, Dan suspects that his patient has cholecystitis. He conducts a focused physical exam and directs James to take vital signs. During the exam, Mr. O'Mara exhibits diffuse right-sided tenderness and a positive Murphy's sign.

En route to St. Joseph's Hospital, Dan has James conduct a detailed physical exam while he watches. At the hospital Dan reports to the emergency department's attending physician, Dr. Cooney, who agrees with his preliminary diagnosis of gallbladder disease. Following an assessment that includes labs and an ultrasound, Dr. Cooney calls for the surgical service. After the call, Dan reviews with James the key points of taking a comprehensive patient history. He explains how it helped him obtain important pieces of information that allowed him to focus the physical exam and led to his correct field diagnosis.

Customer Service Minute

Who's Watching? Imagine this scene in a residential neighborhood in a small town on a Sunday morning. An ambulance, rescue truck, police car, and two or three people who responded in their private vehicles come to the home of a man found in cardiac arrest by his wife. As the crew brings the patient out to the ambulance, neighbors watch from their windows as the crew performs CPR while wheeling their stretcher. Everyone knows the victim. As the ambulance drives away with the victim and his wife, the remaining crews stand in the street talking and joking around. There is some minor horseplay, as most of them are longtime friends. The neighbors are shocked at their behavior following such a tragic event.

Bystanders are a special group of people. They are curious and you have to limit their access to the scene for two reasons: First, they have no right to know what is going on, and second, they probably are not used to watching a crisis unfold, especially if it includes a gory presentation. However, they are watching and judging you as you work, so consider how what you are doing looks to others. Focus on the patient and not on socializing with other responders until after the incident is over and you are back at the station.

Bystanders expect you to restore order and calmness to a chaotic scene. They don't want you to add to the mess. They want to see competent, compassionate, caring field providers in action.

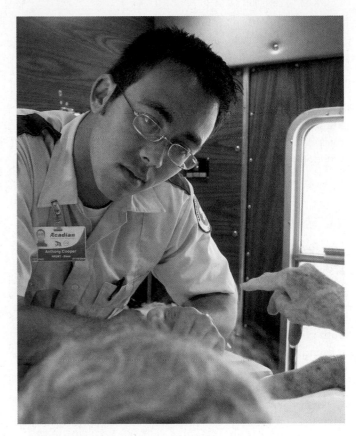

FIGURE 4-1 Listen intently to your patient and respond accordingly. *(© Daniel Limmer)*

Introduction

In the majority of medical cases, you will base your field diagnosis on the patient history. Clearly, the way you conduct the patient interview and the questions you ask will determine how much relevant medical information your patient reveals. In medical cases, obtaining an adequate history of your patient's chief complaint, recent illnesses, and significant past medical history is as important as, if not more important than, the physical exam. The information you gather will direct the physical exam and reveal clues to your patient's problem. Although we present the history by itself in this chapter, you will most likely conduct it simultaneously with parts of the physical exam.

The ability to elicit a good history is the foundation for providing good care to patients you have never met before. To conduct a good interview, you must present yourself as a caring professional and gain your patient's trust in just a very short time. Then you must ask the right questions, listen intently to your patient's answers, and respond accordingly (Figure 4-1). In this chapter, we discuss the components of taking a comprehensive medical history.

We present the medical history in its entirety, as a well-structured, yet flexible, tool having several component procedures that are conducted in order. In reality, your patient's answers will alter the sequence of your questioning, and some of the information in this chapter will not readily adapt itself to prehospital emergency medicine. As you gain clinical experience, however, you will learn which components of the history are appropriate to the particular situations you encounter.

Whether your patient is critical or stable, the situation determines the length and completeness of the interview. For example, complicated medical cases require a close investigation of your patient's chief complaint and past history. For patients with a critical medical condition, you may have time only to elicit a pertinent history while you administer lifesaving treatments. Trauma cases are generally sudden events not precipitated by medical conditions and require only a modified approach to history taking. Let the situation dictate the depth and scope of your history taking.

The interview is the focal point of your relationship with your patients. It establishes the bonding necessary for effective and efficient patient care. By asking a series of well-designed questions, you begin to build a profile of your patients. This comes with time. The more patients you encounter, the better you will become at getting a pertinent history. You also should have a good understanding of their problems and a **differential field diagnosis** (list of causes) to explain their signs and symptoms. Often, learning about your patient's history, medications, and even his lifestyle will reveal clues to your final field diagnosis.

This chapter presents the components of a comprehensive patient history in a systematic order. In practice, you will ultimately select only the components that apply to your patient's situation and status. For example, if you conduct preemployment physical exams for a company, you may use the entire form. On the other hand, if you respond to a gasping patient with acute pulmonary edema, you will focus on the present illness. Common sense and clinical experience will determine how much of the following history to use.

Preliminary Data

For documentation, always record the date and time of the physical exam. Determine your patient's age, sex, race, birthplace, and occupation. This provides a starting point for the interview and establishes you as the interviewer. Who is the source of the information you receive about your patient? Is it the competent patient himself, his spouse, a friend, or a bystander? Are you receiving a report from a first responder, the police, or another health care worker? Do you have the medical record from a transferring facility?

After you have gathered the information, you should establish its reliability, which will vary according to the source's knowledge, memory, trust, and motivation. Again, reconfirm the information with the patient, if possible. This is a judgment call based on your experience. For example, if the patient information you received from a particular EMT first responder has been accurate in the past, you probably will trust it again. On the other hand, if the nurse at a physician's office has repeatedly provided you with erroneous information, you probably will doubt its accuracy.

Chief Complaint

The history begins with an open-ended question about your patient's **chief complaint**. The chief complaint is the pain, discomfort, or dysfunction that caused your patient to request help. In a medical case, it may be a woman's call for help because she has chest pain. In a trauma case, it may be a bystander's call for assistance to a "man down" or a police officer's reporting an injury in an auto collision. Your patient may have called for more than one symptom.

It is important to begin with a general question that allows your patient to respond freely. Ask, for example, "Why did you call us today?" or "What seems to be the problem?" Avoid the tunnel vision that often biases paramedics who focus on dispatch information that may or may not accurately describe the situation. As you interview and assess your patient, the chief complaint will become more specific.[1]

The chief complaint differs from the **primary problem**. Whereas the chief complaint is a sign or symptom noticed by the patient or a bystander, the primary problem is the principal medical cause of the complaint. For example, your patient's chief complaint may be leg pain, whereas the primary problem is a tibia fracture. When possible, report and record the chief complaint in your patient's own words. For example, "I am having a hard time breathing" is better than "the patient has dyspnea." For the unconscious patient, the chief complaint becomes what someone else identifies or what you observe as the primary problem. In some trauma situations, for instance, the chief complaint might be the mechanism of injury, such as "a penetrating wound to the chest" or "a fall from 25 feet."

Patho Pearls

The renowned Canadian physician Sir William Osler said, "Listen to the patient, and he will tell you what is wrong." This advice is as true today as it was 100 years ago. A great deal of information can be determined from a skillful history taking. As you listen to a patient's medical history, try to understand the underlying pathophysiologic processes that might cause the symptoms the patient describes. This will help you to fully comprehend the disease process or processes affecting the patient.

For example, consider the following case. Mrs. J. Franklin is a 72-year-old pensioner, twice widowed, who lives in an older section of town. She summons EMS with what initially seem like vague complaints. She reports to the dispatcher, when queried, that she is "just sick." You arrive and begin an assessment, starting with a pertinent history. The patient reports that her symptoms began about two weeks ago after several family members came to her house with dinner, which included a baked ham. Since that time, she has developed some fatigue, progressive dyspnea, and occasional chest pain. She now reports that she often wakes up at 3:00 A.M. with breathing trouble that resolves when she walks around the room or sleeps with three pillows. She also cannot tie her shoes, and she missed church last Sunday for this very reason. Her medications have remained unchanged and include furosemide, nitroglycerin paste, digoxin, aspirin, and lisinopril.

Clearly, there are physiologic cues in the patient's medical history. The symptoms began with a ham dinner. You learn that she kept the ham and has been eating it daily. The ham is salt cured. Thus, her sodium intake may have increased. Her medications have remained unchanged. Her symptoms seem to indicate worsening heart failure with episodes consistent with both left and right ventricular failure. Her nighttime dyspnea and orthopnea are consistent with left heart failure, whereas her inability to tie her shoes could be due to peripheral edema from right heart failure. The fatigue could be attributed to both. Thus, your physical examination should either support or contradict your history findings.

In fact, it was learned later that the patient's heart failure had always been somewhat tenuous and the sodium load she received from the ham was all that was necessary to cause congestive heart failure. She did well with two days of hospitalization, diuretic administration, and sodium restriction.

Dr. Osler was correct. The history is often the most important part of patient assessment.

Present Problem

Once you have determined the chief complaint, explore each of your patient's complaints in greater detail. Be naturally inquisitive when exploring the events surrounding these complaints. A practical template for exploring each complaint follows the mnemonic OPQRST–ASPN, an acronym for **O**nset, **P**rovocation/**P**alliation, **Q**uality, **R**egion/**R**adiation, **S**everity, **T**ime, **A**ssociated **S**ymptoms, and **P**ertinent **N**egatives.[2] This line of questioning provides a full, clear, chronological account of your patient's symptoms. The present history often provides a clear picture of what happened prior to your arrival and a head start in narrowing down your working field diagnosis.

Onset

Did the problem develop suddenly or gradually? What was your patient doing when the symptoms started? In medical emergencies, investigate your patient's activities at the time of, or shortly before, the signs or symptoms developed. In some cases, especially in trauma, you may have to gather information from a few weeks before the onset of symptoms. For example, the signs and symptoms of a subdural hematoma may not appear until weeks following an injury. Was the patient exercising or exerting himself, or at rest or sleeping? Was he eating or drinking? If so, what? In trauma cases, ensure that a medical problem did not cause the incident. For example, the sudden onset of an illness, such as a seizure or syncope, may have caused a fall.

Provocation/Palliation

What provokes the symptom (makes it worse)? Does anything palliate the symptom (make it better)? In many

Assessment Pearls

Chest pain is a common reason that people summon EMS. However, the causes of chest pain are numerous. In emergency medicine or EMS, we often look to exclude the most serious causes before determining whether chest pain is of a benign origin. Internal organs do not have as many pain fibers as do such structures as the skin and other areas. Pain arising from an internal organ tends to be dull and vague. This is because nerves from various spinal levels innervate the organ in question. The heart, for example, is innervated by several thoracic spinal nerve segments. Thus, cardiac pain tends to be dull and is sometimes described as pressure. It also tends to cause referred pain (i.e., pain in an area somewhat distant to the organ), such as pain in the left arm and jaw. Dull pain that is hard to localize (or to reproduce with palpation) may be due to cardiac disease. One sign often seen with patients suffering cardiac disease is Levine's sign. With Levine's sign, the patient will subconsciously clench his fist when describing the chest pain. Levine's sign is associated with pain of a cardiac origin (e.g., angina or acute coronary syndrome).

illnesses, certain factors, such as motion, pressure, and jarring, may increase or decrease pain, discomfort, or dysfunction. Do eating, movement, exertion, stress, or anything else provoke the current problem?

Positioning also may be a factor. Your patient may wish to curl up and lie on his side to reduce abdominal pain. Congestive heart failure patients will sit bolt upright to ease respiration. They also may sleep with several pillows raising their upper body to relieve paroxysmal nocturnal dyspnea (PND), a sleep-disturbing breathing difficulty caused by fluid that accumulates in the lungs when the patients are supine. Ask your patient how breathing affects the discomfort. Deep breathing may increase the acute abdomen patient's pain. A patient with pleuritic or rib-fracture pain will not breathe deeply, whereas breathing may not affect the pain of angina. Any patient with respiratory pain will breathe with shallower but more frequent breaths.

If your patient took a medication shortly before you arrived, its effect—or lack of effect—may help determine the problem. Drugs such as bronchodilators, hypoglycemic agents, antihypertensives, and anticonvulsants are commonly prescribed and taken at home. Investigate any medication used to relieve a problem and note its effectiveness. Ask about any activity, medication, or other circumstance that either alleviates or aggravates the chief complaint.

Quality

How does your patient perceive the pain or discomfort? Ask him to explain how the symptom feels, and listen carefully to his answer. Does your patient call his pain crushing, tearing, oppressive, gnawing, crampy, sharp, dull, or otherwise? Quote his exact descriptors in your report.

Region/Radiation

Where is the symptom? Does it move anywhere else? Identify the exact location and area of pain, discomfort, or dysfunction. Does your patient complain of pain "here," while holding a clenched fist over the sternum, or does he grasp the entire abdomen with both hands and moan? If your patient has not done so, ask him to point to the painful area. Identify the specific location, or the boundary of the pain if it is regional.

Determine whether the pain is truly pain (occurring independently) or **tenderness** (pain on palpation). Also determine whether the pain moves or radiates. Localized pain occurs in one specific area, whereas radiating pain travels away from the source, in one, many, or all directions. Evaluate moving pain's initial location and progression and any factors that affect its movement.

Note any pain that may be referred from other parts of the body. **Referred pain** is felt in a part of the body away from the source of the disease or problem. The heart and diaphragm are two areas that most commonly produce referred pain. Cardiac problems, such as myocardial infarction or anginal pain, are usually referred to the left arm, with occasional referral to the neck, jaw, and back. Pain associated with irritation of the diaphragm (most commonly caused by blood in the abdomen of the supine patient) generally is referred to the clavicular region.

Severity

How bad is the symptom? *Severity* is the intensity of pain or discomfort felt by your patient. Ask him how bad the pain feels, and then have him compare it with other painful problems he has experienced. Sometimes a patient can describe the severity of the pain on a scale from 1 to 10, with 10 being the worst pain he has ever felt. Also notice the amount of discomfort your patient's condition causes. How easy is it to distract your patient from his concern over the pain? Is your patient very still and resistive to your touch? Is he writhing about? The answers should give you a good idea of the intensity of your patient's pain.

Time

When did the symptoms begin? Is a symptom constant or intermittent? How long does it last? How long has this symptom affected your patient—several days, hours, or just a few minutes or seconds? When did any previous episodes occur? How does this episode's length vary from earlier ones?

Associated Symptoms

What other symptoms commonly associated with the chief complaint in certain diseases can help rule in your field diagnosis? For example, if the chief complaint is chest pain, ask, "Are you short of breath? Are you nauseated? Have you vomited? Are you dizzy or light-headed?" The presence of these symptoms would help support a field diagnosis of cardiac chest pain.

Pertinent Negatives

Are any likely associated symptoms absent? Their absence is as important to the field diagnosis as their presence, because they help rule out a particular disease or injury. Note any element of the history or physical exam that does *not* support a suspected or possible field diagnosis such as congestive heart failure. For example, it is significant if

your patient who complains of chest pain denies shortness of breath, nausea, and light-headedness. It doesn't necessarily rule congestive heart failure out, but it is significant.

Past Medical History

The past medical history may provide significant insights into your patient's chief complaint and your field diagnosis.[3] Look in depth at your patient's general state of health, childhood and adult diseases, psychiatric illnesses, accidents or injuries, surgeries, and hospitalizations. They may reveal general or specific clues that will help you to correctly assess the patient's current problem. Your patient's condition, the situation, and time constraints will determine how much information you can and should gather on the scene. For example, asking about childhood diseases may not be relevant for your acute cardiac or trauma patient.

General State of Health

How does your patient perceive his general state of health? Is he normally in good health? Does he feel energetic for his age and condition? Have there been any major changes in the way he feels about his health lately?

Childhood Diseases

What childhood diseases did your patient have? Did he have mumps, measles, rubella, whooping cough, chickenpox, rheumatic fever, scarlet fever, or polio? Again, this line of questioning's relevance depends on the patient and the situation.

Adult Diseases

Is your patient diabetic? Does he have a history of heart disease, breathing problems, high blood pressure, or similar conditions? A preexisting medical problem may contribute to your patient's current problem or influence his care during the next few hours. To discover significant preexisting medical problems, ask whether your patient has recently seen a physician or been hospitalized. If so, for what condition?

If you discover a preexisting problem, investigate its effects on your patient. When did the problem last affect him? Is your patient on any special diets or prescribed medications or is he restricted in activity? Even with the trauma patient, do not forget that a medical problem may have led to an accident or may complicate the effects of trauma. Also, obtain the name of your patient's physician, as it may be helpful to the emergency department staff.

Current Medications

Is your patient taking any medications? These include over-the-counter medications, prescriptions, home remedies,

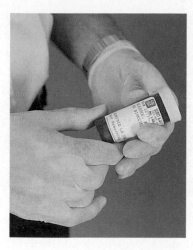

FIGURE 4-2 When practical, take your patient's medications to the hospital with you.

vitamins, and minerals. If so, why is he taking them? Your patient's explanation may not be medically accurate, but it may help to determine underlying conditions. For example, your 65-year-old patient tells you she takes a "water pill." You can safely assume that she takes a **diuretic**, and has a history of renal or cardiac problems.

A medication not taken as prescribed may be responsible for the current medical problem—possibly by under- or overmedication. A recently prescribed medication may cause an allergic or untoward (severe and unexpected) reaction. It also may be out of date and no longer effective. Even for trauma, emergency department personnel will need to know what medications your patient is taking. For example, if your patient takes warfarin, an anticoagulant, it would interfere with the normal clotting process and could actually promote bleeding. If practical, bring your patient's medications to the hospital (Figure 4-2). Is your patient compliant with his medications? If not, why?

Allergies

Does your patient have any known allergies, especially to penicillin, the "caine" family (local anesthetics), tetanus toxoid, or narcotics? These agents are occasionally given in emergency situations. What type of reaction did your patient have to the medication? For example, was it just a mild allergic reaction, with a rash and itching or localized swelling, or was it anaphylactic shock? Knowledge of your patient's allergies may prevent additional complications during the emergency department visit, especially if he becomes disoriented or unconscious during transport. If your patient is short of breath with wheezing, ask about environmental allergies. In cases of possible anaphylaxis, ask about allergies to drugs; to foods such as shellfish, nuts, and dairy products; and to insect bites and stings.

Psychiatric Illnesses

Does your patient have a history of mental illness? Has he ever been diagnosed with depression, mania, schizophrenia, or other problems? Is he being treated for a mental illness? If so, what medications is he taking? Has he ever had thoughts of suicide? Has he ever attempted suicide? Does he have the means available to him to carry out a threat of suicide? Tailor these questions carefully for patients you suspect of having a mental illness.

Accidents or Injuries

Has your patient ever had a serious accident or injury requiring hospitalization? Has he had a previous injury that could be a factor in his current problem? For example, a seemingly minor head injury a week ago may present now as a subdural hematoma in your unconscious elderly patient.

Keep this line of questioning to relevant information only. An old football injury or childhood laceration is probably not influencing your patient's chest pain and respiratory distress today. However, his pneumonectomy (surgical removal of a lung) probably is the reason for the absence of lung sounds on his right side.

Surgeries or Hospitalizations

Has your patient had any other hospitalizations or surgeries not already mentioned? Again, these may offer some insight into your suspected field diagnosis. For example, your patient is an 85-year-old man with a long history of congestive heart failure and no history of chronic lung disease (e.g., asthma, emphysema, bronchitis). He suddenly presents with severe difficulty in breathing and audible wheezing. You should suspect the obvious—a cardiac problem. Don't look for the five-legged cat.

SAMPLE

For trauma patients you will use an abbreviated version of the past history known as SAMPLE. It is a mnemonic for **S**igns and symptoms, **A**llergies, **M**edications, **P**ast history, **L**ast time eaten, and **E**vents leading to the incident. It is a quick and practical history that provides enough relevant information in a trauma emergency.

Family/Social History

Because many disease processes are hereditary, the medical history of immediate family members is important. In the nonemergency setting, you may explore deep into the family tree and chart the medical history of grandparents, parents, aunts, and uncles. In the emergency setting, learning that your 45-year-old patient with chest pain had a father and brother who both died of heart attacks in their late 40s is important information. Look for a family history of diabetes, heart disease, hypercholesterolemia, high blood pressure, stroke, kidney disease, tuberculosis, cancer, arthritis, anemia, allergies, asthma, headaches, epilepsy, mental illness, alcoholism, drug addiction, and any symptoms similar to those of your patient.[4]

Home Situation and Significant Others

Who lives at home with your patient? Ask him about his home life—or lack of one. What is his marital status? Ask about friends, family, and loved ones. Find out whether he has a support network, and whom it includes. Who takes care of him when he needs help? Loneliness and isolation may complicate your patient's physical symptoms.

Daily Life

Ask your patient to describe his typical day. When does he get up? What does he do first? Then what? Such questions reveal a lot about your patient's state of mind and general wellness. Is he busy, active, and motivated to get up in the morning? Does he merely exist from the time he awakens and go through life with no purpose or direction? Is he under high levels of stress from morning to night in a job that requires him to take his problems home with him? Find out what kind of life your patient leads. It may reveal a lot about his illness.

Tobacco

Does your patient use tobacco? If so, what type (cigarettes, cigars, pipe, smokeless, or other), how much, and for how long? To quantify his cigarette smoking history, multiply the number of packs smoked per day by the number of years he has smoked. The result is his pack/year history. For example, if your patient smoked two packs of cigarettes per day for 25 years, he is a 50 pack/year smoker. The higher the number, the more significant the smoking history becomes.

Alcohol, Drugs, and Related Substances

Alcohol and drugs are often contributing factors to, if not the primary cause of, your patient's medical problems (Figure 4-3). Your job is not to pass judgment, but to gather data that will help direct your patient's medical treatment. Remaining nonjudgmental will aid you in your questioning. Start with a general question, such as "How much alcohol do you drink?" If you suspect that a drinking problem may be a factor, you can use the CAGE questionnaire (an alcoholism screening instrument) to determine the

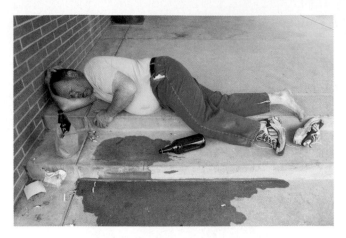

FIGURE 4-3 Alcohol is often a contributing factor in, if not the primary cause of, a patient's medical problems.

presence of alcoholism. Reserve this line of questioning for the chronic patient in a controlled setting. It would be inappropriate in a bar with an unruly, intoxicated patient.

The CAGE Questionnaire

Two or more "yes" answers to the following questions suggest alcoholism and further lines of inquiry.[5]

- Have you ever felt the need to **c**ut down on your drinking?
- Have you ever felt **a**nnoyed by criticism of your drinking?
- Have you ever had **g**uilty feelings about drinking?
- Have you ever taken a drink first thing in the morning as an **e**ye-opener?

Ask about blackouts, accidents, or injuries that happened while drinking. Also ask about alcohol-related job losses, marital problems, and arrests while under the influence of alcohol.

Similarly, ask about drug use: "Do you use marijuana, cocaine, heroin, sleeping pills, or painkillers? How much do you take? How do these drugs make you feel? Have you had any bad reactions?" As your patients realize that you are not judging their substance abuse, they may feel more comfortable telling you about their patterns of use.

Diet

Ask about your patient's normal daily intake of food and drink. Perhaps your 78-year-old retiree just moved to the Arizona desert and underestimated the increased fluid loss as a result of sweating. He does not realize that he needs to increase his daily fluid intake, and now he presents weak and

CONTENT REVIEW

➤ CAGE Questionnaire
- **C**ut down
- **A**nnoyed
- **G**uilty
- **E**ye opener

dizzy from dehydration. Are there any dietary restrictions or supplements? Ask specifically about his use of foods with stimulating effects, such as coffee, tea, cola drinks, and other beverages containing caffeine. For example, your 23-year-old patient with a rapid heartbeat (200 beats per minute) may drink continual cups of coffee each morning at her highly stressful job.

Screening Tests

Ask about certain screening tests that may have been done for your patient. Some examples include a purified protein derivative (PPD) test for suspected tuberculosis, Pap smears and mammograms for female problems, stool testing for occult blood, and cholesterol tests. Record the dates of the tests and their results.

Immunizations

Ask your patient about his immunizations for diseases such as tetanus, pertussis, diphtheria, polio, measles, rubella, mumps, influenza, hepatitis B, and pneumococcal vaccine. For example, ask the parent of a child suspected of having epiglottitis whether he had the *Haemophilus influenzae* B vaccine. *H. influenzae* B is a common cause of epiglottitis and meningitis in children.

Sleep

Ask your patient what time he normally goes to bed and arises. Does he take daytime naps? Does he have problems falling asleep or staying asleep? A sleep disorder could be a contributing factor or a side effect of your patient's problem.

Exercise and Leisure Activities

Does your patient exercise regularly or lead a sedentary existence? Sometimes your patient's lifestyle will support your field diagnosis. For example, a sedentary lifestyle is a major risk factor for cardiac disease.

Environmental Hazards

Ask about possible hazards in the home, school, and workplace. For example, your patient may live or work in an area with high levels of toxic substances. Many health problems can be traced to these environmental causes. Remember that even the average home is stocked with a variety of hazardous materials (e.g., cleaners, bleach, paint thinner).

Use of Safety Measures

In an auto crash, did your patient use a seat restraint system? Were all passengers belted in? Did the air bag deploy?

Such information aids you and the emergency department staff in determining the extent of damage caused by a particular mechanism of injury. For bicycle, inline skate, and skateboard injuries, ask about the use of helmets and knee and elbow pads.

Important Experiences

Ask about your patient's upbringing and home life growing up. How much schooling does he have? Was he in the military? What kinds of jobs has he held? What is his financial situation? Is he married, single, divorced, or widowed? What does he do for fun and relaxation? Is he retired or looking forward to retirement? Again, the answers give you a broader picture of your patient. The sudden loss of a close relative, for example, could be the cause of your patient's insomnia, anorexia, and depression.

Religious Beliefs

Some religions forbid certain treatments and have guidelines regarding the management of illness and injury. For example, some forbid whole-blood transfusions. Knowing whether your patient is guided by these beliefs can help you understand and care for him better. These questions require some expression of sensitivity—or it might be best to ask broadly if he has any limitations in medical care.

The Patient's Outlook

Find out what your patient thinks and how he feels about the present and the future. This can include his physical and mental health, his overall outlook on life, his view of the world, career, family, and so forth. All these factors can contribute to a person's health and well-being and are an important part of taking a comprehensive history.

Review of Body Systems

The review of body systems is a series of questions designed to identify problems your patient has not already mentioned.[6] It is a system-by-system list of questions that are more specific than those asked during the basic history. Again, the patient's chief complaint, condition, and clinical status determine how much, if any, of the review of body systems you will use. For example, if your patient complains of chest pain, you may want to review the respiratory, cardiac, gastrointestinal, and hematologic systems. If your patient complains of a headache, you may want to review the **HEENT** (**h**ead, **e**yes, **e**ars, **n**ose, and **t**hroat), neurologic, peripheral vascular, and psychiatric systems. Let your patient lead you through the history. The following sampling includes a few of the many questions that you might ask.

General

What is your patient's usual weight, and have there been any recent weight changes? Has he had weakness, fatigue, fever, chills, or night sweats?

Skin, Hair, Nails

Has your patient noticed any new rashes, lumps, sores, itching, dryness, color change, or changes in nails or hair? Could cosmetics or jewelry have caused these problems?

Head, Eyes, Ears, Nose, and Throat (HEENT)

Has your patient had headaches, recent head trauma, or loss of consciousness? How is his vision? Does he wear glasses or contact lenses? When was his last eye exam, and have there been any changes in his vision? Has he experienced any of the following: pain, redness, excessive tearing, double vision, blurred vision, photophobia, spots, specks, flashing lights? Has he ever had glaucoma or cataracts?

How is his hearing? Does he use hearing aids? Has he ever experienced ringing in the ears (**tinnitus**), hearing loss, vertigo, earaches, infection, or discharge? Does he have frequent colds, nasal stuffiness, nasal discharge, hay fever, nosebleeds, nasal obstruction, and/or sinus problems? Has he experienced any changes in his sense of smell?

Does he wear dentures? When was his last dental exam? Describe the condition of his teeth and gums. Do his gums bleed? Does he get a sore tongue, dry mouth, frequent sore throats, or hoarseness? Does he have lumps or swollen glands? Has he ever had a goiter, neck pain, difficulty swallowing, or stiffness? Has he experienced any changes in his sense of taste?

Chest and Lungs

Has your patient ever had wheezing, coughing up of blood (**hemoptysis**), asthma, bronchitis, emphysema, pneumonia, TB, or pleurisy? When was his last chest X-ray? Is he coughing now? If so, can you describe the sputum (color, amount, consistency)?

Heart and Blood Vessels

Has your patient ever had heart trouble, high blood pressure, rheumatic fever, heart murmurs, chest pain or discomfort, palpitations, shortness of breath (**dyspnea**), shortness of breath while lying flat (**orthopnea**), or peripheral edema? Has he ever been awakened from sleep with shortness of breath (**paroxysmal nocturnal dyspnea**)? Has he ever had an ECG or other heart tests? Has your patient ever had intermittent calf pain while walking (**intermittent claudication**), leg cramps, varicose veins, or blood clots?

Lymph Nodes

Has your patient noticed any enlargement or tenderness in his lymph nodes?

Gastrointestinal System

Has your patient ever had trouble swallowing, heartburn, loss of appetite, nausea/vomiting, regurgitation, vomiting of blood (**hematemesis**), or indigestion? How often does he move his bowels? Describe the color and size of his stools. Have there been any changes in his bowel habits? Has he had rectal bleeding or black, tarry stools, hemorrhoids, constipation, or diarrhea? Has he had abdominal pain, food intolerance, or excessive belching or passing of gas? Has he had jaundice, liver or gallbladder problems, or hepatitis?

Genitourinary System

How often does your patient urinate? Has he ever had excessive urination (**polyuria**), excessive urination at night (**nocturia**), burning or pain while urinating, blood in the urine (**hematuria**), urgency, reduced caliber or force of urine flow, hesitancy, dribbling, or incontinence? Has he ever had a urinary tract infection or passed a kidney stone?

Male Genitalia

Has your patient ever had a hernia, discharge from or sores on the penis, testicular pain or masses? Has he ever had a sexually transmitted disease? If so, how was it treated? Has he experienced any erectile dysfunction?

Female Genitalia

At what age did your patient have her first menstrual period? Describe the regularity, frequency, duration, and amount of bleeding of her periods. When was her last menstrual period? Does she bleed between periods or after intercourse? Has she ever had difficulty with her period (**dysmenorrhea**) or premenstrual tension? At what age did

---

Assessment Pearls

Estimating Gestational Age Occasionally, you will encounter a pregnant patient who cannot provide information that will help you determine the approximate gestational age (e.g., last menstrual period or sonogram). One way to estimate the gestational age is to measure the fundal height. To do this, get a cloth or soft tape measure marked in centimeters. Place the start of the tape on the symphysis pubis bone and measure the distance to the topmost part of the uterus (the fundal height). On average, every centimeter is approximately 1 week of gestation. Thus, a reading of 24 cm correlates to 24 weeks. Please note, however, that this measurement is least accurate early in pregnancy and at the very end of pregnancy, when the fetus's head descends into the pelvis.

she become menopausal? Were there symptoms or bleeding? Has she ever had any vaginal discharge, lumps, sores, or itching? Has she ever had a sexually transmitted disease? If so, how was it treated? How many times has she been pregnant? How many deliveries? Any abortions (spontaneous or induced)?

Some health care personnel use the G-P-A-L system to document a patient's history of pregnancy:

- **Gravida** How many times pregnant?
- **Para** How many viable births?
- **Abortions** How many abortions (including miscarriages)?
- **Living** How many living children?

Has your patient ever had complications of pregnancy? Does she use birth control? If so, what type? If postmenopausal, is she on hormone replacement therapy?

Musculoskeletal System

Has your patient ever experienced muscle or joint pain, loss of motion, swelling, redness, heat, deformity, stiffness, arthritis, gout, or backache? Describe the location or symptoms.

Neurologic System

Has your patient ever experienced any of the following: fainting, blackouts, memory loss, seizures, speech difficulty, vertigo, weakness, loss of coordination, paralysis, numbness or loss of sensation, tingling, "pins and needles," twitches, tremors, or other involuntary movements?

Hematologic System

Has your patient ever been anemic? Has he experienced fatigue lately? Has he ever had a blood transfusion? If so, did he have a reaction to it? Does he bruise or bleed easily?

Endocrine System

Has your patient ever had thyroid trouble? Did he ever experience heat or cold intolerance, skin changes, swelling of the hands and feet, or excessive sweating? Does he have diabetes? Has he ever had excessive thirst, hunger, or urge to urinate? Has he experienced any changes in body and facial hair?

Psychiatric History

Is your patient nervous? Is he under much stress and tension? Has he ever been depressed? Has he noticed mood changes? Has he ever thought of committing suicide or homicide? Has he experienced irritability, difficulty concentrating, sleep disturbances, or fatigue on waking?

Clinical Reasoning

As a paramedic, you must gather, evaluate, and synthesize much information in very little time. You will obtain this information using your senses (sight, smell, hearing, and touch) during the history and physical exam. Analyzing these data will involve the total of your education, training, and clinical experience. For example, as you enter a patient's home, the sound of his gasping for breath with audible wheezes startles you. Having heard wheezing before and having learned in class that it results from a variety of problems will help you to make what is called a *differential diagnosis*. The differential diagnosis is a preliminary list of possible causes for your patient's problem. For example, a differential diagnosis for diffuse wheezing might include asthma, emphysema, bronchitis, and acute pulmonary edema. Now you conduct a history and physical exam and arrive at a field diagnosis, or impression.

Your next step will involve applying your clinical experience and exercising independent decision making as you develop and implement a management plan. For example, your gasping and wheezing patient is an elderly man who presents with severe difficulty breathing. He has a history of cardiac and pulmonary disease, and you are not sure which problem precipitated this episode. You gather information and make an initial field diagnosis of congestive heart failure. You immediately administer medications (nitroglycerin, CPAP, morphine) to reduce cardiac preload, ease the workload of the heart, and increase tissue oxygenation. You prepare for endotracheal intubation and mechanical ventilation in case CPAP fails. This decision to administer potentially life-threatening drugs requires you to think clearly and work effectively under pressure. Few prehospital situations create more pressure than a patient struggling to breathe.

The ability to think under pressure and make decisions cannot be taught; it must be developed. As a paramedic, you will be a team leader on emergency scenes. In that role, you must make sound, reasonable decisions regarding your patient's care. Several aspects of this program will help you to develop this essential skill. In the classroom, you will work on case histories. In the labs, you will practice patient scenarios on moulaged victims. In the hospital, you will assess and help manage real patients in the emergency department and critical care units. In the field internship, you will assess and manage patients in the streets. In all these settings, you will begin developing clinical judgment.

Fundamental Knowledge and Abilities

First, you must have an excellent working knowledge of anatomy and physiology and of the pathophysiology of your patient's disease or injury. To assess and manage a patient with difficulty breathing, for instance, you must know which organs and body systems are involved in breathing. You must understand the process of normal breathing and each body system's role in that effort. You must recall the factors that inhibit normal breathing and recognize the signs and symptoms of respiratory distress.

For example, a patient might wheeze because of lower airway obstruction from secretions, bronchoconstriction, edema, or any combination of these conditions. All reduce the inner diameter of the airways, restricting airflow and making movement of air in and out of the lungs difficult. Managing this patient would require knowledge of the respiratory and cardiovascular causes of wheezing, because their treatments are vastly different. Respiratory causes for generalized wheezing include asthma and bronchitis, which you would manage with bronchodilators. Cardiac causes for wheezing include congestive heart failure, which you would manage with CPAP and vasodilators. Without a good working knowledge of these diseases, you might make a mistaken and potentially devastating field diagnosis.

Gathering Data

You also must be able to focus on many specific data. When you conduct a patient assessment, you will evaluate all relevant information while focusing on specific important findings. You will be inundated with information requiring you to establish relationships and form conclusions. Your patient who presents with difficulty breathing and wheezing in the previous example would require an in-depth history and focused examination of his cardiac and respiratory systems. You also would assess other systems relative to his chief complaint (HEENT, musculoskeletal, neurologic, and lymphatic), while remaining focused on the primary problem (cardiorespiratory). Although his chief complaint is difficulty breathing, his primary problem might originate in the cardiovascular, musculoskeletal, immune, hematologic, or neurologic system.

Forming a Differential Diagnosis

You must be able to organize the information you obtain and form concepts from it. Initially, you elicit your patient's chief complaint and begin to formulate a differential field diagnosis. As you conduct the history and a clearer picture of your patient's problem emerges, you narrow your differential field diagnosis to the most probable disease. For example, your patient has severe difficulty breathing and inspiratory stridor. Your differential field diagnosis might include foreign body obstruction, epiglottitis, respiratory burns, anaphylaxis, laryngeal trauma, and throat cancer. Then you learn that he is hoarse and febrile, has had a sore throat for 2 days, and in the past 6 hours has had increas-ing difficulty swallowing. You now suspect epiglottitis. This ability to formulate a working field diagnosis is essential for paramedics.

Sorting through the Ambiguities

You must be able to identify and deal with medical ambiguity. Many patients present with vague signs and symptoms. It is not unusual for a patient to complain of "just not feeling right." He will provide you with an imprecise story and you will be unable to arrive at a specific field diagnosis. In these cases, your field diagnosis will have to be generalized: "abdominal pain" or "general illness." Often it will be almost impossible to definitively determine the underlying problem without laboratory results, X-rays, and other tests.

You must be able to differentiate between relevant and irrelevant data. You will have to sift the important data from the many bits of information you receive during your patient assessment. A positive family history for sudden cardiac death is relevant for your patient with chest pain; for your patient with a fractured arm, it is not. Pupil and extraocular movement exams are relevant for trauma and for patients with an altered mental status; for a patient with asthma or arthritis, they are not. When you radio the medical direction physician, you will report critical information only. Likewise, in your written documentation you will record relevant information and omit the rest.

Recognizing Patterns

You must be able to analyze and compare similar and contrasting situations. What were the similarities among your last three stroke patients? Did all three have facial drooping, slurred speech, and unilateral paralysis? Did they all have a history of hypertension? Can you depend on any patterns of presentation for future calls such as this? Have some patient presentations been unusual? Have any patients presented with signs of stroke but ultimately had a different diagnosis? For example, your patient is a 45-year-old woman who presents with right-sided facial drooping. Your initial impression may be stroke, but further investigation reveals no other neurologic deficits. You now change your impression to Bell's palsy, caused by inflammation of the facial nerve (CN-VII). You must be able to recall the factors that help rule in or rule out a particular disease or injury.

Defending Your Decisions

You must be able to explain your decisions and construct logical arguments. Often, the emergency physician will want to know what you were thinking when you made your field diagnosis. You must be able to express yourself rationally while you make your case.

These are the times when you demonstrate your professionalism to other health care providers. Observe the following conversation:

Physician: Why did you think your patient had Bell's palsy and not a stroke? How can you rule out a stroke in the field?

Paramedic: Well, she had paralysis on the entire right side of her face, indicating a lesion of the seventh cranial nerve, rather than the lower facial paralysis of a stroke. All other neuro tests were negative.

Physician: OK, I agree, good job!

Through interactions such as this, you establish credibility with the emergency physician. The next time you contact him regarding a patient, he is more apt to trust your assessment and judgment.

Summary

Before you can treat your patient appropriately, you must thoroughly assess him to determine what the primary problem is. The patient's chief complaint will begin to lead you in the right direction—but remember, the chief complaint is only a symptom of the actual problem. Obtaining a comprehensive history and physical exam will provide you with the information necessary to begin a treatment regime.

Each situation is different and requires the paramedic to think critically and remain open-minded while progressing through the assessment. Remaining open-minded also means that you must ask open-ended questions and avoid leading questions. You want to hear what the patient has to say in his own words, not in words that were given to him through questioning.

As you progress through your career, you will develop a script for nearly all interactions with patients. This script will become like second nature for you and will help you to approach any assessment systematically. Inside the script you will have mnemonics and acronyms, such as SAMPLE or OPQRST–ASPN, to help you assess the patient thoroughly.

A thorough history can include everything from current events to family and social history. Obtaining a comprehensive history seems cumbersome and lengthy at first, but with practice come smooth transitions between lines of questioning, along with the ability to treat your patient as you are asking questions. Keep in mind, though, that the most important step you can perform is to document the answers to your questions as you receive them. This proves especially true in critical situations in which you are multitasking. You may remember to ask the patient a question but not stop long enough to hear the answer. Writing the patient's responses on a notepad—or even on your glove—helps you to acknowledge the response and record the information for the receiving facility.

You Make the Call

You respond to a skilled nursing facility for a patient with an altered mental status. You arrive to find an elderly woman being cared for by fire department personnel, and two nursing facility staff members standing nearby. You get a handoff report from a first responder, who tells you that the woman appears confused and has no immediate life threatening problems with airway, breathing, or circulation. As you approach, you see that the patient has bilateral hearing aids and appears to be speaking in short repetitive sentences. As you introduce yourself, the woman interrupts you and says "You'll have to speak up young man . . . I have trouble hearing!"

1. What potential challenges does this patient present with regard to history taking? List at least three, and describe your strategies for effectively overcoming these challenges.

See Suggested Responses at the back of this book.

Review Questions

1. When you couple the physical assessment findings with the patient's medical history, you are able to derive a list of _____
   a. clinical diagnostics.
   b. field prognoses
   c. chief complaints
   d. differential field diagnoses.

2. The pain, discomfort, or dysfunction that caused your patient to request help is known as the

   _____
   a. primary problem.
   b. nature of the illness.
   c. differential diagnosis.
   d. chief complaint.

3. You are assessing a patient who complains of cardiac-type chest pain that is felt in the jaw and down the left arm. This pattern of pain is known as

   _____
   a. sympathetic pain.
   b. tenderness.
   c. referred pain.
   d. associated pain.

4. Your patient has smoked 2 packs of cigarettes each day for the past 35 years. He is a _____ pack/year smoker.
   a. 35   c. 730
   b. 70   d. 25,550

5. The CAGE questionnaire is used as an evaluation tool to assess a patient with what type of history?
   a. Alcoholism   c. Allergies
   b. Lung disease   d. Pregnancy

6. What interviewing mnemonic should be used for each presenting problem a patient has?
   a. SAMPLE
   b. DCAP–BTLS
   c. OPQRST–ASPN
   d. AEIOU–TIPS

7. The mnemonic GPAL is used to evaluate a patient's

   _____
   a. alcoholism.
   b. allergies.
   c. pregnancy history.
   d. endocrine dysfunction.

Match the following elements of the present illness of the patient with a chief complaint of chest pain with their respective examples:

1. O   **a.** Pain is 6 on a scale of 1–10
2. P   **b.** Patient also complains of shortness of breath and nausea
3. Q   **c.** Pain had a sudden onset
4. R   **d.** Pain began 2 hours ago
5. S   **e.** Pain worsens while lying down
6. T   **f.** Patient denies dizziness
7. AS   **g.** Pain goes through to the back
8. PN   **h.** Pain is heavy and vise-like

See Answers to Review Questions at the back of this book.

References

1. *Expert 10-Minute Physical Exams.* 3rd ed. St. Louis: Mosby Lifeline, 1997.
2. *Assessment Made Incredibly Easy.* 5th ed. Springhouse, PA: Springhouse Corporation, 2008.
3. Id.
4. Seidel, H. M. *Mosby's Guide to Physical Examination.* 8th ed. St. Louis: Mosby, 2006.
5. Bates, B., L. S. Bickley, and R. A. Hoekelman. *A Guide to Physical Examination and History Taking.* 11th ed. Philadelphia: Lippincott Williams & Wilkins, 2005.
6. Epstein, O., et al. *Clinical Examination.* 3rd ed. St. Louis: Mosby, 2003.

Further Reading

Coulehan, J. L. and M. R. Block. *The Medical Interview: Mastering Skills for Clinical Practice*. 5th ed. Philadelphia: F.A. Davis, 2006.

Limmer, D. D., J. J. Mistovich, and W. S. Krost. *Beyond the Basics: The Art of Critical Thinking*. (Available at http://www.emsworld. com/print/EMS-World/Beyond-the-Basics–The-Art-of-Critical-Thinking- Part-1/1$7434. Accessed July 20, 2015.)

Lipkin, M., Jr., S. M. Putnam, and A. Lazare. *The Medical Interview: Clinical Care, Education, and Research*. New York: Springer, 1996.

Maggiore, W. A. "Escape Faulty Thinking: How to Minimize the Influence of Bias in Patient Assessment." *JEMS* 33 (2008): 117–125.

Silvestri, S., S. G. Rothrock, D. Kennedy, et al. "Can Paramedics Accurately Identify Patients Who Do Not Require Emergency Department Care?" *Prehosp Emerg Care* 6 (2002): 387–390.

Sullivan, D. L. and C. Chumbley. "Critical Thinking: A New Approach to Patient Care." *JEMS* 35(4) (2010): 48–53.

Willms, J. L., H. Schneiderman, and P. S. Algranati. *Physical Diagnosis: Bedside Evaluation of Diagnosis and Function*. Baltimore: Williams & Wilkins, 1994.

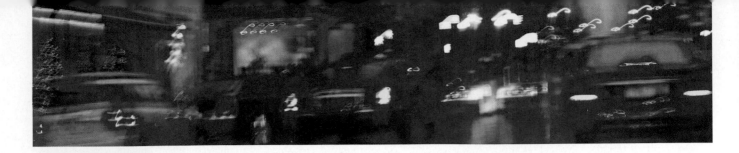

Chapter 5

Secondary Assessment

Richard A. Cherry, MS, EMT-P

STANDARD
Assessment

COMPETENCY
Integrate scene and patient assessment findings with knowledge of epidemiology and patho-physiology to form a field impression. This includes developing a list of differential diagnoses through clinical reasoning to modify the assessment and formulate a treatment plan.

 ## Learning Objectives

Terminal Performance Objective: After reading this chapter, you should be able to perform a secondary assessment suited to individual patients' needs.

Enabling Objectives: To accomplish the terminal performance objective, you should be able to:

1. Define key terms introduced in this chapter.

2. Briefly discuss the purpose and general approach to physical examination of the secondary assessment.

3. Identify and describe the physical assessment techniques of inspection, palpation, percussion, and auscultation to the physical examination process.

4. Interpret the findings obtained through inspection, palpation, percussion, and auscultation.

5. Discuss how to perform a general survey, to include assessing the patient's mental status, general appearance, and vital signs.

6. Describe how to use physical assessment techniques to identify and integrate findings from the anatomic region exam into the patient's primary and differential diagnosis.

7. Discuss alterations to the secondary assessment and physical exam techniques the paramedic should be aware of when caring for pediatric and geriatric age groups.

8. Identify the components of, and how to perform a reassessment according to the patient's age and condition.

9. Given a scenario, discuss strategies for completing the secondary assessment on a patient under the care of a paramedic.

KEY TERMS

Case Study

The overnight crew at Station 51 tonight consists of paramedic Matt Giffer and his EMT-Basic partner, Ron Arme. Early into their shift, they are called to a "man down" at Cirrincione's, a popular Italian restaurant featuring Sicilian cuisine. On arrival they find Robert Dalton, an agitated male in his early 70s who just can't seem to stand up. Mr. Dalton is alert and oriented. He complains of general weakness and of being unable to stand without wobbling or to walk a straight line.

Matt begins to elicit a history from Mr. Dalton's wife. She claims that he has been having these problems off and on for the past few days, but that this is worse. Mr. Dalton denies any chest pain, shortness of breath, dizziness, or nausea. His past history includes coronary artery disease, hypertension, and congestive heart failure. He takes nitroglycerin as needed, furosemide, aspirin, digoxin, and a potassium supplement. He and his wife have not yet eaten tonight. Matt tells his partner to get the stretcher and continues his assessment, which includes a focused physical exam and vital signs.

Because they have a 35-minute ride to McGivern General Hospital, Matt decides to perform a more detailed secondary assessment en route. His patient appears to be an otherwise healthy 72-year-old man. He is well dressed and well groomed. His vital signs are blood pressure, 150/86 mmHg; heart rate, 88, strong and regular; respirations, 18; skin: warm, dry, and pink. Matt finds no evidence of head trauma. His patient's ears, nose, and throat are normal. He shows no facial drooping or slurred speech. His pupils are equal and reactive to light and accommodation. Visual acuity is normal. Extraocular muscles are intact. Matt notes nystagmus with his patient's left lateral gaze. He finds no palpable nodes. His patient's trachea is midline, and his chest and abdomen appear normal. His distal extremities are warm and pink. Deep tendon reflexes are 21 in the upper extremities and 11 in the lower. His peripheral pulses are strong.

Matt decides to conduct a complete neurologic examination. His patient's mental status is normal. He is alert and oriented to person, place, and time. His responses are appropriate and timely, and he does not drift off the topic or lose interest. His posture is somewhat slumped, and he has trouble maintaining his balance when standing. He also complains of difficulty buttoning his shirt. He has no tremors or fasciculations. His facial expressions are appropriate for the situation. His speech is inflected, clear and strong, fluent and articulate, and he can vary his volume. He expresses his thoughts clearly and speaks spontaneously with a clear and distinct voice. His present state of uncoordinated movement and imbalance agitates him, yet he organizes his thoughts and speaks logically and coherently.

Satisfied that Mr. Dalton's mental status is normal, Matt continues with the motor function exam. Mr. Dalton's general posture is slumped to the left. He has no tremors except at the very end of fine motor movements. His overall muscle bulk, tone, and strength appear normal.

Matt then asks his patient to perform a series of tests aimed at evaluating coordination. First, he asks him to tap the distal joint of his thumb with the tip of his index finger as rapidly as possible. Next he asks him to place his hand palm up on his thigh, quickly turn it over, palm down, and then repeat this movement as rapidly as possible for 15 seconds. Mr. Dalton cannot perform these tests with his left hand. He cannot perform point-to-point testing on his left side, and he has tremors at the far point. Finally, he cannot perform the heel-to-shin movement on his left side.

Convinced that his patient is having a left cerebellar infarct, Matt contacts McGivern General Hospital and gives his report to Dr. Markum, a very impressed emergency physician. Computed tomography and magnetic resonance imaging results confirm Matt's report.

Customer Service Minute

Professional Respect. Have you ever responded to a physician's office for a patient in cardiac arrest, only to find no one doing anything? Have you ever been in a doctor's office with a COPD patient in severe respiratory distress and have the doctor order you to withhold oxygen? Have you ever responded to a nursing home for an unconscious patient only to find that the patient had been unresponsive since yesterday? If you have been in EMS for more than a week, you have surely encountered one of these typical scenarios. We often pick up patients at nursing homes, doctor's offices, and other health care clinics. Sometimes you find a critical patient, but not much has been done prior to your arrival.

Treat everyone with respect and be professional, no matter what happened before you got there. Understand the constraints of their system. They are probably not trained or equipped to manage patients with life-threatening emergencies. If they were, you might be out of a job. Just be nice and focus on your patient. After the call, offer to provide some in-service training aimed at working together to improve the care of your patients. Demonstrate your capabilities, explain your protocols, and help them help you in the future.

Introduction

The purpose of the secondary assessment is to conduct a focused physical examination to investigate areas that you suspect are involved in your patient's primary problem. During the secondary assessment, you will investigate the physical findings associated with major body systems, such as the cardiovascular, respiratory, and neurologic systems. You will also assess major anatomic regions, such as the eyes, ears, nose, and throat. Just as we covered the entire history in the "History Taking" chapter, we present the entire physical exam in this one.

Again, if you practice in a setting other than a prehospital one, such as conducting preemployment physicals for a company, you might perform the entire physical examination outlined here. On an emergency run, however, you limit the exam to only the aspects that you decide are appropriate. In the chapter "Patient Assessment in the Field," we discuss how to tailor your exam to the situation and provide some examples.

The General Approach

How you approach your patient—both in the emergency setting and elsewhere—will set the stage for an efficient and effective patient assessment. Most patients are apprehensive about a physical examination. They feel exposed and vulnerable, and they fear painful procedures. This anxiety is multiplied in an emergency. You must recognize your patient's apprehension and take steps to alleviate it. Display confidence and skill while you complete your history and physical exam.

If you assess your patient's complaints systematically and perform your duties efficiently, he should feel safe. Then add the personal touches of active listening, a reassuring voice, and gestures that convey your sincere compassion and interest. Most patients will respond favorably. Let your patient know that you are not just checking off items on a diagnostic list; you are conducting a personal examination of his problems.

When we do something repetitively, we tend to develop patterns. This is true with physical exams. You should establish a personal system or order in which you assess patients. Following your own personal system or pattern will help ensure that you do not leave out part of

Cultural Considerations

The physical exam process often includes viewing parts of the body that are generally shielded from the view of strangers. Because of this, some patients may be particularly sensitive about revealing various aspects of the body to a stranger—even a paramedic. The way in which you approach a patient for physical assessment must take into consideration the patient's cultural beliefs or customs.

In some cultures, especially certain Arab cultures, it is forbidden for a woman to reveal her face or body to a man who is not her husband. This constraint certainly makes a detailed physical exam difficult. Sometimes, in fact, an examination cannot be completed because of patient refusal. In some instances, an examination may be allowed only if the examiner is of the same gender as the patient. Likewise, seemingly innocent comments by rescuers—such as "You have a pretty face. Let me take a look at your head"—can be insulting or offensive. It implies that flattery can convince these patients to consent to something that is not allowed by their culture or religion, or both.

If you work in an area where there is considerable cultural diversity, it is important to understand the cultural beliefs and practices of the groups you may encounter. More important, you must respect these beliefs and customs. In turn, the patients will respect you.

the exam. In fact, having a system or established pattern is often a medical–legal defense. If you document that you always perform your physical exam the same way, it shows a jury or judge that there is less of a chance that you missed something during your assessment.

This is not to say, however, that you should never modify your exam. Everyone modifies the exam for children and special situations. Even then, though, you tend to develop a subroutine that you follow. Again, such a system ensures that an important part of the physical examination is not missed.

Proficiency will come only with clinical practice. In time, you will become adept at focusing the exam on your patient's chief complaint and present illness. In the emergency setting, no matter how nervous and apprehensive you may be, never let your patient see anything but a calm, professional, confident demeanor. This will help alleviate his anxiety about disclosing personal information to, and being examined by, a nonphysician.

Try to remain objective, even when confronted by alarming or disgusting information. A bad bedsore, a perverted sexual story, or a foul-smelling gastrointestinal discharge can test even the most experienced clinician's composure. Simply thinking about how embarrassed your patient must be may help you keep your own poise.

Practice and clinical experience will dictate your ability to apply the skills you learn in this chapter to real situations. The techniques you use will vary from patient to patient depending on the history, your patient's stability, his ability to communicate, and the potential for unrecognized illness.

Physical Exam Techniques

Four techniques—inspection, palpation, percussion, and auscultation—are the foundation of the formal physical exam.[1] Each can reveal information essential to a comprehensive patient assessment.

Inspection

Inspection is the process of informed observation (Figure 5-1). A simple, noninvasive technique that clinicians often take for granted, it is also one of their most valuable tools in appraising patient condition. With a keen eye, you can evaluate your patient's condition in great detail.

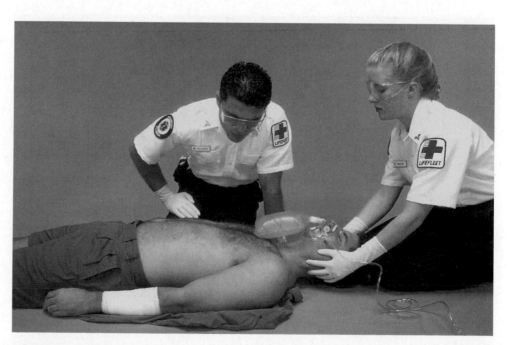

FIGURE 5-1 Inspect your patient's body for signs of injury or illness.

Inspection begins when you first meet your patient and continues while you take his history. Often, this first impression forms the basis for your history, because you will judge your patient's clinical status immediately. Notice how he presents himself. Is he conscious and alert or unconscious and flaccid? Is he lying on the floor, sitting upright, or limping badly on one foot? Is he breathing normally or gasping for each breath? You can learn a great deal about your patient's neurologic, musculoskeletal, and respiratory systems just by careful observation. Watch for changes in his emotional and mental status throughout the history and physical exam.

During the formal physical exam, consciously evaluate each body area, looking for discoloration, unusual motion, or deformity. Pay special attention to areas in which you most expect to find signs and where the patient complains of symptoms. For example, if your patient struck his chest against a bent steering wheel, you would expect to see chest wall abnormalities. Remember that you may not notice the skin color changes that follow a significant contusion until after your patient arrives at the emergency department.

Effective inspection depends on good lighting, adequate time, and a curiosity for looking beyond the obvious. During your inspection, draw on your past clinical experiences to identify the signs of illness and injury. Knowing what you are looking for is essential. Do not hurry. Give yourself enough time to inspect and then to process what you see. Inspection is an ongoing process that should not end until you transfer your patient to emergency department staff. Finally, although you must respect your patient's modesty and dignity, never allow clothing to obstruct your examination.

Palpation

Palpation is usually the next step in assessing your patient, although sometimes you will inspect and palpate your patient simultaneously. Palpation involves using your sense of touch to gather information. With your hands and fingers, you can determine a structure's size, shape, and position. You also can evaluate its temperature, moisture, texture, and movement. You can check for growths, swelling, tenderness, spasms, rigidity, pain, and crepitus. When you become skilled at this procedure, you can detect a distended bladder, an enlarged liver, a laterally pulsating abdominal aorta, or the position of a fetus.

Certain parts of your hands and fingers are better than others for specific types of palpation. For example, the pads of your fingers are more sensitive than the tips for detecting position, size, consistency, masses, fluid, and crepitus; therefore, you would use them to palpate lymph nodes or rib fractures (Figure 5-2).[2] The palm of your hand is better for sensing vibrations such as fremitus. Because its skin is thinner and more sensitive, the back of your hand or fingers is better for evaluating temperature.

Palpation may be either deep or light. You control its depth by applying pressure with your hand and fingers. Because deep palpation may elicit tenderness or disrupt tissue or fluid, you should always perform light palpation first. Use light palpation to assess the skin and superficial structures. Press in approximately 1 centimeter. Apply the same gentle pressure you use to feel a pulse. Too much pressure dulls your sensitivity and can injure your patient.

To assess visceral organs, such as those in the abdomen, use deep palpation. Apply pressure by placing the fingers of the opposite hand over the sensing fingers and gently pressing in about 4 centimeters. This will increase your sensitivity to any masses, guarding, or other abdominal pathology. Feel for areas of warmth that might reflect injury before significant edema or discoloration occur. Observe how your patient responds with facial expressions while you palpate tender areas. Even if he is unconscious, he may respond to pain with facial expressions or purposeful (pulling or pushing away) or purposeless (abnormal posturing) motion.

Palpation begins the hands-on portion of the physical assessment of your patient. Three commonsense tips will help make it therapeutic and respectful:

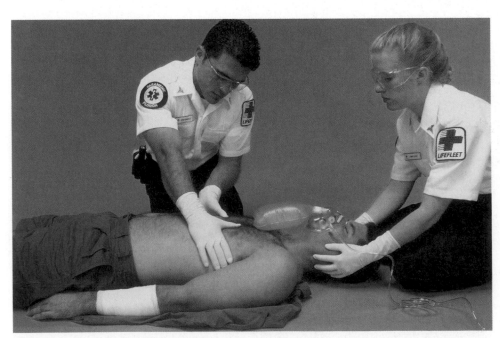

FIGURE 5-2 Palpate with the pads of your fingers to detect masses, fluids, and crepitus.

Keep your hands warm, keep your fingernails short, and be gentle to avoid discomfort or injury to your patient.

Percussion

Percussion is the production of sound waves by striking one object against another. In this technique, you strike a knuckle on one hand with the tip of a finger on the opposite hand. The impact causes vibrations that produce sound waves from 4 to 6 centimeters deep in the underlying body tissue. We hear these sound waves as percussion tones. The density of the tissue through which the sound must travel determines the degree of percussion. The denser the medium, the quieter the tone. The tone's resonance or lack of resonance indicates whether the underlying region is filled with air, air under pressure, fluid, or normal tissue. Listen to each sound and evaluate its meaning (Table 5-1).

Move across the area that you are percussing and compare the sounds with what you know to be normal there. For example, in the chest you expect to hear the resonant sound of a healthy lung filled with air and tissue. In a pneumothorax or emphysema, however, you may hear the hyperresonant sound of air trapped in the chest. In a hemothorax, you may hear the dull sound of blood in the same area.

There are three basic types of percussion: direct, indirect, and blunt. Direct percussion involves tapping directly on your patient's skin with your fingertip. You simply tap sharply and release your finger immediately. This method is best used when percussing your patient's frontal and maxillary sinuses.

The second and most often used method is indirect percussion. Place one hand on the area of the body you wish to percuss. Use a finger of that hand (usually the middle finger) as the striking surface. Sharply tap the distal knuckle of that finger with the tip of your other middle finger (Figure 5-3). The tap should come from snapping the wrist, not the forearm or shoulder. Snap the finger back quickly to avoid dampening the sound. When percussing the chest, make sure the finger lies between the ribs and parallel to them. In this way, you will percuss the tissue underneath the ribs, not the ribs themselves.

The third type of percussion is the blunt method, best used for detecting pain and inflammation. You simply

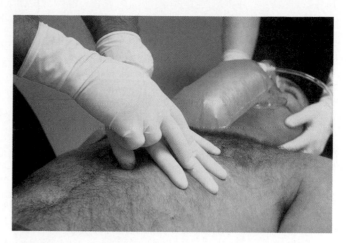

FIGURE 5-3 Percuss your patient to evaluate vibrations and sounds.

strike your patient's skin with the ulnar side of your fist with just enough force to elicit tenderness but not cause undue pain. This is often used in the costovertebral angle when examining a patient for a kidney infection.

A wall in your home is a good place to practice your percussion skills. As you percuss the air-filled area between wall studs, you will hear a hollow, resonant sound. Wall spaces filled with insulation will sound less resonant. When you percuss over a wall stud, you will notice a flatter, dull sound. You can apply this principle to the percussion of body cavities. Compare the sounds on the affected side with those on the unaffected side. The key is knowing what is normal, so above all you must practice percussion on healthy people in order to recognize abnormalities in sick or injured patients.

Unfortunately, at most emergency scenes, especially those in the street, noise prevents percussing your patient effectively. Your clinical experience and common sense will tell you when to use this valuable assessment technique.

Auscultation

Auscultation involves listening for sounds produced by the body, primarily the lungs, the heart, the intestines, and major blood vessels. It is difficult to master. You may hear some sounds clearly, such as stridor, the high-pitched squeal of a partially obstructed upper airway.

Table 5-1 Percussion Sounds

Sound	Description	Intensity	Pitch	Duration	Location
Tympany	Drumlike	Loud	High	Medium	Stomach
Hyperresonance	Booming	Loud	Low	Long	Hyperinflated lung
Resonance	Hollow	Loud	Low	Long	Normal lung
Dull	Thud	Medium	Medium	Medium	Solid organs
Flat	Extremely dull	Soft	High	Short	Muscle, atelectasis

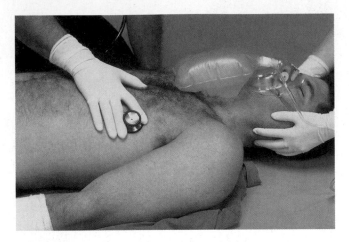

FIGURE 5-4 Auscultate body sounds with the stethoscope.

Most, however, require a stethoscope. You should perform auscultation in a quiet environment. Unfortunately, this is not always practical in emergency services. Hearing the low-amplitude heart and lung sounds against on-scene noise or in-transit background noise may be especially difficult.

To auscultate, hold the endpiece of your stethoscope between your second and third fingers and press the diaphragm firmly against your patient's skin (Figure 5-4). If you are using the bell side, place it evenly and lightly on the skin. Avoid touching the tubing with your hands or allowing it to rub any surfaces. Make sure the earpieces point anteriorly before you put them in your ears.

Listen for the presence of sound and its intensity, pitch, duration, and quality. When reporting and recording lung sounds, always note abnormal sounds (crackles, wheezes), their locations (bilateral, right lower lobe, bases), and their timing during the respiratory cycle (inspiratory, end-expiratory). Sometimes, closing your eyes helps you concentrate on the sounds by eliminating visual stimuli. Try to isolate and concentrate on one sound at a time.

Generally, auscultate after you have used other assessment techniques. The only exception is the abdomen, which you should auscultate before palpation and percussion because those procedures can alter peristalsis. A paramedic should be proficient in auscultating blood pressure, lung sounds, heart sounds, bowel sounds, and arterial

In the Field

The Tools of Your Trade: *The Stethoscope*

The **stethoscope** is a basic paramedic tool used to auscultate most sounds (Figure 5-5). It transmits sound waves from the source through an endpiece and along rubber tubes to the ear. One side of the endpiece is a rigid diaphragm that best transmits high-pitched sounds, such as heart sounds and blood pressure sounds. The diaphragm also screens out low-pitched sounds, such as lung sounds and bowel sounds.

The other side of the endpiece is a bell that uses the skin as a diaphragm. The sounds that the bell transmits vary with the amount of pressure exerted. For example, with light pressure, the bell picks up low-pitched sounds; with firm pressure, it acts as a diaphragm and transmits high-pitched sounds.[3] Whether you use the bell or the diaphragm depends on which sounds you are auscultating. To hear blood pressure or heart sounds, for instance, use the diaphragm; to hear lung or bowel sounds, use the bell side.

Accurate auscultation depends in part on the quality of your instrument. Your stethoscope should have the following important characteristics:

- A rigid diaphragm cover
- Thick, heavy tubing that conducts sound better than thin, flexible tubing
- Short tubing (30 to 40 cm) to minimize distortion
- Earpieces that fit snugly—large enough to occlude the ear canal—and are angled toward the nose to project sound toward the eardrum
- A bell with a rubber-ring edge to ensure good contact with the skin

For your patient's comfort, warm the endpiece of your stethoscope with your hands before auscultating.

Electronic stethoscopes are becoming more popular because they digitally enhance body sounds in the noisy prehospital setting. Although manufacturers use a variety of techniques, basically they all convert acoustic sound waves to electrical signals, amplify them, and process them for optimal listening. Because the sounds are transmitted electronically, an electronic stethoscope can be a wireless device, can be a recording device, and can provide noise reduction, signal enhancement, and both visual and audio output.

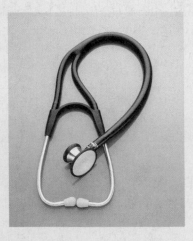

FIGURE 5-5 Use a stethoscope to auscultate most sounds.

Pediatric Pearls

Conducting a physical examination of a sick or injured child can challenge any clinician. Your success will depend on several factors. First, you must be familiar with the anatomic differences between children and adults. Second, you must understand the physical and psychological developmental stages of the different age groups. Most important, you must practice these skills daily.

Children are not just small adults, and you cannot treat them as if they were. Children are naturally apprehensive of strangers and new things. A sick or injured child is a frightened child. He fears pain, separation from his family, and unfamiliar surroundings. Dealing with these fears paves the way for a successful encounter with the child and his parents. You are a stranger. In uniform, you become even more ominous. Gaining your pediatric patient's trust becomes a vital part of your assessment. Unless he requires emergency critical care, take time to establish a rapport with him. This will help to ensure continuous cooperation (Figure 5-6).

Although different age groups have specific fears and characteristics, the following general rules apply to pediatrics as a whole: Remain calm and confident. Be direct and honest about what you are doing, especially if you are performing a painful procedure. If possible, do not separate the child from his parents. Instead, elicit their help in obtaining the history and allow them to help hold the child while you conduct your exam.

The more invasive the procedure, the later in the exam you should perform it—unless, of course, your patient is critically ill or injured. (Never delay important procedures or techniques on

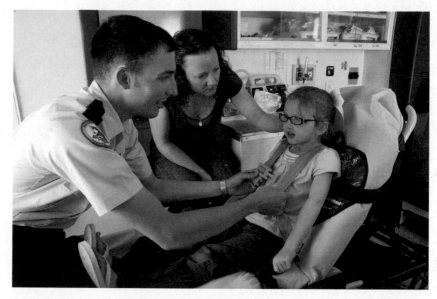

FIGURE 5-6 Have parents nearby or have them hold young children while you examine them.

the critically ill or injured child.) If your patient begins crying and carrying on, the more difficult, if not impossible, the rest of your exam will be. Finally, provide continuous reassurance and feedback to your patient and his family members. This helps reduce everyone's anxiety over what is wrong, what you are doing, and what comes next.

Position yourself at the child's eye level, use a soft voice, and smile a lot. Often a small toy, such as a teddy bear, can distract your patient while you examine him. If you are using diagnostic equipment, allow the child to handle it while you explain how it works. Make sure your movements are slow and deliberate, and explain everything you are doing.

bruits. As with any other physical assessment tool, you cannot detect abnormalities unless you know what is normal. Take every opportunity to auscultate lung, heart, arterial, and bowel sounds regularly.

The General Survey

A general survey is the first part of a comprehensive physical exam. It begins with noting your patient's mental status, his general appearance, and his vital signs.

Mental Status

Level of Consciousness

First, assess your patient's level of response.[4] Is he alert and awake? Does he understand your questions? Are his responses appropriate and timely, or does he drift off the topic easily or lose interest? If you detect an abnormality, continue with more specific questions. Is he drowsy, but does he answer questions appropriately before falling

asleep again? Does he open his eyes and look at you but give slow, confused responses? Sometimes you must arouse your patient repeatedly by gently shaking him or shouting his name. If he does not respond to your verbal cues, assess him with painful stimuli. Is he arousable for short periods but not aware of his surroundings, or is he unconscious and totally unarousable?

If your patient is not apparently awake, speak to him in a loud voice. If he does not respond to your verbal cues, shake him gently. If he still does not respond, apply a painful stimulus, such as pinching a tendon, rubbing his sternum, or rolling a pencil across a nail bed. Note and document his response. Use the AVPU scale as in the primary assessment.

Appearance and Behavior

If your patient is awake and alert, observe his posture and motor behavior. Does he lie in bed or prefer to walk around? His posture should be erect and he should look at you. A slumped posture and a lack of facial expression may indicate depression. Excessive energetic movements or constantly

Table 5-2 Posture and Behavior

Motor Activity	Suggested Meaning
Tense posture, restlessness, fidgeting	Anxiety
Crying, hand-wringing, pacing	Agitation, depression
Hopeless, slumped posture, slowed movements	Depression
Singing, dancing, expansive movements	Mania

watchful eyes suggest tension, anxiety, or a metabolic disorder. Watch the pace, range, and character of his movements. Are they voluntary? Are any parts immobile? Do his posture and motor activity change with the environment? Some possible findings are listed in Table 5-2.

Observe your patient's grooming and personal hygiene. How is he dressed? Are his clothes clean, pressed, and properly fastened? Is his appearance appropriate for the season, climate, and occasion? Poor grooming and personal hygiene in the previously well-groomed person may suggest an emotional problem, a psychiatric disorder, or an organic brain disease. Patients with obsessive–compulsive behavior, on the other hand, may exhibit excessive attention to their appearance. Note your patient's hair, teeth, nails, skin, and beard. Are they well groomed? Compare one side with the other. One-sided neglect may suggest a brain lesion.

In addition, observe your patient's facial expressions. Are they appropriate? Do they vary when he talks with others and when the topic changes, or is his face immobile throughout the interaction? Can he express happiness, sad-

Pediatric Pearls

Evaluate the child's general appearance and behavior. Ask the parents whether his behavior seems normal. Observe his body position and muscle tone, keeping in mind the normal physical and psychological developmental stages of children. Ask yourself two questions: Does your patient look and act like a normal child in the same age group? Do his actions appear normal to you and to his parents? It is best to leave children in a parent's arms or have the parent nearby while you examine them (Figure 5-6).

Infants (Newborn–1 Year). In the newborn or young infant, the arms and legs will flex slightly and move equally (Figure 5-7). Infants recognize their parents' faces and voices at about 2 months. They are normally alert and like to look around. They also like to be held and kept warm. They are frightened by loud noises and bright lights and may be soothed by having something to suck on. They are somewhat easy to assess because they are not very strong. At 4 to 6 months, they begin to sit up,

and they can do so without assistance by 8 months. They are easily distracted by a toy or shiny object. They are very distressed by separation from their parents. Because they will not understand what you are doing or why you are there, they probably will resist being examined. It is best to examine any child under the age of 1 from toe to head.

Toddlers (1–3 Years). Toddlers should be able to walk by their 18th month (Figure 5-8). They love to disagree with everyone and everything, and they trust no one but their parents. They are the most difficult age group to examine, even when they are not sick or hurt. They do not want you to touch them, so be prepared

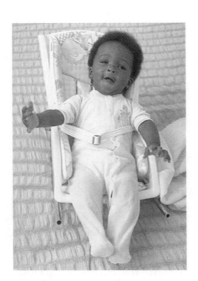

FIGURE 5-7 Infant (newborn–1 year).

(© Michal Heron)

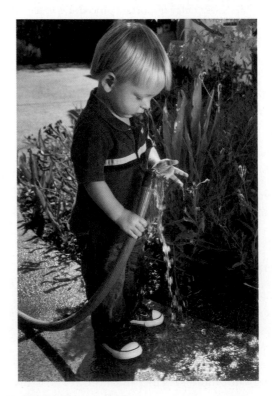

FIGURE 5-8 Toddler (1–3 years).

to take opportunities to assess areas as they become available. You may want to limit your assessment of the very ill or injured toddler to the most important areas. For example, focus on the chest and lungs of any child in respiratory distress. Do the vital areas first, before the child becomes agitated and makes the rest of your exam nearly impossible. Toddlers do like to be distracted with toys; if possible, make a game of the examination. In addition, because toddlers are beginning to sense their dignity, always respect their modesty.

Preschoolers (3–6 Years). Preschoolers (Figure 5-9) are particularly distrusting of strangers. Talk with them, gain their trust, and answer their questions honestly. Always prepare them if something you are going to do may hurt. Tell them it may hurt and that it's all right to cry. They have a great fear of being hurt and of the sight of their own blood. They fear mutilation of their bodies, and the slightest injury may result in a temporarily hysterical child. Always cover a preschooler's wounds quickly, so he won't have to look at them. Often, injured or sick children in this age group feel guilty about their problem, as if it is their fault, regardless of the circumstances. Approach them slowly and offer a calming reassurance that they will be all right.

School-Age (6–12 Years). School-age children (Figure 5-10) will cooperate with you if you gain their trust. They want to participate and to remain somewhat in control. Allow them to participate in the exam and to make treatment choices whenever possible. They have a basic understanding of their bodies, but they still fear separation, pain, and punishment. Modesty becomes more important, and they will not like being examined. Talk honestly with them about what you are doing and prepare them for what will come next as you proceed.

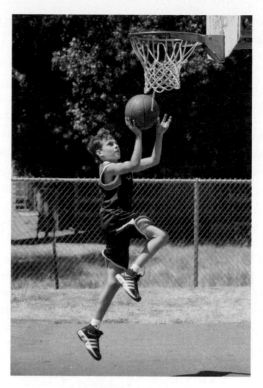

FIGURE 5-10 School-age child (6–12 years).

Adolescents (13–18 Years). Adolescents (Figure 5-11) can be treated much the same as adults. Because a teenager's modesty is extremely important, have a person of the same sex examine this patient, if possible. Otherwise, conduct the physical exam just as you would for an adult patient.

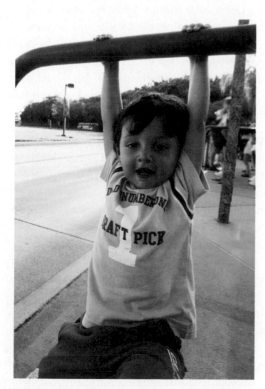

FIGURE 5-9 Preschooler (3–6 years).

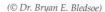
(© Dr. Bryan E. Bledsoe)

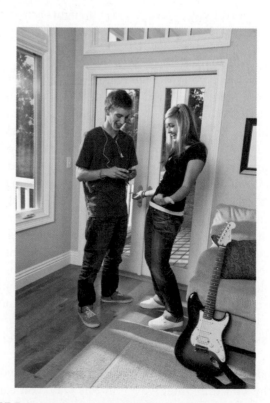

FIGURE 5-11 Adolescent (13–18 years).

ness, anger, or depression? Patients with Parkinson's disease have facial immobility, a masklike appearance.

Speech and Language

Note your patient's speech pattern. Normally, a person's speech is inflected, clear, strong, fluent, and articulate, and varies in volume. It should express thoughts clearly. Is your patient excessively talkative or silent? Does he speak spontaneously, or only when you ask him a direct question? Is his speech slow and quiet, as in depression? Is it fast and loud, as in a manic episode? Does he speak clearly and distinctly? Does he have **dysarthria** (defective speech caused by motor deficits), **dysphonia** (voice changes caused by vocal cord problems), or **aphasia** (defective language caused by neurologic damage to the brain)? With expressive aphasia, his words will be garbled; with receptive aphasia, his words will be clear but unrelated to your questions. Your patient with aphasia may have such difficulty talking that you mistakenly suspect a psychotic disorder.

Mood

Observe your patient's verbal and nonverbal behavior for clues to his mood. Note any mood swings or behaviors that suggest anxiety or depression. Is he sad, elated, angry, enraged, anxious, worried, detached, or indifferent? Assess the intensity of your patient's mood. How long has he been this way? Is his behavior normal for the circumstances? For example, anxiety is normal for someone having a heart attack; if your heart attack patient did not act frightened and concerned, that would be abnormal. If your patient is depressed, is he suicidal? If you suspect the possibility of suicide, ask him directly, "Have you ever thought of committing suicide? Are you currently thinking of committing suicide?"

Thoughts and Perceptions

Assess how well your patient organizes his thoughts when he speaks. Is he logical and coherent? Does he shift from one topic to an unrelated topic without realizing that the thoughts are not connected? These "loose associations" are typical in schizophrenia, manic episodes, and other psychiatric disorders. Does he speak constantly in related areas with no real conclusion or end point? Such "flight of ideas" is most often associated with mania. Does he ramble with unrelated, illogical thoughts and disordered grammar? You may see this "incoherence" in severe psychosis. Does he make up facts or events in response to questions? You may see this "confabulation" in amnesia. Does he suddenly lose his train of thought and stop in mid-sentence before completing an idea? Such blocking occurs in normal people but is pronounced in schizophrenia.

Assess the thought content of your patient's responses as they occur during the interview; for example, "You said you thought you were allergic to your mother. Can you tell me why you think that way?" In this way, you can ask about your patient's unpleasant or unusual comments.

Allow him the freedom to explore these thoughts with you. Is your patient driven to try to prevent some unrealistic future result (compulsion)? Does he have a recurrent, uncontrollable feeling of dread and doom (obsession)? Does he sense that things in the environment are strange or unreal (feelings of unreality)? Does he have false personal beliefs that other members of his group do not share (delusions)? Compulsions and obsessions are neurotic disorders, whereas delusions and feelings of unreality are psychotic disorders.

Determine whether your patient perceives imaginary things. Does he see visions, hear voices, smell odors, or feel things that are not there? Ask him about these false perceptions just as you would ask about anything else. For example, ask "When you see the pink elephants, what are they doing?" Decide whether your patient is misinterpreting what is real (illusions) or seeing things that are not real (hallucinations). Both illusions and hallucinations may occur in schizophrenia, posttraumatic stress disorders, and organic brain syndrome. Auditory and visual hallucinations are common in psychedelic drug ingestion, whereas tactile hallucinations suggest alcohol withdrawal.

Insight and Judgment

During the interview, you will most likely evaluate your patient's insight and judgment. Does he understand what is happening to him? Does he realize that what he thinks and how he feels are part of the illness? Patients with psychotic disorders may not have insight into their illness. Judgment refers to your patient's ability to reason appropriately. Does your mature patient respond appropriately to questions concerning his family and personal life? Ask him what he would do if he cut himself shaving. Proper judgment means that your patient can evaluate the data and provide an adequate response. Impaired judgment is common in emotional problems, mental retardation, and organic brain syndrome.

Memory and Attention

Assess your patient's orientation. Does he know his name? Person disorientation suggests trauma, seizures, or amnesia. Does he know the time of day, day of the week, month, season, and year? Time disorientation may suggest anxiety, depression, or organic brain syndrome. Does he know where he is, where he lives, the name of the city and state? Place disorientation suggests a psychiatric disorder or organic brain syndrome. Your patient should be oriented to person, time, and place and respond appropriately to your questions.

To assess your patient's ability to concentrate, use the following three exercises. First, have him repeat a series of numbers back to you (digit span). Normally, a person can repeat at least five numbers forward and backward. Then, ask him to start from 100 and subtract seven each time (serial sevens). A normal person can complete this in 90 seconds with fewer than four errors. Finally, ask your patient to spell a common five-letter word backward (spelling backward). Poor performance in these tests may suggest delirium, dementia, mental retardation, loss of calculating ability, anxiety, multiple sclerosis, fibromyalgia, fetal alcohol syndrome, previous brain injury, medication toxicity, or depression. Obviously, in these cases you're not going to make a definitive diagnosis. Your job is to assess and report the findings.

Memory can be divided into three grades: immediate, recent, and remote. First, test your patient's immediate memory. Ask him to repeat three or four words that have no correlation, such as desk, toothbrush, six, and blue. This tests immediate recall and is similar to digit span. Next, test your patient's recent memory by asking him what he had for lunch or to repeat something he told you earlier in the interview. Make sure the information you ask for is verifiable. Finally, test for remote memory by asking about facts such as his wife's name, son's birthday, or his Social Security number. Ask him to describe the house in which he grew up or the schools he attended. Long-term and short-term memory problems may be due to amnesia, anxiety, or organic causes.

Finally, test your patient's ability to learn new things. Give him the names of three or four items, such as man, chair, grass, and hot dog. Ask him to repeat them. This tests registration and immediate recall. About 5 minutes later, ask him to repeat them. Normally, he will be able to name all four. Note his accuracy, his awareness of whether he is correct, or whether he tries to confabulate by making up new words.

General Appearance

A thorough evaluation of your patient's appearance can provide a great deal of valuable information about his health. Note his level of consciousness, posture, and any obvious signs of distress, such as sitting upright gasping for each breath or slumped to one side. Is his motor activity normal, or does he have noticeable tremors or paralysis? Observe his general state of health, dress, grooming, and personal hygiene. Obvious odors can also provide significant information.

Signs of Distress
Is your patient in distress? For example, does he have a cardiac or respiratory problem, as evidenced by labored breathing, wheezing, or a cough? Is he in pain, as evidenced by wincing, sweating, or protecting the painful area? Is he anxious, as evidenced by his facial expression, cold moist palms, or nervous fidgeting?

Apparent State of Health
Is your patient healthy, robust, and vigorous? Or is he frail, ill looking, or feeble? Does he have an obvious abnormality? Base your evaluation of his general state of health on

your observations throughout the interview and physical examination.

Vital Statistics
Vital statistics—weight and height—are used widely in clinical medicine. Accurately measuring your patient's weight and height with a scale, however, is not a practical prehospital assessment procedure. You will occasionally estimate your patient's weight to administer medications for which the dose is weight dependent. You also may use a **Broselow tape** to measure your infant patient's length. The Broselow tape provides information concerning drug dosages, airway management adjuncts, and intravenous calculations based on your patient's height.

General Stature
Is your patient lanky and slender, short and stocky, muscular and symmetrical? Does he have any obvious deformities or disproportionate areas? Is he extremely thin or obese? If he is obese, is the fat evenly distributed or is it concentrated in his trunk? Has he gained or lost weight recently?

Sexual Development
Is your patient's sexual maturity appropriate for his or her age and gender? Consider such indicators as voice, facial and body hair, and breast size.

Skin Color and Obvious Lesions
Is your patient's skin pale, suggesting decreased blood flow or anemia? Does he have central (lips, oral mucosa) or peripheral (nail beds, hands) cyanosis, the bluish color resulting from decreased oxygenation of the tissues? Does he have the yellow color of jaundice or high carotene levels? Note any rashes, bruises, scars, or discoloration.

Posture, Gait, and Motor Activity
Observe your patient's posture and presentation. Is he sitting straight up and forward, bracing his arms (tripoding)? This suggests a serious breathing problem, such as acute pulmonary edema or airway obstruction. Does one side of his body droop and seem immobile, suggesting a stroke? Does he sit quietly or does he seem restless? Does he have tremors or other involuntary movements?

Dress, Grooming, and Personal Hygiene
Does your patient dress appropriately for the climate and situation? Are his clothes clean and properly fastened? Are they conventional for his age and social group? Abnormalities in dress might suggest the cold intolerance of hypothyroidism or the hiding of a skin rash or needle marks, or they might simply reflect personal or cultural preference. Look at his shoes. Are they clean? Do they have holes, slits, open laces, or other alterations to accommodate painful foot conditions, such as gout, bunions, or edema? Does he wear a slipper, or slippers, instead of shoes? Is he wearing unusual jewelry, such as a copper bracelet for arthritis or a medical

Table 5-3 Identifying Odors

Odor	Possible Causes
Urine or ammonia	Dehydration, incontinence, urinary tract infection
Fruity breath	Diabetic ketoacidosis
Bitter almonds on breath	Cyanide poisoning
Bad breath	Throat infection, dental problems, poor hygiene
Body odor	Infection, poor hygiene
Fishy vaginal odor	Infection
Fecal breath	Bowel obstruction

information tag? Do his grooming and hygiene seem appropriate for his age, lifestyle, occupation, and social status? Does his lack of concern over appearance (overgrown nails and hair, for instance) suggest a long illness or depression?

Breath or Body Odors

Does your patient have any unusual or striking breath or body odors? The acetone breath of a diabetic, the bitter-almond breath of cyanide poisoning, the putrid smell of bacterial infection, or the obvious smell of alcohol may give important clues to the underlying problem. Avoid tunnel vision when you smell alcohol, which often masks other serious illnesses such as liver failure or injuries such as a subdural hematoma. Table 5-3 lists some common odors encountered in the field.

Facial Expressions

Watch your patient's facial expressions throughout your interaction. His face should reflect his emotions during the interview and physical exam. The patient with hyperthyroidism may stare intently. The Parkinson's patient's face may appear immobile.

Vital Signs

Taking your patient's vital signs provides a baseline measurement of his respiratory, circulatory, and perfusion sta-

Pediatric Pearls

Especially in the emergency setting, note whether your pediatric patient looks toxic, or sick. A toxic child appears not to recognize or respond to his parents. He may look tired and have a decreased respiratory effort, and may have mottled skin or a generalized rash. He may be gray or cyanotic and just look very sick, usually from some type of bacterial process. These children, who present with the signs and symptoms of respiratory failure or shock, usually require rapid transport while you provide aggressive resuscitation procedures (advanced airway management, oxygenation and ventilation, intravenous access, and rapid fluid administration).

tus. These measurements are the primary indicators of your patient's health. Measure them early in the physical examination and, in emergency situations, repeat them often and look for trends. For example, in a serious head injury, watch for your patient's systolic blood pressure to rise, his pulse pressure to widen, and his pulse rate to fall. These trends suggest an increase in intracranial pressure, a serious medical emergency. Conversely, a falling blood pressure with an increasing pulse rate may indicate shock.

As a paramedic, you should become an expert at taking vital signs on patients of every age. Let us look at the methods we use to measure our patient's respiration, circulation, and perfusion.

Respiration

Because oxygen and carbon dioxide exchange is essential to sustain life, **respiration** must occur continuously and must be effective. The lungs supply the arteries with oxygen and maintain the blood's pH by eliminating or retaining carbon dioxide. These two functions occur during respiration. Continuously observe your patient's respiratory rate, effort, and quality. Look for subtle signs of distress. Recognize when your patient requires rapid intervention, such as aggressive airway management, positive pressure ventilation, and oxygenation. These interventions often will make the difference between life and death.

Your patient's **respiratory rate** is the number of times he breathes in 1 minute. In general, the normal respiratory rate for a healthy adult at rest is 12 to 18 breaths per minute.[5] Rapid breathing (**tachypnea**) can be the result of hypoxia, shock, head injury, or anxiety. Slow breathing (**bradypnea**) can be caused by drug overdose, severe hypoxia, or central nervous system insult. Very rapid or very slow breathing rates require rapid intervention to ensure that the adequate exchange of gases continues. The importance of accurately obtaining and recording the respiratory rate cannot be over-emphasized. Never "guesstimate."

A change in respiratory rate is often the first physical exam finding you will observe with an emergency condition. People involuntarily change their respiratory rate when they know it is being measured. Thus, if they are aware that you are measuring the respiratory rate, you will end up with an inaccurate reading. To avoid this, you must distract or mislead the patient. Make the patient think you are still measuring his pulse rate. Place your hand on his wrist and measure the pulse rate for 15 to 30 seconds. After you have determined the pulse rate, leave your hand in place and then measure the respiratory rate for at least 30 seconds (Procedure 5-1a). This should give you an accurate measurement.

Your patient's **respiratory effort** indicates how hard he works to breathe. Normal inhalation involves using the respiratory muscles (diaphragm and intercostals) to increase the chest's inner diameter. It is an active process

Procedure 5-1 Taking Vital Signs

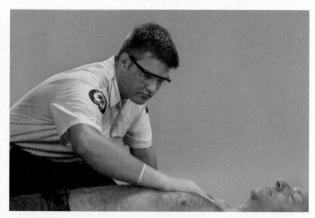

5-1a Count your patient's respirations.

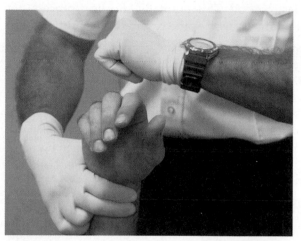

5-1b Assess the pulse as an indicator of circulatory function.

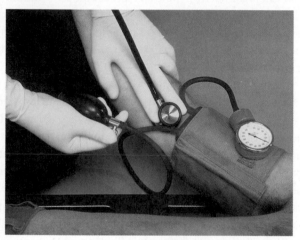

5-1c Assess blood pressure with a sphygmomanometer and stethoscope.

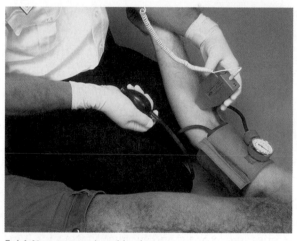

5-1d If you cannot hear blood pressure with a stethoscope, use an ultrasonic Doppler device.

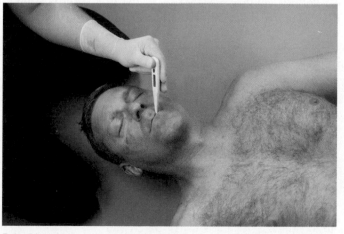

5-1e Use a battery-operated oral thermometer to take your patient's temperature.

that requires energy. The increasing space creates negative pressure, like a vacuum, that draws air into the lungs. Exhalation is the passive process of the respiratory muscles' elastic recoil. This normally effortless process can become difficult with some respiratory conditions. For example, an airway obstruction may compromise inhalation. The resultant increased breathing effort is evident in accessory muscle use, retractions, and possibly abnormal breath sounds.

Diseases such as asthma and emphysema, in which the smaller airways collapse and trap air in the distal airways, may obstruct exhalation. Exhalation then becomes an active process that leads to respiratory distress and failure. Some injuries can decrease the respiratory effort. Rib fractures, for example, will cause a decrease in chest wall expansion because it hurts to breathe. A pneumothorax decreases effective gas exchange because the air enters the pleural space instead of the alveoli. Children become tired and decrease their respiratory effort, making their condition even worse. Evaluating your patient's respiratory effort will provide invaluable information about his respiratory status.

The **quality of respiration** refers to its depth and pattern. The depth, or **tidal volume**, of respiration is the amount of air your patient moves in and out of his lungs in one breath. The normal depth for a healthy adult at rest should be approximately 500 mL, just enough to cause the chest to rise. The tidal volume may increase during exercise or anxiety. It may decrease in the presence of a rib injury, when every breath hurts.

Assess your patient's respiratory depth by inspecting and palpating the chest wall for symmetrical chest expansion, by feeling and listening for air movement and noise from the nose and mouth, and by auscultating for lung sounds. The depth may be shallow, normal, or deep. Once again, to recognize inadequate respiratory depth, you must know what is normal. The respiratory pattern should be regular. Variations in respiratory pattern can be associated with specific diseases (Table 5-4). Some irregular patterns,

Pediatric Pearls

Because a child's airway is so much smaller than an adult's, a minor obstruction can create an acute respiratory problem. Watch the child's face for signs of distress and increased respiratory effort, such as nasal flaring. Children in acute respiratory distress will appear anxious and not interested in their surroundings. Also watch for retractions and head bobbing. Listen for stridor, wheezing, and grunting as further signs of severe breathing problems. As the child speaks, listen for hoarseness (upper airway obstruction) or moaning (decreasing level of consciousness). These findings always require appropriate intervention and rapid transport. Remember, a crying or screaming child has a patent airway.

such as Cheyne-Stokes, may indicate serious brain or brainstem problems.

Pulse

As the heart ejects blood through the arteries, a pulse wave results. Each pulse beat corresponds to a cardiac contraction and results from the ejected blood's impact on the arterial walls. The pulse is a valuable indicator of circulatory function. Your patient's pulse rate, rhythm, and quality indicate his hemodynamic (circulatory) status and the critical nature of his condition.

Pulse rate refers to the number of pulsations felt in 1 minute. It can be slow (bradycardic), normal, or fast (tachycardic). **Pulse rhythm** refers to the pulse's pattern and the equality of intervals between beats. It can be regular, regularly irregular, irregularly irregular, or grossly chaotic. Irregular pulse rates may be caused by extra beats, skipped beats, or pacemaker problems and usually indicate a cardiac abnormality. The rhythm's effect on cardiac output determines whether intervention is necessary. **Pulse quality** refers to the pulse's strength. Terms such as *bounding* or *thready* are used to describe the pulse's quality.

The normal pulse rate for an adult is 60 to 100 beats per minute. Rates below 60 are bradycardic; rates above 100 are tachycardic. **Bradycardia** may indicate an increase in parasympathetic nervous system stimulation. It might also be

Table 5-4 Breathing Patterns

Condition	Description	Causes
Eupnea	Normal rate and pattern	Normal finding
Tachypnea	Increased rate	Fever, anxiety, exercise, shock
Bradypnea	Decreased rate	Sleep, drugs, metabolic disorder, head injury, stroke
Apnea	Absence of breathing	Deceased patient, head injury, stroke
Hyperpnea	Deep respirations	Stress, diabetic ketoacidosis (DKA)
Cheyne-Stokes	Gradual increases and decreases in respirations with periods of apnea. Rapid, deep respirations (gasps) with short pauses between sets	Increasing intracranial pressure, brainstem injury. Spinal meningitis, many CNS causes, head injury
Kussmaul's	Tachypnea and hyperpnea	Renal failure, metabolic acidosis, DKA

the result of a head injury, hypothermia, severe hypoxia, or drug overdose. Bradycardia is a common finding in the well-conditioned athlete, but it may be found in almost anyone. Treat bradycardia only if it compromises your patient's cardiac output and general circulatory status.

Tachycardia usually indicates an increase in sympathetic nervous system stimulation as the body compensates for another problem, such as blood loss, fear, pain, fever, drug overdose, or hypoxia. It is an early indicator of shock and may indicate ventricular tachycardia, a life-threatening cardiac dysrhythmia.

The pulse's quality can be weak, strong, or bounding. Weak, thready pulses indicate a decreased circulatory status, such as shock. Strong, bounding pulses may indicate high blood pressure, heat stroke, or increasing intracranial pressure. The pulse location may be another indicator of your patient's clinical status. The presence of a carotid pulse generally means that his systolic blood pressure is at least 60 mmHg. The presence of peripheral pulses indicates a higher blood pressure; their absence suggests circulatory collapse. Practice locating each of the pulse locations (Figure 5-12). As with other vital signs, take your patient's pulse frequently in the emergency setting and note any trends.

To take the pulse of a conscious adult or large child, the most accessible and commonly used location is the radial artery. With the pads of your first two or three

Peripheral Pulse Sites

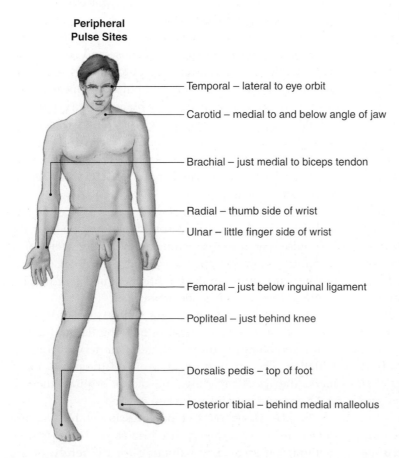

Temporal – lateral to eye orbit
Carotid – medial to and below angle of jaw
Brachial – just medial to biceps tendon
Radial – thumb side of wrist
Ulnar – little finger side of wrist
Femoral – just below inguinal ligament
Popliteal – just behind knee
Dorsalis pedis – top of foot
Posterior tibial – behind medial malleolus

FIGURE 5-12 Know each pulse location.

Pediatric Pearls

In infants and small children, use the brachial artery or auscultate for an apical pulse. Remember that auscultating an apical pulse does not provide information about your patient's hemodynamic status. To locate the brachial artery, feel just medial to the biceps tendon. Auscultate the apical pulse just below the left nipple.

fingers, compress the radial artery onto the radius, just below the wrist on the thumb side (Procedure 5-1b). In the unconscious patient, begin by checking his carotid pulse. To locate the carotid pulse, palpate medial to and just below the angle of the jaw. Locate the thyroid cartilage (Adam's apple) and slide your fingers laterally until they are between the thyroid cartilage and the large muscle in the neck (sternocleidomastoid).

First, note your patient's pulse rate by counting the number of beats in 1 minute. If his pulse is regular, you can count the beats in 15 seconds and multiply that number by 4. If his pulse is irregular, you must count it for a full minute to obtain an accurate total. Also note the pulse's rhythm and quality.

Blood Pressure

Blood pressure is the force of blood against the arteries' walls as the heart contracts and relaxes. It is equal to cardiac output times the systemic vascular resistance. Any alteration in the cardiac output or the vascular resistance will alter the blood pressure.

An important indicator of your patient's condition, blood pressure is measured during both systole and diastole. **Systolic blood pressure** (the higher numeric value) measures the maximum force of blood against the arteries when the ventricles contract. **Diastolic blood pressure** (the lower numeric value) measures the pressure against the arteries when the ventricles relax and are filling with blood. The diastolic blood pressure is a measure of systemic vascular resistance and correlates well with changes in vessel size. The sounds of the blood hitting the arterial walls are called the **Korotkoff sounds**.

Many factors may influence your patient's blood pressure. Anxiety, for example, may cause it to rise. His position (sitting, lying, standing) also may affect the measurement. If your patient has recently been smoking, exercising, or eating, you must wait at least 5 to 10 minutes to allow his blood pressure to return to a resting level before you measure it. Because of these many intangibles, you should never use blood pressure as the single indicator of your patient's condition. Always correlate it with his other clinical signs of end-organ **perfusion**, such as level of response, skin color, temperature, and condition, as well as peripheral pulses.

The average blood pressure in the healthy adult is approximately 120/80 mmHg. Women usually will have a lower blood pressure until menopause. **Pulse pressure** is the difference between the systolic and diastolic pressures. For example, a blood pressure of 120/80 represents a pulse pressure of 40 mmHg. A normal pulse pressure is generally 30 to 40 mmHg. In certain conditions, such as pericardial tamponade or tension pneumothorax, the pulse pressure will narrow. In others, such as increasing intracranial pressure or fever, the pulse pressure will widen. Again, take your physiologically unstable patient's blood pressure as often as every 5 minutes to chart trends.

What is normal? This question has no easy answer. Generally, systolic blood pressure in adults ranges from 100 to 135 mmHg, diastolic from 60 to 80 mmHg. **Hypertension** in adults is defined as a pressure higher than 140/90 mmHg. A blood pressure of 130/70, however, may represent hypertension if a patient's usual pressure is 90/60 or **hypotension** if his usual pressure is 170/90. The numbers are not as important as detecting trends and assessing end-organ perfusion. Define hypotension not by numbers, but by whether perfusion is adequate to sustain life.

Hypertension can result from cardiovascular disease, kidney disease, stroke, or head injury, in which it is a classic sign of increasing intracranial pressure. It may be a predisposing factor to, and preexist in, stroke or cardiovascular disease. Did the hypertension occur before or after the condition? Hypotension usually indicates shock resulting from cardiac insufficiency (cardiogenic shock), low blood volume (hypovolemic shock), or massive vasodilation (neurogenic shock). Orthostatic hypotension is a decrease in your patient's blood pressure when he stands or sits up.

If you suspect shock owing to blood or fluid volume loss and you do not suspect a spinal injury, perform an orthostatic vital sign test. Take your patient's pulse and blood pressure while he is supine. Then have him sit up and dangle his feet, then stand. In 30 to 60 seconds, retake his vital signs. The healthy patient's vital signs should not change. The test is positive either if his pulse rate increases 10 to 20 beats per minute or if his systolic blood pressure drops 10 to 20 mmHg. (Research suggests that an increase in heart rate is a more sensitive indicator of hypovolemia than a decrease in systolic blood pressure.) This finding is common in patients suspected of having hypovolemia.

To measure your patient's blood pressure, first choose the arm you will use. Remove any clothing that covers the upper arm; do not take the blood pressure over clothing, if possible. Look for a dialysis shunt in patients with renal failure. Do not take a blood pressure in that arm. Use the correct size cuff to obtain an accurate measurement. Its width should be one-half to one-third the circumference of your patient's arm. For most adults, unless they are obese or extremely slim, the large-size cuff (15 cm wide) will suffice. If your patient has an obese arm, use a larger cuff. If the larger cuff is still too small, use your patient's forearm and place your stethoscope over the radial artery.

For all patients, use a cuff that covers approximately two-thirds of the upper arm or thigh. Using a cuff that is too wide, too narrow, too long, or too short will result in an inaccurate measurement. Most ambulances should have an assortment of various sizes of blood pressure cuffs. Forearm readings are often more accurate than standard readings in the morbidly obese patient.

Place the arm in a slightly flexed position, palm up and fingers relaxed. Support the upper arm at the level of your patient's heart. Turn the control valve counterclockwise to open it; squeeze all the air out of the bladder before applying the cuff. Locate the brachial artery by palpating on the medial side of the antecubital space until you feel a pulse. Place the lower edge of the cuff 1 inch above the antecubital space. Find the center of the bladder (usually marked on the cuff with an arrow), and place it directly over the artery. Fasten the cuff so it is smooth and fits tightly enough to obtain an accurate reading. If you have difficulty inserting a finger between the cuff and your patient's arm, it is snug enough. Also make sure the rubber tubing is clear of the cuff. Check the placement of the manometer so you can see it easily.

Palpate the radial artery. With your other hand, turn the control valve completely clockwise and squeeze the bulb rapidly to inflate the cuff to approximately 30 mmHg over the point at which the radial pulse disappears. Place your stethoscope directly over the brachial artery and hold it firmly in place without pressing on the artery (Procedure 5-1c). Turn the control valve counterclockwise slowly and steadily to deflate the cuff at a rate of 2 to 3 mmHg per heartbeat. Deflating too slowly or too rapidly will cause an inaccurate reading.

As you deflate the cuff slowly, watch the manometer and listen for the Korotkoff sounds. When you hear the first pulse beat, note the reading on the manometer dial or mercury column. This is the systolic pressure. Continue deflating the cuff until the pulsations diminish or become muffled. This is the diastolic pressure.

If you do not obtain a reading, wait 30 seconds to allow the blood pressure to normalize before inflating the cuff again. Sometimes you can palpate the artery during the deflation. The point at which you feel the pulse return marks the systolic reading. You cannot evaluate the diastolic pressure with the palpation method.

To take your patient's blood pressure with a Doppler device, follow the same procedure as for the palpation method, but instead of palpating for the return of the pulse, place the Doppler device over the palpated artery

In the Field

The Tools of Your Trade: *The Sphygmomanometer*

The circumstances and the patient care setting determine what type of equipment you use to measure blood pressure (Figure 5-13). Intensive care unit staffs commonly use intraarterial pressure devices for critically ill patients who need continuous monitoring. When a noisy environment makes auscultation difficult or when the sounds are especially weak, a Doppler device that amplifies the sounds is useful. You can find these devices in emergency departments, newborn nurseries, and labor and delivery suites.

By far, the most popular devices used in physician's offices, clinics, and emergency vehicles are the electronic blood pressure monitors either as stand-alone units or as part of a ECG monitor/defibrillator. But the most reliable device is one that has been around for centuries—the **sphygmomanometer**.

A sphygmomanometer includes a bulb, a cuff, and a manometer. The cuff has an airtight, flat, rubber bladder enclosed within a fabric cover. Cuffs are available in various sizes and designs. Flexible tubing attaches the rubber bulb to the cuff. Squeezing the bulb pumps air into the cuff's bladder. A control valve allows you to inflate and deflate the cuff. To inflate the cuff, close the valve by turning it clockwise; to deflate the cuff, open the valve by turning it counterclockwise.

The manometer is a pressure gauge with a scale calibrated in millimeters of mercury (mmHg). Each line represents 2 mmHg. The heavy lines are 10 mmHg of mercury apart. The aneroid manometer displays the scale on a circular dial. As the pressure in the bladder changes, the needle moves and indicates the pressure reading at a given moment. When you use an aneroid sphygmomanometer, keep the dial in plain sight. The aneroid types lose their calibration, so you will need to calibrate them periodically against a mercury-type device.

The mercury sphygmomanometer displays the scale along a glass tube connected to a reservoir of mercury. As pressure in the cuff increases, the mercury in the tube rises. When using a mercury sphygmomanometer, keep the scale at eye level and vertical. Available as portable, wall-mounted, or floor units, mercury sphygmomanometers are more accurate than aneroid ones, but they are impractical for prehospital use.

Although initial blood pressures should be taken with a sphygmomanometer and stethoscope, noninvasive blood pressure devices are used extensively in the field. Often, they are a feature of your ECG monitor or are handheld devices. As with any other patient-monitoring device, pay close attention to the manufacturer's instructions on its use.

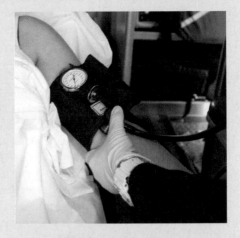

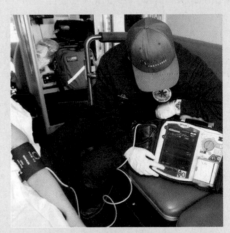

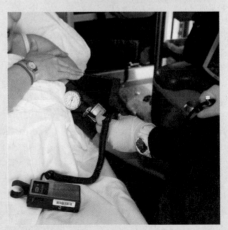

FIGURE 5-13 Use a blood pressure device suited to the circumstances. Shown: aneroid sphygmomanometer, digital electronic, and Doppler device.

(All photos: © Dr. Bryan E. Bledsoe)

and listen for the "whooosh" of flowing blood indicating the systolic measurement (Procedure 5-1d). Record the blood pressure on your patient's chart. Include the systolic and diastolic pressures (for instance, 134/78), the arm used (right/left), and your patient's position (lying, sitting, standing).

Body Temperature

The body works hard to maintain a temperature of approximately 98.6°F (37°C). This temperature reflects the balance between heat production and heat loss through the skin and respiratory system. Even a slight variance can mean that significant events are happening within the body or on

Assessment Pearls

On most encounters, patients who have chronic obstructive pulmonary disease (COPD) are easy to identify. First, they will tell you that they have emphysema or chronic bronchitis. Often, the physical exam will reveal findings suggestive of the disease (e.g., barrel chest, wheezing, accessory muscle usage). However, the presentation of COPD is not always so clear. One clinical indicator of emphysema that you can check for during your physical exam is pulsus paradoxus. Normally, the patient's systolic blood pressure will fall during inspiration. Under normal conditions, this fall is less than 10 mmHg. However, patients with COPD (and other conditions) will have an exaggerated fall in systolic blood pressure (greater than 10 mmHg) during inspiration. To check for pulsus paradoxus, inflate the blood pressure cuff until it is above the patient's systolic pressure. Place your stethoscope over the brachial artery and listen for the Korotkoff sounds (blood pulsing through the vessel) as the cuff is deflated at a rate of approximately 2 to 3 mmHg per heartbeat. The peak systolic pressure during expiration should be identified and reconfirmed. The cuff is then slowly deflated to determine the pressure at which the Korotkoff sounds are again audible during both inspiration and expiration. When the difference in this reading exceeds 10 mmHg during quiet respiration, pulsus paradoxus is present. In addition to COPD, pulsus paradoxus is associated with asthma, pericardial tamponade, hypovolemia, and pericardial effusions.

In the Field

The Tools of Your Trade: *The Thermometer*

A variety of methods can provide accurate temperature readings. You can use glass thermometers to take oral, rectal, or axillary temperatures. A rectal thermometer is the preferred device for children younger than 6 years old and for patients with an altered level of consciousness. An axillary temperature reading is the least accurate of these three methods.

The type of glass thermometer you use determines how long you must leave it in place to get an accurate reading. To take your patient's temperature orally with a glass thermometer, place the thermometer under his tongue for at least 3 to 4 minutes. It may provide a false reading if your patient has swallowed liquid or smoked within 15 to 30 minutes. To use a rectal thermometer, lubricate it well and then insert it 1.5 inches into the rectum; leave it in place for at least 2 to 3 minutes. If you use an axillary thermometer, it must remain under your patient's armpit for at least 10 minutes.

If your service uses electronic thermometers, become familiar with them and follow the manufacturer's instructions for their use (Procedure 5-1e). For example, when using the tympanic membrane device, place the speculum into the ear canal, push the button and hold it for 2 to 3 seconds, then remove the device. The temperature is then displayed on a digital readout.

the body from environmental factors. Assess your patient's temperature to approximate his internal core temperature.[4]

An increase in body temperature (**hyperthermia**) can result from environmental extremes, infections, drugs, or metabolic processes. Ordinarily, the body's cooling mechanisms maintain a steady core temperature. In an extremely hot and humid environment or in cases such as heat stroke, the cooling mechanisms can fail and the core temperature will rise despite an internal thermostat that wants to maintain a normal temperature.

Fever, on the other hand, results when the body tries to make its internal environment inhospitable to invading organisms. It often presents with a history of illness. The skin is somewhat dry until the fever breaks and the body's cooling mechanisms begin to take effect. As the body temperature rises, it begins to threaten body processes, specifically those of the brain. A temperature of up to 102°F (38°C) increases metabolism markedly. As body temperature rises above 103°F (39°C), the neurons of the brain may denature. At temperatures above 105°F (41°C), brain cells die and seizures may occur.

Extreme cold also affects body temperature. When peripheral vasoconstriction and shivering mechanisms can no longer balance heat production and loss, core temperature drops (**hypothermia**). At a body temperature of 93°F (34°C), normal body warming mechanisms begin to fail. As the core temperature drops below 90°F (32°C), shivering stops, heart sounds diminish, and cardiac irritability increases. If the temperature drops much below 70°F (21°C), your patient will present with a deathlike appearance and, possibly, irreversible asystole (absence of heartbeat). Because of their low fibrillation threshold, always handle hypothermic patients gently when assessing and moving them.

Have you ever had a patient tell you that one side of his body was cold? Have you had trouble determining whether one foot was cooler than the other (indicative of peripheral vascular disease)? A simple trick to help with this is the crossover test. Place one of your hands on the body part to be tested for warmth and your other hand on the opposite (contralateral) body part. After 30 to 60 seconds, cross each hand over to the opposite side. If there's an equal amount of warmth bilaterally, there will be no discernible difference in temperature. You will find that even subtle temperature differences can be discerned in this manner.

Capillary Refill

Checking for capillary refill time involves pinching the finger and letting go, to allow blood to refill the area, and timing it. In warm weather, it should take less than 2 seconds to refill in a healthy adult. Because smoking, medications, ambient room temperature, cool or cold weather, or chronic conditions of the elderly may affect capillary refill, you should always also consider the other indicators of circulatory function. In infants and young children, capillary refill is a reliable indicator of circulatory function.[6]

Oral Mucosa Color

The oral mucosa color is a reliable indicator for central circulation and oxygenation. It should appear pinkish-red, smooth, and moist. Early signs of central deoxygenation will include lip and oral mucosa pallor and cyanosis.

Anatomic Region Examination

After you complete the general survey, you will examine the body regions and systems in more detail. Again, the specific situation and your experience and common sense will determine whether you conduct a thorough examination, as you would when performing physicals for an insurance company, or narrow the focus of your examination, as you might in an emergency setting.

Skin

Anatomy and Physiology

The skin is the largest organ in the human body, making up 15 percent of our total body weight. The skin performs many important functions. It protects the body against foreign substance invasion and minor physical trauma. It provides a watertight barrier to keep body fluids in and environmental fluids out. It excretes sweat, urea, and lactic acid and regulates body temperature through radiation, conduction, convection, and evaporation. It provides sensory perception through nerve endings and specialized receptors. It helps regulate

blood pressure by constricting skin blood vessels, and it repairs surface wounds by exaggerating the normal process of cell replacement.

The skin consists of two layers that lie atop the subcutaneous fat: the epidermis and the dermis (Figure 5-14). The thickness of each layer varies with age and body site. The outer layer, the epidermis, is composed mostly of dying and dead cells that are shed constantly and replaced from beneath by new cells. It is avascular (has no blood vessels), so blood vessels from the underlying dermis must supply its nutrition. The dermis is rich in blood supply and nerve endings. It also contains some hair follicles and sebaceous glands that secrete oil called sebum. This oil lubricates the epidermis and helps make the watertight seal. The subcutaneous tissue under the dermis contains fat, sweat glands, and hair follicles.

The two types of sweat glands are eccrine glands and apocrine glands. Eccrine glands, also known as merocrine glands, open onto the skin surface and help control body temperature through water excretion. They are widely distributed but are most heavily concentrated in the axilla and genital areas. Apocrine glands are found exclusively in the armpits and genital region, and they open into hair follicles. These glands respond to emotional stress. During adolescence, the apocrine glands enlarge and actively increase the axillary sweating that causes adult body odor. Also during this period, the sebaceous glands increase

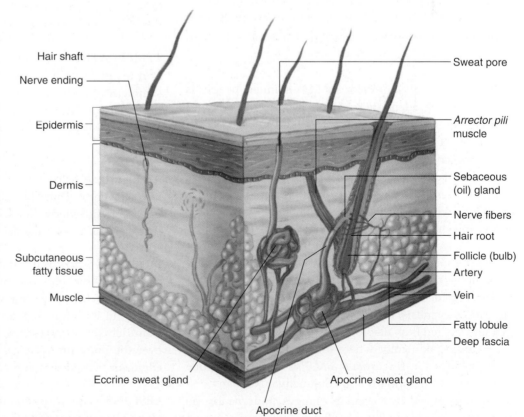

FIGURE 5-14 The skin.

CONTENT REVIEW
➤ Skin Characteristics to
   Assess
   • Color
   • Moisture
   • Temperature
   • Texture
   • Mobility and turgor
   • Lesions

their activity, giving the skin an oily appearance. This predisposes the teenager to acne problems.

As we age, sebaceous and sweat gland activity decreases. As a result, the skin becomes drier and produces less perspiration. The epidermis thins and flattens, and the dermis loses some of its vascularity. The skin wrinkles as it loses turgor. In warmer climates, the skin can become thickened, yellowed, and furrowed and take on a weather-beaten appearance. Elderly people develop a variety of spots on the thin skin of the backs of their hands and forearms. Whitish, depigmented marks are known as *pseudoscars*. Purple spots (purpura) caused by minor capillary bleeding may appear and fade after a few weeks.[5]

Assessment

Although you will observe your patient's skin throughout your assessment, a comprehensive physical exam must also include a concentrated inspection of all areas of the skin. The skin provides data on a variety of systemic problems, in addition to skin-related disorders. Examining the skin requires good light and a keen eye. The characteristics of normal skin vary with your patient's racial, ethnic, and familial backgrounds. Evaluate its color, moisture, temperature, texture, mobility and turgor, and any lesions. Always wear protective gloves if your patient has any areas of open skin, exudative lesions, or rashes.[7]

COLOR   Normal skin color in light-skinned people is pink, indicating adequate cardiorespiratory function and vascular integrity. This means that the capillaries in the skin are well oxygenated. The bright red oxyhemoglobin in the oxygen-rich blood circulating through the capillary beds gives the epidermis its pink appearance. A pale color suggests decreased blood flow through the skin. This is typical in hypothermia, hypovolemia, and compensatory shock, in which blood flow through the distal capillary beds is severely diminished. It also is common in anemia, in which your patient's red blood cell count is low. As the hemoglobin loses its oxygen to the tissues, it changes to the darker, blue deoxyhemoglobin. Increased deoxyhemoglobin causes cyanosis, a bluish skin color. Cyanosis means that less oxygen is available at the tissue level.

Evaluate skin color where the epidermis is thinnest. This includes the fingernails and lips and the mucous membranes of the mouth and conjunctiva. Note any discoloration caused by vascular changes underneath the skin. Petechiae are small, round, flat, purplish spots caused by capillary bleeding from a variety of etiologies. Ecchy-

Assessment Pearls

Assessing skin abnormalities in dark-skinned people can be a challenge. Try the following techniques:

Jaundice: Look for a yellow color in the sclera and hard palate.

Erythema: Look for an ashen color in the sclera, conjunctiva, mouth, tongue, lips, nail beds, palms, and soles.

Pallor: Feel for warmth in the affected area.

Petechiae: Look for tiny purplish dots on the abdomen.

Cyanosis: Look for a dull, dark coloring in the mouth, tongue, lips, nail beds, palms, and soles.

Rashes: Feel for abnormal skin texture.

Edema: Look for decreased color and feel for tightness.

mosis is a blue-black bruise resulting from trauma or bleeding disorders. Jaundice first appears in the sclera and then, in the late stages of liver disease, all over the skin. If only your patient's palms, soles, and face are yellow, he may have carotenemia, a harmless nutritional condition caused by eating a diet high in carrots and yellow vegetables or fruits.

MOISTURE   Inspect and palpate the skin for dryness, increased sweating, and excessive oiliness. Dry skin, common during the cold winter months and in the elderly, may be the result of other conditions. Excessive oiliness, especially where the sebaceous glands are concentrated in the face, neck, back, chest, and buttocks, may suggest acne or hyperthyroidism. Increased sweating may indicate a sympathetic nervous system response to anxiety, fear, or exertion.

TEMPERATURE   Use the backs of your fingers to feel the skin temperature in several different locations. Compare symmetrical body areas. Generalized warming or cooling suggests an environmental, infectious, or thyroid problem. Localized warmth may indicate bleeding or swelling.

TEXTURE   Feel your patient's skin. Is it rough or smooth? Are there large patches or small areas of scaling? Observe the skin's thickness. Thin and fragile skin is a sign of debilitating disease in the elderly. Thick skin often occurs with eczema and psoriasis. Inspect the palms and soles for calluses.

MOBILITY AND TURGOR   Test the skin's turgor and elasticity by picking up a fold of skin over a bony prominence and then releasing it. Normal skin immediately returns to its original state. Poor turgor (tenting) results from dehydration. Test the skin's mobility by moving it over the bony prominence. Decreased mobility suggests edema or scleroderma, a progressive skin disease.

LESIONS   A skin lesion is any disruption in normal tissue. Skin lesions are classified as vascular, involving a blood vessel (Figure 5-15); primary, arising from previously normal

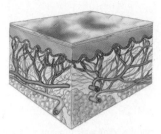

Purpura – Reddish-purple blotches, diameter more than 0.5 cm

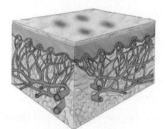

Petechiae – Reddish-purple spots, diameter less than 0.5 cm

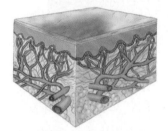

Ecchymoses – Reddish-purple blotch, size varies

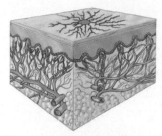

Spider angioma – Reddish legs radiate from red spot

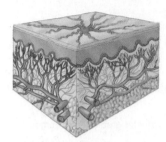

Venous star – Bluish legs radiate from blue center

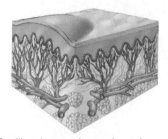

Capillary hemangioma – Irregular red spots

FIGURE 5-15 Vascular skin lesions.

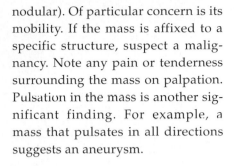

nodular). Of particular concern is its mobility. If the mass is affixed to a specific structure, suspect a malignancy. Note any pain or tenderness surrounding the mass on palpation. Pulsation in the mass is another significant finding. For example, a mass that pulsates in all directions suggests an aneurysm.

Hair

Anatomy and Physiology

Hair is a tactile sensory organ, while also playing a role in sexual stimulation and attraction. It covers the entire body, except the palms, soles, and parts of the sex organs. Hair develops from the base of the hair follicle, where it is nourished by the papilla, a vast capillary network. An involuntary arrector pili muscle fiber attaches to the base of the hair shaft. When these arrectores pilorum contract, the hair stands erect and goosebumps appear on the skin.

The two types of hair are vellus and terminal. Vellus hair is short, fine, and lacking pigment (similar to "peach fuzz"). Terminal hair is coarser, thicker, and pigmented. It appears on the eyebrows and scalp, in the armpits and groin of both sexes, and on the faces and bodies of men.

With aging, the hair turns gray from a decrease in pigmentation and its growth declines. A transition from terminal to vellus hair on the scalp causes baldness in both men and women. The opposite occurs in the nares and ears of men, where terminal hair replaces vellus hair. Both genders generally experience a decrease in body hair as they age. Loss of the lateral third of the eyebrow is also normal in the elderly.[5]

Assessment

Inspect and palpate the hair, noting its color, quality, distribution, quantity, and texture. Is there hair loss? Is there a pattern to the loss? Patients undergoing chemotherapy for cancer may experience generalized hair loss. Failure to develop normal hair growth during puberty may indicate a pituitary or hormonal problem. Abnormal facial hair growth in women (hirsutism) also may indicate a hormonal imbalance.

Part the hair in several places and palpate the scalp (Figure 5-18). A normal scalp is clean with no scaling,

skin (Figure 5-16); or secondary, resulting from changes in primary lesions (Figure 5-17). Skin lesions can take any shape, color, or arrangement. Note their anatomic location and distribution. Are they generalized or localized? Do they involve exposed surfaces or areas that fold over? Do they relate to possible irritants, such as wristbands, bracelets, or necklaces? Are they linear, clustered, circular, or dermatomal (following a sensory nerve pathway)? What type are they? Inspect and feel all skin lesions carefully.

Skin tumors are another variety of skin lesion. These include basal cell and squamous cell carcinomas, malignant melanomas, Kaposi's sarcoma in AIDS, actinic keratosis, and seborrheic keratosis.

When you detect a skin lesion, use anatomic landmarks to describe its exact location on the skin's surface. Describe its shape in terms such as oval, spherical, irregular, or tubular. Sometimes sketching an outline of the lesion is helpful. Record the size of the mass in centimeters, carefully measuring its length, width, and depth. Describe the consistency of the mass exactly as it feels to you (for instance, soft, firm, edematous, cystic, or

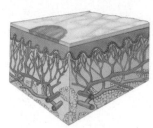

Macule – Flat spot, color varies from white to brown or
from red to purple, diameter less than 1 cm

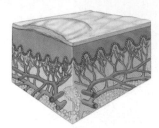

Plaque – Superficial papule, diameter more than 1 cm,
rough texture

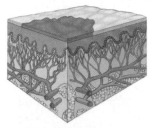

Patch – Irregular flat macule, diameter greater than 1 cm

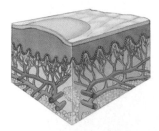

Wheal – Pink, irregular spot varying in size and shape

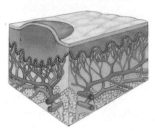

Papule – Elevated firm spot, color varies from brown to
red or from pink to purplish red, diameter less
than 1 cm

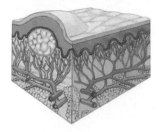

Nodule – Elevated firm spot, diameter 1–2 cm

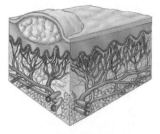

Tumor – Elevated solid, diameter more than 2 cm,
may be same color as skin

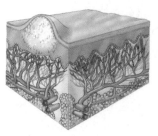

Pustule – Elevated area, diameter less than 1 cm,
contains purulent fluid

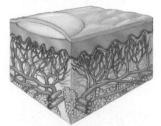

Vesicle – Elevated area, diameter less than 1 cm,
contains serous fluid

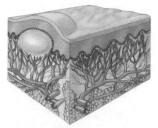

Cyst – Elevated, palpable area containing liquid
or viscous matter

FIGURE 5-16 Primary
skin lesions.

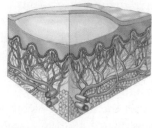

Bulla – Vesicle with diameter more than 1 cm

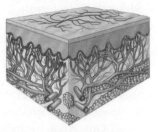

Telangiectasia – Red, threadlike line

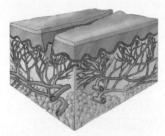

Fissure – Linear red crack ranging into dermis

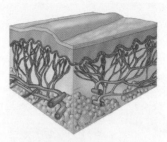

Scar – Fibrous, depth varies, color ranges from white to red

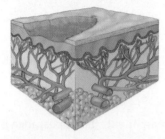

Erosion – Depression in epidermis, caused by tissue loss

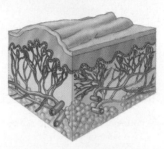

Keloid – Elevated scar, irregular shape, larger than original wound

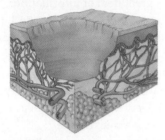

Ulcer – Red or purplish depression ranging into dermis, caused by tissue loss

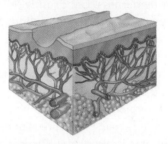

Excoriation – Linear, may be hollow or crusted, caused by loss of epidermis leaving dermis exposed

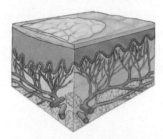

Scale – Elevated area of excessive exfoliation, varies in thickness, shape, and dryness, and ranges in color from white to silver or tan

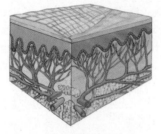

Lichenification – Thickening and hardening of epidermis with emphasized lines in skin, resembles lichen

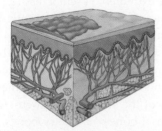

Crust – Reddish, brown, black, tan, or yellowish dried blood, serum, or pus

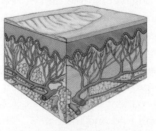

Atrophy – Skin surface thins and markings disappear, semitransparent parchment-like appearance

FIGURE 5-17 Secondary skin lesions.

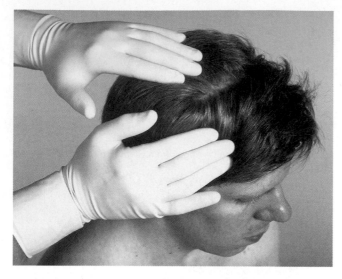

FIGURE 5-18 Inspect and palpate your patient's hair and scalp.

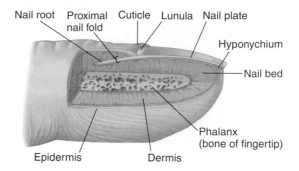

FIGURE 5-19 The nail.

lesions, redness, lumps, or tenderness. Dandruff is characterized by mild flaking, psoriasis by heavy scaling, and seborrheic dermatitis by a greasy scaling. Try to differentiate the flaking of dandruff from the nits (eggs) of lice. Dandruff flakes off the hair easily, whereas nits attach themselves firmly to the hair shaft.

Feel the hair texture. In white people, a soft hair texture is normal; in black people, a coarser texture is normal. Very dry, brittle, or fragile hair is abnormal. Inspect and palpate the eyebrows. Note the quality and distribution of the hair and any scaling of the underlying skin.

When assessing hair, remember that the normal quantity and distribution of hair is related to gender and racial group. For instance, men have more trunk and body hair than women. Native American men have less facial and body hair than male Caucasians. In addition, Caucasians have more abundant and coarser body hair than Asians.

Nails

Anatomy and Physiology

Nails are found at the most distal ends of fingers and toes and are primarily for protection. Nails are strong, yet flexible, and provide a sharp edge for scratching, scraping, and clawing. They are made up of the nail plate, the nail bed, the proximal nail fold, and the nail root (Figure 5-19). Fingernails grow approximately 0.1 mm daily, slightly faster in the summertime. Thus, looking at an intact nail will provide information about the past three months or so of your patient's life.

The angle between the proximal nail fold and the nail plate should be less than 180 degrees. The nail plate lies on a highly vascular nail bed that gives the nail a pink appearance. Nail edges should be smooth and rounded. The nail plates should be smooth, flat, or slightly curved and should feel hard and uniformly thick. As we age, nail growth diminishes because of decreased peripheral circulation.

The nails, especially the toenails, become hard, thick, brittle, and yellowish.[5]

Assessment

In the multiple-trauma patient, the appearance of fingernails is of little consequence. In a medical patient, however, the nails can provide a great deal of information.

Inspect and palpate the fingernails and toenails. Observe the color beneath the transparent nail. Normally it is pink in Caucasians and black or brown in blacks. Note whether the nails appear blue-black, purple, brown, or yellow-gray. Look for lesions, ridging, grooves, depressions, and pitting (Table 5-5). Depressions that appear in all nails are usually caused by a systemic disease.

Gently squeeze the nail between your thumb and forefinger to test for adherence to the nail bed. A boggy (soft and pliable) nail suggests the clubbing seen in systemic cardiorespiratory diseases. The condition of the fingernails also can provide important insight into your patient's self-care and hygiene. Check the toenails for any deformity or injury, such as being ingrown.[4]

Head

Anatomy and Physiology

The scalp consists of five layers of tissue. You can remember their names with the convenient acronym SCALP: **S**kin, **C**onnective tissue, **A**poneurosis, **L**oose tissue, and **P**eriosteum. The scalp is extremely vascular, as it protects and insulates the skull and sensitive brain tissue. When injured, it can bleed profusely.

The skull consists of the cranium and the face. The cranium comprises the frontal, parietal, temporal, occipital, ethmoid, and sphenoid bones and is covered by the scalp (Figure 5-20). The bones of the skull fuse at their sutures. The face includes the nasal bones, maxillary bones, lacrimal bones, zygomatic bones, the palate, the inferior nasal concha, and the vomer (Figure 5-21). The facial bones have air-filled compartments called *sinuses* and have cavities for the eyes, mouth, and nose (Figure 5-22).

The movable mandible joins the skull at the temporomandibular joint (TMJ). The TMJ is in the depression just

Table 5-5   Abnormal Nail Findings

Condition	Description
Clubbing	Clubbing occurs when normal connective tissue and capillaries increase the angle between the plate and proximal nail to greater than 180 degrees. The distal phalanx of each finger is rounded and bulbous. The proximal nail feels spongy. This is caused by the chronic hypoxia found in cardiopulmonary diseases and lung cancer.
Paronychia	This is an inflammation of the proximal and lateral nail folds. It may be acute or chronic. The folds appear red and swollen and tender. The cuticle may not be visible. People who frequently immerse their hands in water are susceptible.
Onycholysis	The nail bed separates from the nail plate. It begins distally and enlarges the free edge of the nail. There are many causes, including hyperthyroidism.
Terry's nails	These appear as a mostly whitish nail with a band of reddish-brown at the distal nail tip. This may be seen in aging and with people suffering from liver cirrhosis, congestive heart failure, and diabetes.
White spots	Trauma to the nail often results in white spots that grow out with the nail. They often follow the curvature of the cuticle and can be the result of overzealous manicuring.
Transverse lines	These are white lines that parallel the lunula, rather than the cuticle. They may appear following a severe illness. They appear from under the proximal nail folds and grow out with the nail.
Psoriasis	These appear as small pits in the nails and may be an early sign of psoriasis.
Beau's lines	These are transverse depressions in the nails and are associated with severe illness. As with the transverse white lines, they form under the nail fold and grow out with the nail. You may be able to estimate the timing or length of an illness by the location of the line. The presence of these lines on more than one nail often indicates that, sometime during the past 2 to 3 months, the patient had a serious systemic illness. During severe illness, the nails grow slowly, thus forming the lines.

in front of the ear. It allows you to open and close your mouth and to jut your jaw forward. A variety of muscles gives the face its contour and general shape. Although facial characteristics vary according to race, gender, and body build, the skull and face should appear symmetrical.[5]

Assessment

You can also examine the skull when you inspect and palpate the scalp and hair. Look for any wounds or active bleeding. The scalp is extremely vascular and lacks the protective vasospasm mechanism that helps control

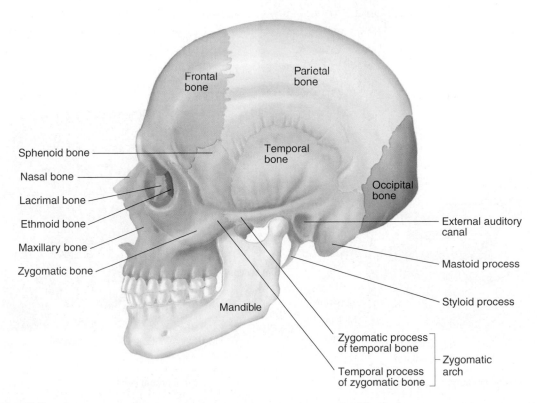

FIGURE 5-20 The skull.

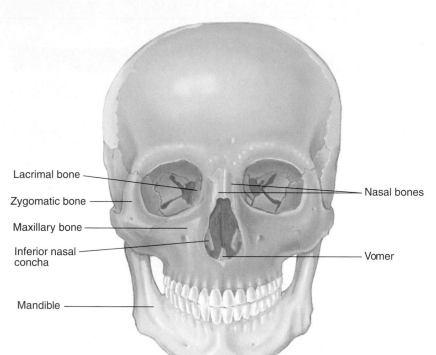

FIGURE 5-21 The facial bones.

Lacrimal bone

Zygomatic bone

Maxillary bone

Inferior nasal concha

Mandible

Nasal bones

Vomer

detect uncontrolled bleeding from the scalp, apply a direct pressure dressing immediately. A simple scalp laceration can cause a life-threatening hemorrhage.

Observe the general size and contour of the skull. Palpate the cranium from front to back (Procedure 5-2a). It should be symmetrical and smooth. Note any tenderness or deformities (depressions or protrusions). An indentation in the skull may suggest a depressed skull fracture. Note any areas of unusual warmth. Palpate the skull for open wounds, depressions, protrusions, lack of symmetry, and any unusual warmth. Use cupped hands and do not probe with your fingers.

If you feel a depression, stop palpating it, because this risks pushing a broken piece of bone into the brain. If you find an impaled object, stabilize it in place with bulky dressings. If your patient presents with an altered mental status and any abnormality in the structure of the skull, consider this a serious emergency and expedite transport while you continue your assessment and treatment.

bleeding. Thus, even the most minor lacerations tend to bleed profusely. Inspect the scalp for lacerations that are hidden under hair matted with clotted blood. Look for blood flowing into the hair, and examine your gloved fingers periodically for blood or other body fluids. If you

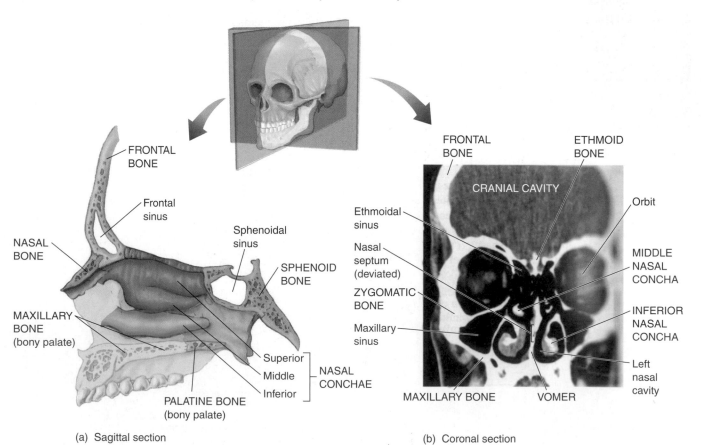

(a) Sagittal section

(b) Coronal section

FIGURE 5-22 The sinuses and cavities of the skull (a) sagittal view (b) coronal CT view.

Procedure 5-2 Examining the Head

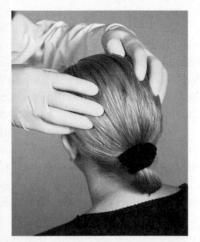

5-2a Palpate the cranium from front to back.

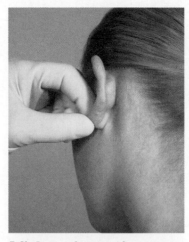

5-2b Inspect the mastoid process.

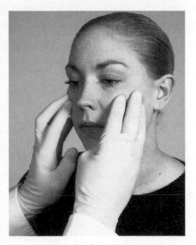

5-2c Palpate the facial bones.

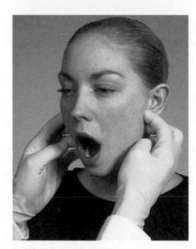

5-2d Palpate the TMJ.

Inspect the face. Is it symmetrical? Are there any involuntary movements? Note any masses or edema. Observe the bony orbits of the eye for periorbital ecchymosis, a bluish discoloration also known as "raccoon eyes." Also check the mastoid process for discoloration (Procedure 5-2b). These are classic signs of a basilar skull fracture. Discoloration normally will not appear on the scene but will present hours after the injury occurs. Palpate the facial bones for stability and note any crepitus or loose fragments (Procedure 5-2c). Note whether your patient's facial expressions change appropriately with his mood.

Evaluate the TMJ. Place the tip of your index finger into the depression in front of the tragus (the cartilaginous projection just in front of the ear's outer opening) and ask your patient to open his mouth (Procedure 5-2d). The tips of your fingers should drop into the joint space. Palpate the joint for tenderness, swelling, and range of motion. Sometimes, you may hear a clicking or snapping. This is neither

unusual nor problematic unless it is accompanied by pain, swelling, and crepitus. Test for range of motion by asking your patient to open and close his mouth, jut and retract his jaw, and move it from side to side.[8] Finally, assess the skin of the face for color, pigmentation, texture, thickness, hair distribution, and lesions.

Eyes

Anatomy and Physiology

The eyes comprise external and internal parts. The external eye consists of the eyelid, conjunctiva, lacrimal gland, ocular muscles, and the bony skull orbit (Figure 5-23). The lacrimal glands, in the temporal region of the superior eyelid, produce tears that moisten the eye. The eyelids distribute the tears over the eye's surface. They also regulate the amount of light entering the eye and protect it from foreign bodies. The eyelashes extend from the eyelid's border. The

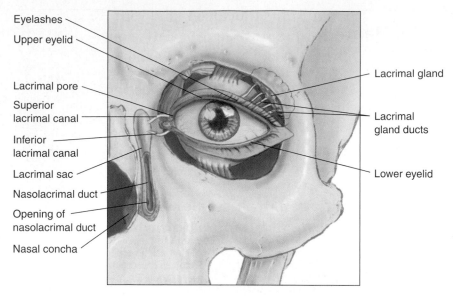

FIGURE 5-23 The external eye.

conjunctiva is a thin membrane that covers the anterior surface of the eye and the inside of the eyelid. It protects the eye from foreign bodies. The ocular muscles (Figure 5-24) control eye movement and are innervated by three cranial nerves (CNs): the oculomotor (CN-III), trochlear (CN-IV), and abducens (CN-VI).

The internal eye consists of the sclera, cornea, iris, lens, and retina (Figure 5-25). The sclera—the white of the eye—is a dense, avascular structure that gives physical shape to the eyeball. The cornea separates the watery fluid in the anterior chamber from the external environment. It also permits light

to enter the lens and reach the retina. The iris is a circular, contractile muscle; its pigment produces the color of the eye. The opening in the center of the iris is the pupil. The iris controls the amount of light reaching the retina by constricting and dilating. It is innervated by the optic nerve (CN-II), which senses light, and by the oculomotor nerve (CN-III), which constricts the pupil.

The lens is a cellular structure immediately behind the iris. It is convex and transparent, allowing images to focus onto the retina. The retina is the sensory network of the eye. It transforms light rays into electrical impulses that the optic nerve transmits to the brain. Besides the optic nerve, the ophthalmic artery and vein provide necessary circulation to and from the eye. Accurate vision depends on these components functioning effectively.[5]

Assessment

The ideal environment for an eye exam is a quiet room, free from distractions, in which you can control the lighting and make your patient comfortable.[6] First, test for visual acuity. Place your patient 20 feet from a **visual acuity wall chart** or have him hold a **visual acuity card** 14 inches from his face. Ask him to cover one eye with a card and begin reading the lines (Procedure 5-3a). Record the visual acuity

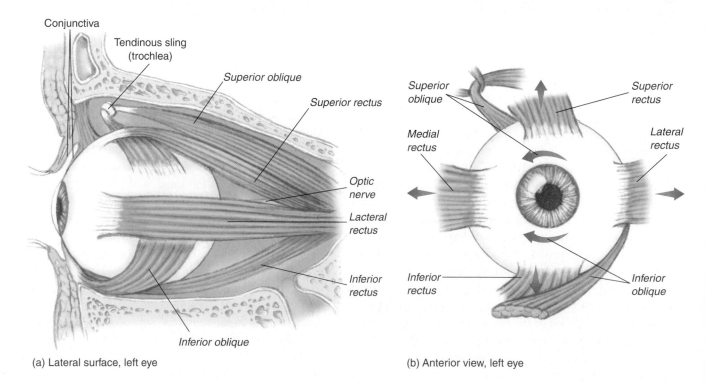

(a) Lateral surface, left eye

(b) Anterior view, left eye

FIGURE 5-24 The extraocular muscles: (a) sagittal view (b) anterior view.

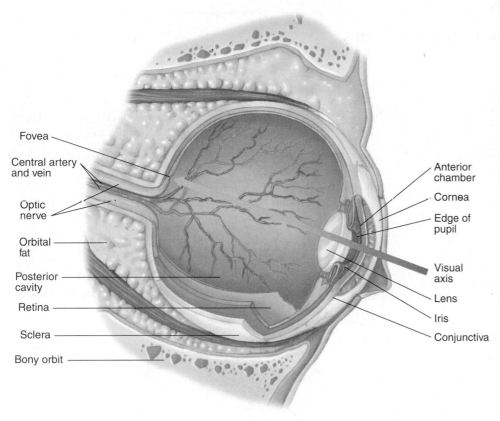

Fovea

Central artery and vein

Optic nerve

Orbital fat

Posterior cavity

Retina

Sclera

Bony orbit

Anterior chamber

Cornea

Edge of pupil

Visual axis

Lens

Iris

Conjunctiva

FIGURE 5-25 The internal eye.

grade next to the smallest line in which he can read at least half the letters.

The result is written as a fraction. The first number represents the distance away from the chart. The second number is the distance from which a normal eye could read the line. Normal is 20/20. A result of 20/70 means that a normal eye could read the line from 70 feet away but your patient could read it only from 20 feet. If no chart is available, you can have your patient count your raised fingers, read from a distance something you have printed, or distinguish light from dark. This type of exam is routinely conducted as part of a comprehensive physical exam in a clinic setting.

Test the visual fields by confrontation. Sit directly in front of your patient. Have him cover his left eye while you cover your right eye. Ask him to look at your nose. Extend your left arm to the side and slowly bring it toward you. Ask your patient to say when he first sees your finger. Use your own peripheral vision as a guide. If he sees your finger when you do, his visual field is grossly normal in that direction. Do this test in all four quadrants (left and right, up and down). Then perform the same test with the other eye (Procedure 5-3b). Any abnormalities suggest a defect in peripheral vision.

Some common abnormalities include a horizontal defect (loss of vision in the upper or lower half of an eye), a blind eye, bitemporal hemianopsia (loss of vision in the outside half of each eye), left or right homonymous hemi-

anopsia (loss of vision in the right half of both eyes or the left half of both eyes), or homonymous quadrantic defect (loss of vision in the same quadrant of both eyes). Record the area of defect as illustrated in Figure 5-26.

Examine the external eyes. Place yourself directly in front of your patient. Inspect his eyes for symmetry in size, shape, and contour. Do they look alike? Do they protrude (proptosis)? Are they properly aligned? Note the eyelids' position relative to the eyeballs. They should cover the upper quarter of the iris. Are the eyes totally exposed or do the eyelids droop (ptosis)? Have your patient close his eyes. Do they close completely? Do you see any edema, inflammation, or mass? Note the eyelid's color. It should be pink, indicating good central oxygenation. If the lid is pale, your patient could be in shock or anemic. If cyanotic, he could have central hypoxemia. Are there any lesions?

Carefully observe the lids' shape and inspect their contours for any growths. If you see any drainage, note its color and consistency. Do the eyelashes turn inward to scrape against the eyeball, or outward to prevent the complete closure of the eye? Are they clean and free from debris? Is there a stye (reddened swelling of the inner eyelid)? Quickly assess the regions of the lacrimal sacs and glands for swelling, excessive tearing, or dryness of the eyes.

Ask your patient to look up while you pull down both lower eyelids to inspect the sclera and conjunctiva (Procedure 5-3c). Be careful not to put pressure on the eyeball.

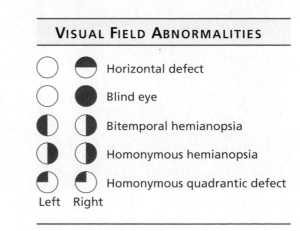

VISUAL FIELD ABNORMALITIES

Horizontal defect

Blind eye

Bitemporal hemianopsia

Homonymous hemianopsia

Homonymous quadrantic defect

Left Right

FIGURE 5-26 Visual field abnormalities.

Procedure 5-3 Examining the Eyes

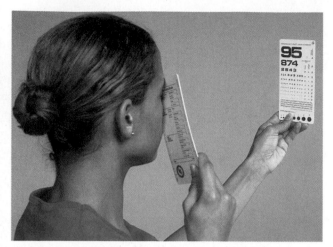

5-3a Use a visual acuity chart to test visual acuity.

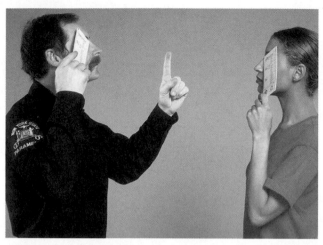

5-3b Test peripheral vision.

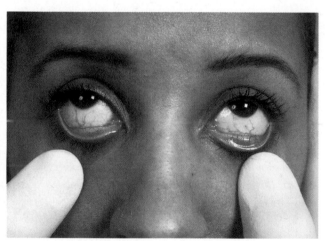

5-3c Inspect the external eye.

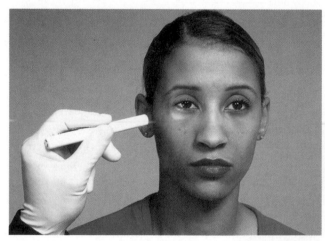

5-3d Test the pupil's reaction to light.

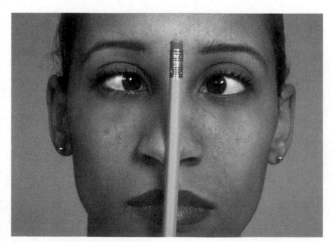

5-3e Test for accommodation.

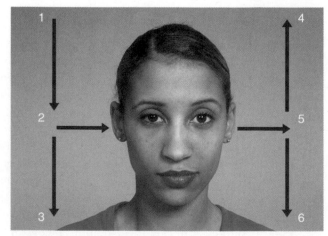

5-3f Move your finger in an H pattern to test your patient's extra-ocular muscles.

(Continued)

Procedure 5-3 *Continued*

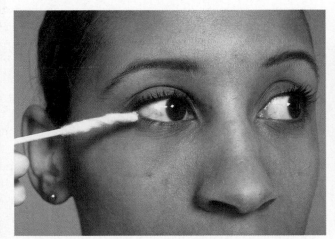

5-3g Check the corneal reflex.

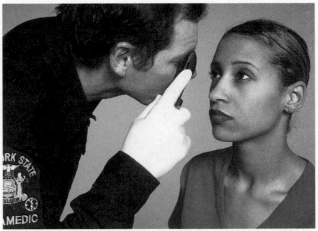

5-3h Visualize the interior eye with an ophthalmoscope.

Ask your patient to look left and right, up and down. The conjunctiva should be clear and transparent, with no redness or cloudiness. Redness or a cobblestone appearance suggests an allergic or infectious conjunctivitis. Bright red blood in a sharply defined area surrounded by normal tissue, not extending into the iris, indicates a hemorrhage under the conjunctiva. Look for any nodules, swelling, or discharge. The normal sclera is white. A yellow sclera suggests the jaundice of liver disease. With an oblique light source, inspect each cornea for opacities. Also check the lens for opacities that you may see through the pupil. Inspect the iris when you inspect the cornea. Shine the light directly from the lateral side and look for a crescent-shaped shadow on the medial side of the iris. Because the iris is flat, the light should cast no shadow. A shadow could suggest glaucoma, caused by a blockage that restricts aqueous humor from leaving the anterior chamber. This increases intraocular pressure and threatens your patient's eyesight.

Inspect the size, shape, and symmetry of the pupils. Are they unusually large (excessive dilation) or unusually small (excessive constriction)? Are they equal? Some patients (20 percent) have unequal pupils, a condition known as *anisocoria*. If the difference in the pupils' size is less than 2 millimeters and they react normally to light, anisocoria is benign.

To test the pupils, first shine a light into one eye and observe that eye's reaction (Procedure 5-3d). This tests the eye's direct response. The pupil should constrict. Repeat this test for the other eye. Now shine a light into one eye and observe the other eye's reaction. This tests the eye's consensual response. Both eyes should react simultaneously to the light. Repeat this test for the other eye.

Normal pupils react to light briskly. A sluggish pupil suggests pressure on the oculomotor nerve (CN-III) from increased intracranial pressure. Bilateral sluggishness may indicate global hypoxia to the brain tissue or an adverse drug reaction. Constricted pupils suggest an opiate overdose, whereas fixed and dilated pupils usually mean brain death.

Have your patient focus on an object in the distance. Then, ask him to focus on an object right in front of him. As he focuses on the near object, his pupils should constrict (near response). Have your patient follow your finger or a pen, pencil, or similar object as you move it from a distance to the bridge of his nose (Procedure 5-3e). His eyes should converge on the object as the pupils constrict (accommodation).

Finally, check the cardinal positions of gaze. Have your patient follow your finger as you move it in an H pattern in front of him (Procedure 5-3f). This tests the integrity of the extraocular muscles. Normal eye movements to follow your finger will be conjugate (together). *Nystagmus* is a fine jerking of the eyes; it may be normal if noted at the far extremes of the test. Check the corneal reflex by touching the eye gently with a strand of cotton and watch for your patient to blink (Procedure 5-3g).

The ophthalmoscopic exam (Procedure 5-3h) may be quite challenging. It requires a significant amount of practice to master this physical exam skill. First, it is necessary to become familiar with your equipment. Locate the aperture, the indicator of diopters, and lens disk. If you or your patient wears glasses, you may remove them unless you or your patient has marked nearsightedness or severe astigmatism. Contact lenses may remain in place.[9]

First, darken the room to the extent possible. Because you will not likely be dilating the patient's pupils, select the narrowest beam of light possible. Dim the light of the ophthalmoscope to minimize pupillary constriction. Begin the exam with the lens disk at zero diopters. Keep your index finger on the lens disk so you can adjust the disk as necessary to focus on the various structures during the exam. Use the same eye as the eye you are examining (i.e., use your right eye to examine the patient's right eye and use your left eye to examine the patient's left eye). Ask your patient to focus on a stationary object straight ahead and slightly above his neutral plane of vision.

Examine the eye in the following manner: Standing laterally and slightly above your patient, look at the eye

In the Field

The Tools of Your Trade: *The Ophthalmoscope*

An **ophthalmoscope** (Figure 5-27) is a medical instrument used to examine the internal eye structures, especially the retina, located at the back of the eye. Although it is most often used to diagnose eye conditions, you can discover information that may be relevant to other medical and traumatic events.

The ophthalmoscope is basically a light source with lenses and mirrors. It has a handle, which houses the batteries, and a head, which includes a window through which you visualize the internal eye; an aperture dial, which changes the width of the light beam; a lens dial to bring the eye into focus; and a lens indicator, which identifies the lens magnification number (i.e., 0 to +40 or 0 to –20). You examine the eye by looking through a monocular eyepiece into the eye of your patient. You can view different depths of the eye at different magnifications by rotating a disk of varying lenses within the instrument itself.

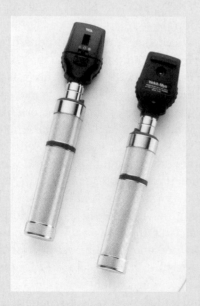

FIGURE 5-27 An ophthalmoscope is used to visualize the interior of your patient's eyes.

from about 6 to 15 inches away and aim your light about 15 to 25 degrees nasally. At this distance, you should note a red "reflex" while looking through the pupil. The red reflex is simply a reflection of the retina back through the pupil. Absence of the red reflex is commonly secondary to cataracts. Less commonly, it may indicate a detached retina, an artificial eye, or, in children, a retinoblastoma.

Place your non-examining hand on the patient's shoulder or on the patient's forehead to gain a sense of proprioception so you can tell how far away you are from the patient. If your hand is on the patient's forehead, you may assist the patient in keeping his eyelid open by holding the lid up with your thumb near the eyelashes. While keeping the red reflex in view, slowly move toward your patient's eye while the patient continues to fix his gaze on an object in the distance. Adjust the lens disk as needed to focus on the retina. Farsighted patients will require more "plus" diopters (black or green numbers), whereas nearsighted patients will require more "minus" diopters (red numbers) to keep the retina in focus.

Try to keep both your eyes open and relaxed. The optic disk should come into view when you are about 1.5 to 2 inches from the eye while you are still aiming your light 15 to 25 degrees nasally. If you are having difficulty finding the disk, look for a branching (bifurcation) in a retinal blood vessel. Usually the bifurcation will point toward the disk.

Follow the vessel in the direction of the bifurcation and you should arrive at the optic disk. The disk should appear as a yellowish-orange to pink round structure. Within the center of the disk there should be a central physiologic cup, which normally appears as a smaller, paler circle. The cup should be less than half the diameter of the disk. An enlarged cup may indicate chronic open-angle glaucoma. Indistinct borders or elevation of the optic disk may indicate papilledema, which is a marker of increased intracranial pressure.

Next, look at the arteries and veins of the retina. The arteries are usually brighter and smaller than the veins. Spontaneous venous pulsations are normal. Abnormalities of the retina such as hemorrhages, arteriovenous (AV) nicking, and cotton wool spots may indicate local or systemic disease such as retinal vein occlusion, hypertension, or many other conditions.

Finally, look at the fovea and surrounding macula. This area is where vision is most acute. It is located about two disk diameters temporal to the optic disk. You may also find the macula by asking the patient to look directly into the light of your ophthalmoscope. Prepare for a fleeting glimpse as this area is very sensitive to light and may be uncomfortable for your patient to maintain. A "cherry red" macula with surrounding pallor of tissue in the setting of acute painless monocular visual loss indicates a central retinal artery occlusion. Irreversible damage occurs within 90 minutes of complete occlusion. Unfortunately, these patients rarely respond to therapy.

Ears

Anatomy and Physiology

The ear has three components: the outer ear, the middle ear, and the inner ear (Figure 5-28). The outer ear consists of the auricle, the ear canal (external acoustic meatus), and the lateral surface of the tympanic membrane (eardrum). The auricle is the visible, skin-covered cartilage that extends outward from the skull. It comprises the helix (the prominent outer rim), the antihelix (the inner rim), the lobe (which contains no cartilage), the concha (the deep cavity containing the opening to the ear canal), and the tragus (the protuberance that lies just in front of the concha).

Behind the ear lies the mastoid process of the temporal bone. It functions as an attachment for the sternocleidomastoid muscle and is palpable just behind the earlobe. The mastoid bone contains air-filled cells that are continuous with the middle ear. This is why an inner ear infection (otitis) often presents with tenderness in the mastoid area. The ear canal opens behind the tragus and is approximately 2 to 3 centimeters long in adults. Hair and sebaceous glands that produce wax (cerumen) line the distal third of the canal. At the end of the ear canal, the translucent tympanic membrane separates the ear canal from the middle ear.

The middle ear, an air-filled cavity in the temporal bone, begins with the medial surface of the tympanic membrane. It contains three small bones known as ossicles (the malleus, the incus, and the stapes) that transmit and amplify sound from the tympanic membrane to the inner ear. The irregularly shaped malleus connects directly to the medial surface of the tympanic membrane at the umbo. It pulls the eardrum inward, making it concave. A "cone of light" is visible here during otoscopy. A light shined on the translucent eardrum makes the middle ear somewhat visible. The eustachian tubes help move mucus from the middle ear to the nasopharynx. They also help equalize the pressure between the outside air and the middle ear during swallowing, sneezing, and yawning.

The inner ear cavity contains the vestibule, the semicircular canals, and the cochlea. The cochlea is a coiled structure that transmits sound to the acoustic nerve (CN-VIII). Hearing involves air conduction of vibrations from the environment to the tympanic membrane. These vibrations are transmitted through the eardrum to the ossicles and to the cochlea, which translates them into nerve impulses. The acoustic nerve transmits these nerve impulses to the brain. The labyrinth within the inner ear helps us maintain our balance by sensing the position and movement of our head. It also is innervated by the acoustic nerve.[5]

Assessment

Begin the examination by simply observing the ears from in front of your patient.[10] Something that "just doesn't look right" warrants further investigation. In particular, look for symmetry. Then examine each ear separately. Inspect each auricle for size, shape, symmetry, landmarks,

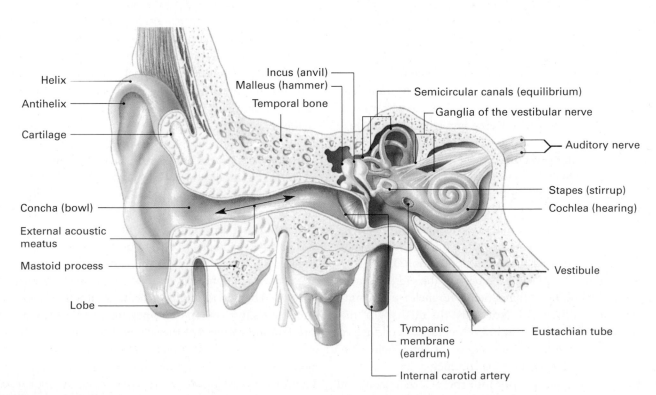

FIGURE 5-28 The ear.

color, and position on the head. Observe the surrounding area for deformities, lumps, skin lesions, tenderness, and erythema (redness). Lumps on or near the ear may indicate a benign process, such as cutaneous cysts or keloids, a malignant process such as squamous cell or basal cell carcinoma, or a local sign of a systemic process such as gout or rheumatoid arthritis.

Pull the helix upward and outward and note any tenderness or discomfort (Procedure 5-4a). Press on the tragus and on the mastoid process (Procedure 5-4b). Pain or tenderness in any of these areas suggests infection such as otitis or mastoiditis. Discoloration in this area is known as Battle's sign, a common, but late, finding in a basilar skull fracture. An earache may arise from the ear itself or be referred from another place through adjoining and shared sensory nerve pathways. Sources of referred pain may include sinus problems, an infected tooth or abscess, temporomandibular joint pain, the common cold, a sore throat, and the cervical spine.

Inspect for discharge (otorrhea) from the ear canal (Procedure 5-4c). The discharge may contain mucus, pus, blood, or cerebrospinal fluid that may have leaked from the skull through a fracture in its base. Injuries to the ear itself can result from blunt trauma to the side of the head, causing temporary or permanent damage to the outer or middle ear. A ruptured eardrum can result from sticking a sharp object into the ear canal or from a pressure wave caused by an explosion.

Evaluate your patient's hearing by occluding one canal. Whisper very softly into the other ear (Procedure 5-4d). Begin by exhaling completely before you speak, to minimize the intensity of your whisper. Use words such as "baseball" that have equally accented syllables. Gradually increase the intensity of your voice until the patient is able to hear you. Do the same for the other ear and evaluate symmetry.

To test for conductive and sensorineural hearing loss, you can use a tuning fork (typically 512 Hz) to perform the Rinne and Weber tests. The Rinne test will differentiate a conductive from a sensorineural hearing loss. First, place the base of the slightly vibrating tuning fork behind the patient's ear. When the patient can no longer hear the vibration, put the tuning fork up to his ear with the tip of the fork closest to the ear and the "U" of the tuning fork facing forward. Under normal circumstances, the patient should still be able to hear the vibrations, indicating that air conduction is greater than bone conduction. The Weber test is performed by placing the base of the vibrating tuning fork at the middle of the patient's forehead or the middle of the top of the head. Normally, the intensity of the sound will be heard equally in both ears. If a conductive hearing loss is present, the intensity of the sound will actually be greater in the ear with the conductive loss.

To examine more deeply into the external canal, an **otoscope** is used. A speculum is placed on the end of the

otoscope to facilitate entry into the canal. Use the largest size speculum that will fit easily into the canal. As a general guideline, a 4-millimeter speculum is sufficient for the examination of most adults. Again, grasp the auricle gently but generously and pull upward and outward. This motion will help align the external canal and facilitate your view of the eardrum (tympanic membrane) in much the same way that the "sniffing position" aligns the structures of the airway and facilitates your view of the vocal folds (Procedure 5-4e).

Hold the otoscope between your thumb and fingers of your other hand. Brace your hand against the patient's face so you will move in tandem with any sudden or unexpected patient movement. Gently advance the speculum into the canal. Be careful not to touch the sensitive walls of the canal with your speculum. Visualize the canal itself. A thickened, red, itchy canal wall occurs in chronic otitis externa. Obstruction of the canal from earwax (cerumen impaction) is a common cause of correctible hearing loss. The cerumen may have to be cleared before you can visualize the tympanic membrane. You may see fine hairs in the canal. Continue advancing the speculum until you are just past the point where the hairs end. At this point you should have a good view of the tympanic membrane.

In a normal eardrum, you will see a "cone of light" reflection at the anterior and inferior aspects of the drum. Check the tympanic membrane for color. Normally, the membrane should be pearly white to pinkish gray. Redness (erythema) of the membrane is common in crying children but may be secondary to an infectious process such as acute otitis media. A chalky white area of the drum with irregular borders indicates scarring or sclerosis, which may occur after frequent episodes of otitis media. This is somewhat common and rarely clinically significant. Next, examine the integrity of the drum itself. Look for perforations, which often occur after infections. People with chronic infections may have undergone a procedure to make a hole in the eardrum to allow for draining. A tube (myringotomy tube), which is often brightly colored, is often left in place. Without the tube, the hole would close. If there is a tube in place, make sure it is not obstructed.

Because the tympanic membrane is translucent, you may be able to see through the membrane. In a normal ear, you should see landmarks, or protrusions, occurring from the middle ear bones (ossicles) pushing on the tympanic membrane from behind. In the setting of inflammation, these normal landmarks may be lost. Clear or amber-colored fluid behind the drum indicates a serous effusion. Air-fluid levels, which appear somewhat like bubbles, may be present, indicating that there is both air and fluid behind the drum. A serous effusion may be caused by a viral infection or by sudden changes in pressure (barotrauma). Blood behind the eardrum (hemotympanum) may appear as a purple or bluish discoloration and indicates local trauma,

Procedure 5-4 Examining the Ears

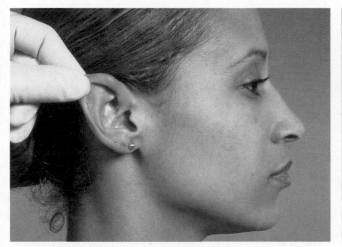

5-4a Examine the external ear.

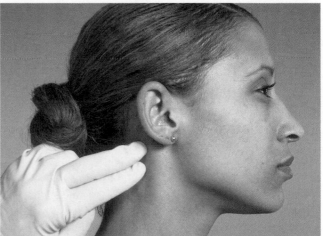

5-4b Press on the mastoid process.

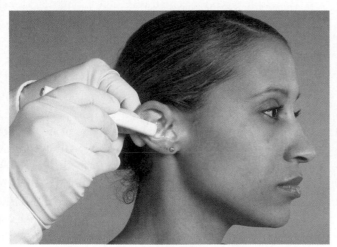

5-4c Inspect the ear canal for drainage.

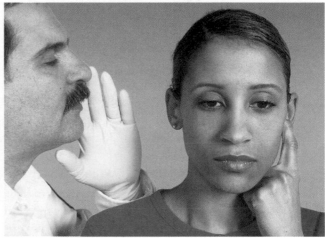

5-4d Whisper into your patient's ear.

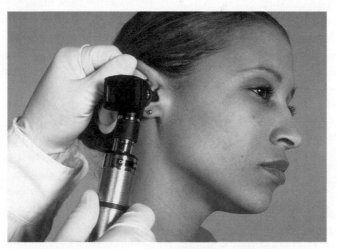

5-4e Visualize the inner ear canal and tympanic membrane.

In the Field

The Tools of Your Trade: *The Otoscope*

An otoscope is a medical device that is used to visualize the ear canal and tympanic membrane (Figure 5-29). Health care providers use otoscopes to screen for illness during regular checkups and also to investigate when a symptom involves the ears. With an otoscope, it is possible to see the outer ear and middle ear. You can also use an otoscope to examine a patient's nares (avoiding the need for a separate nasal speculum) and (with the speculum removed) upper throats.

Like the ophthalmoscope, an otoscope consists of a handle and a head. The head contains an electric light source and a low-power magnifying lens. The front end of the otoscope has an attachment for disposable plastic ear speculums, which are available in different sizes. Many models have a detachable sliding rear window that allows you to insert instruments through the otoscope into the ear canal, such as for removing earwax (cerumen), but this is not in the scope of your practice. Most models also have the capability to push air through the speculum; these are called *pneumatic otoscopes*. This puff of air allows an examiner to test the mobility of the tympanic membrane.

Many otoscopes found in doctors' offices are wall mounted. The one you use will probably be portable. Wall-mounted otoscopes are attached by a flexible power cord to a base, which is its source of electric power and a place to hold

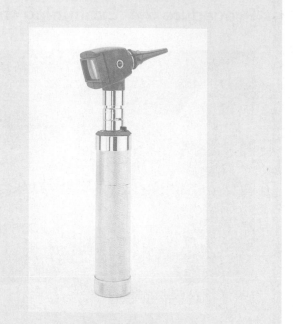

FIGURE 5-29 An otoscope enables you to inspect the ear canal and tympanic membrane.

the otoscope when it is not in use. Portable models are powered by rechargeable batteries found in the handle. Otoscopes are often sold with ophthalmoscopes as a diagnostic set.

---

barotrauma, or a basilar skull fracture. In the setting of purulent otitis media you may be able to visualize pus behind the tympanic membrane.

Your otoscope may come with a bulb that will allow you to insufflate a small puff of air into the canal to detect movement of the tympanic membrane. Squeezing the bulb lightly instills air into the canal, normally making the drum move away from you. Releasing the bulb will remove air,

Pediatric Pearls

Assess the outer ear for position. The top of the ear should be on a horizontal line with the outer corner of the eye. As a child grows, the anatomy of the external ear canal changes. In infancy, the canal curves downward, so you should pull down the auricle to see the tympanic membrane at the distal end of the canal. As the child grows, the canal starts to move up and backward, and the ear is relatively higher and farther back on the head. Remember to pull the auricle upward and backward to afford the best view with the otoscope. Brace your hand against the child's skull to prevent injury from sudden movement.

Choose the largest speculum that will fit comfortably into the child's ear. Tilt the child's head away from you. Hold the otoscope firmly in one hand and, with your free hand, pull the ear appropriately to straighten the ear canal. Slowly insert the speculum 1 to 2 centimeters into the canal. Observe the amount, texture, and color of wax and the presence of foreign bodies. Inspect the tympanic membrane for color, light reflex, and bony landmarks. Repeat the same steps for the other ear.

pulling the drum toward you. The "cone of light" should also move as you alter the air pressure within the canal. This is an excellent way to evaluate for the presence of serous otitis media, which will prevent normal movement of the membrane. Acute otitis media will often diminish the response of the drum to fluctuations in air pressure as well.

Nose

Anatomy and Physiology

The external nose comprises the nasal bones and cartilage covered by skin. The nares are the anterior openings in the nose. A cartilaginous bony septum divides the left and right nasal cavities. The turbinates, or conchae, are bony ridges on the medial surface of the nose (Figure 5-30). They create a turbulence to help clean, warm, and humidify the inspired air. Coarse nose hair, the turbinates, and the highly vascular and mucus-producing membrane make up the respiratory system's initial filtration system. The mucous membrane is comprised of mucus-producing glands and cells that moisten the inner respiratory tract.

The paranasal sinuses are air-filled extensions of the nasal cavities in the frontal, maxillary, ethmoid, and sphenoid bones (Figure 5-31). They are lined with mucous membranes and with cilia, fine hairlike projections that move secretions along pathways opening into the oral and nasal cavities. The sinuses help insulate the sensitive brain

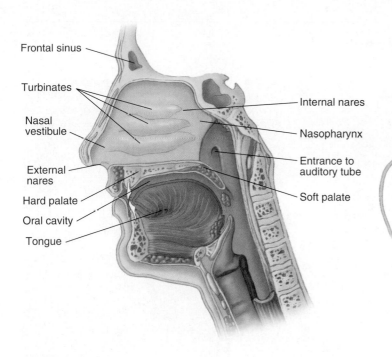

Frontal sinus

Turbinates

Nasal vestibule

External nares

Hard palate

Oral cavity

Tongue

Internal nares

Nasopharynx

Entrance to auditory tube

Soft palate

FIGURE 5-30 The nose.

and provide the vocal resonance that is conspicuously absent during a bad head cold.[5]

Assessment
Check your patient's nose from the front and from the side and note any deviation in shape or color.[10] Also note any nasal flaring, an indication of respiratory distress. Palpate the external nose for depressions, deformities, and tenderness (Procedure 5-5a).

To inspect the nose's internal structures, tilt your patient's head back slightly. Insert the speculum of your otoscope and check the nasal septum for deviation and perforations (Procedure 5-5b). Erosions suggest intranasal cocaine abuse. Examine the nasal mucosa for evidence of

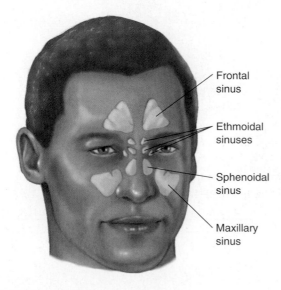

Frontal sinus

Ethmoidal sinuses

Sphenoidal sinus

Maxillary sinus

FIGURE 5-31 The paranasal sinuses.

drainage and note the color, quantity, and consistency of the discharge. Rhinitis (a runny nose) may produce a watery, clear fluid, as seen in seasonal allergies. If the discharge appears thick and yellow, suspect an infection. Epistaxis (a nosebleed) may be caused by trauma or a septal defect.

Test for nasal obstruction by occluding one side of the nose and having your patient breathe through the other side (Procedure 5-5c). It is normal for one side to be more patent than the other. A deviated septum, foreign body, excessive secretions, or mucosal edema may cause abnormal obstructions.

Inspect and palpate the frontal and maxillary sinuses for swelling and tenderness. To palpate the frontal sinus, press your thumbs upward, deep under the orbital ridges (Procedure 5-5d); to palpate the maxillary sinuses, press up under the zygomatic arches (cheeks) (Procedure 5-5e). You also can tap on each area for similar symptoms. Swelling or tenderness suggests a sinus infection or obstruction.[6]

Mouth
Anatomy and Physiology
The lips mark the entrance to the mouth and play a role in the articulation of speech. The mouth houses the tongue, the gums (gingiva), and the teeth (Figure 5-32). The roof of the mouth is formed by the hard palate and the soft palate. The uvula is the peninsular extension of the soft palate that hangs in the back of the mouth. The oral cavity, lined with buccal (cheek/mouth) mucosa, is rich in mucous membranes. The parotid glands, just in front of the ears, and the submandibular glands, just beneath the mandible, secrete digestive enzymes and saliva into the oral cavity (Figure 5-33). The sublingual glands secrete enzymes just beneath the tongue. You can easily palpate these glands under the chin.

The tongue, a large, mobile muscle covered by mucous membranes, has many functions. It helps in chewing by keeping food on the teeth, and it assists in swallowing by moving the food into the oropharynx. It also contains the taste buds and is essential in forming words when we speak.

A highly vascular mucosa lines the gingiva, giving it a pink color. The teeth are anchored in bony sockets; only their white enamel-covered crowns are visible. An adult normally has 32 permanent teeth, including incisors, canines, premolars, and molars.

The pharynx consists of three distinct areas: the nasopharynx (behind the nasal cavity), the oropharynx (back of the throat), and the laryngopharynx (just above the

Procedure 5-5 Examining the Nose

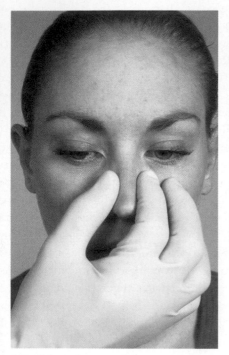

5-5a Palpate the external nose.

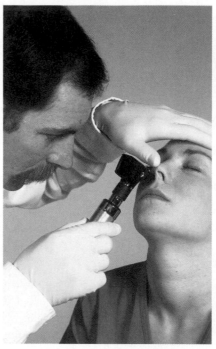

5-5b Inspect the internal nose with an otoscope.

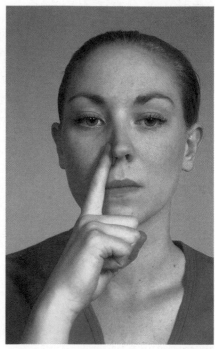

5-5c Inspect the nose for nasal obstruction.

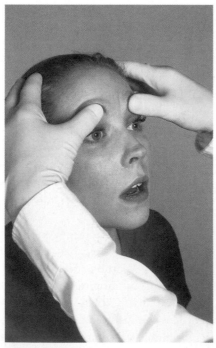

5-5d Palpate the frontal sinus.

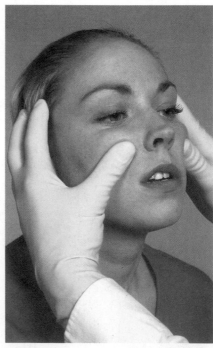

5-5e Palpate the maxillary sinus.

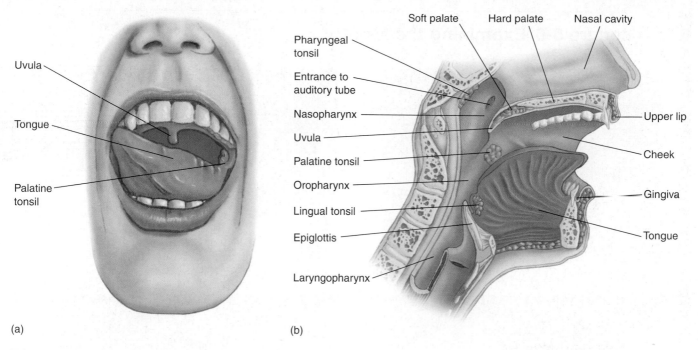

FIGURE 5-32 The mouth.

epiglottis). At the back of the throat on either side, the tonsils help separate the oropharynx (food processing) from the nasopharynx (air passage).[5]

Assessment

Assess the mouth from anterior to posterior, starting with the lips.[10] Note their condition and color. They should be pink, smooth, and symmetrical and devoid of lesions, swelling, lumps, cracks, or scaliness. Gently palpate the lips with the jaw closed (Procedure 5-6a) and note any lesions, nodules, or fissures, especially at the corners. Observe the undersurfaces of the upper and lower lips

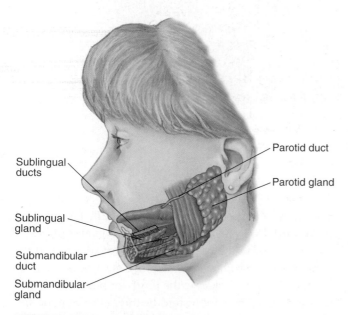

FIGURE 5-33 The salivary glands.

(Procedure 5-6b). They should be wet and smooth. Look for any of the lip abnormalities listed in Table 5-6.

To examine the mouth, you will need a bright light and a tongue blade. Holding the tongue blade like a chopstick will give you good downward leverage. Examine the oral mucosa for color, ulcers, white patches, and nodules. The oral mucosa should appear pinkish-red, smooth, and moist. Note the color of the gums and teeth. The gums should be pink with a clearly defined margin surrounding each tooth. Inspect the teeth for color, shape, and position. Are any missing or loose? Suspect periodontal disease if the gums are swollen, bleed easily, and are separated from the teeth by large crevices that trap food. Use a tongue blade to move the lateral lip to one side while you examine the buccal mucosa and parotid glands (Procedure 5-6c). Note the buccal mucosa's color and texture.

Ask your patient to stick his tongue straight out and then to move it from side to side. Coating of the tongue indicates dehydration. Note its color and normally velvety surface. Hold the tongue with a 2-inch × 2-inch gauze pad and

Table 5-6 Lip Abnormalities

Lips	Cause
Dry, cracked lips	Dehydration, wind damage
Swelling/edema	Infection, allergic reaction, burns
Lesions	Infection, irritation, skin cancer
Pallor	Anemia, shock
Cyanosis	Respiratory or cardiac insufficiency

Procedure 5-6 Examining the Mouth

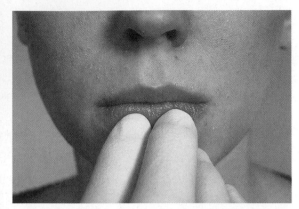

5-6a Palpate the lips.

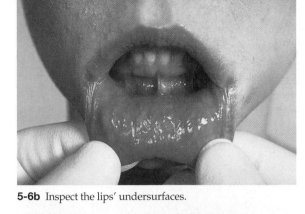

5-6b Inspect the lips' undersurfaces.

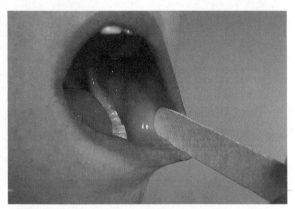

5-6c Examine the buccal mucosa.

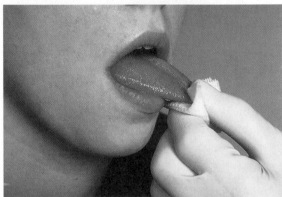

5-6d Inspect the tongue using a gauze pad and a gloved hand.

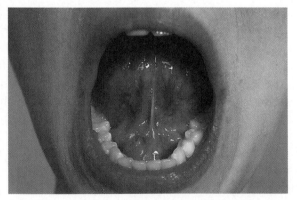

5-6e Inspect under the tongue.

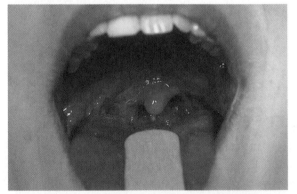

5-6f Have your patient say "aaahhh" while you examine the soft palate and uvula.

a gloved hand to manipulate it for inspection (Procedure 5-6d). Make sure to inspect the sides and bottom of the tongue because malignancies are more likely to develop there, especially in patients over age 50 who smoke, chew tobacco, or drink alcohol (Procedure 5-6e). The undersurface should be smooth and pink; often you can see the bluish discoloration of dilated veins or the yellowish tint of early jaundice. Inspect the floor of the mouth, the submandibular ducts, and the fold over the sublingual gland.

Now examine the normally white hard palate and the normally pink soft palate (Procedure 5-6f). Check them for texture and lesions. Observe the posterior pharyngeal wall. Press the blade down on the middle third of the tongue and have your patient say "aaahhh." Examine the posterior

Pediatric Pearls

Inspect the child's mouth much the same as you would for the adult. A young child's mouth is small, whereas the tongue is relatively large, so examining the child's oral cavity will be a challenge. Examine the nose using the nasal speculum and penlight or the appropriate attachment to the otoscope. To examine the mucous membrane, tip the child's head back and use the otoscope to inspect for color or swelling.

pharynx, the palatine tonsils, and the movement of the uvula. Inspect the tonsils for color and symmetry. Look for exudate (pus), swelling, ulcers, or drainage. The uvula should move straight up with no deviation.

Note any odors from your patient's mouth. The smell of alcohol, feces (bowel obstruction), acetone (diabetic ketoacidosis), gastric contents, or the bitter-almond smell of cyanide poisoning may all provide important clues to your patient's problem. Also look for any fluids or unusual matter in your patient's mouth. For example, coffee-grounds-like material suggests an upper gastrointestinal (GI) bleed. Pink-tinged sputum indicates acute pulmonary edema, whereas green or yellow phlegm suggests a respiratory infection. Pay special attention to anything in your patient's mouth that can eventually obstruct his upper airway, including dentures or missing teeth.[6]

Neck

Anatomy and Physiology

The neck houses many life-sustaining structures. It contains the spinal cord, blood vessels delivering blood to (via the carotid arteries) and from (via the jugular veins) the brain, and the conduits for air passage (larynx/trachea) into the lungs and food passage (esophagus) into the stomach. Any major disruption of these vital structures can cause rapid deterioration or immediate death. Especially during an emergency, examining the neck can be a critical part of your patient assessment.

From anterior to posterior, the thyroid gland, larynx and trachea, esophagus, and spinal column lie in the midline. The thyroid cartilage is the visible and palpable Adam's apple in the anterior neck midline (Figure 5-34). Just below it lie the cricoid cartilage and the rings of the trachea. The thyroid gland sits on both sides of the trachea, with its isthmus crossing the trachea.

Between the thyroid cartilage and the large sternocleidomastoid muscles, the common carotid arteries extend toward the brain.

The internal jugular veins are next to the carotids and are not visible. The external jugular veins extend diagonally across the surface of the sternocleidomastoid muscles and are clearly visible when they are distended or the patient is lying down. The lymph system helps drain fluid from the head and face and assists in fighting infection. A long chain of lymph nodes runs along the side of the neck, behind the ears, and under the chin (Figure 5-35). The nodes are palpable only when inflamed.

Assessment

Briefly inspect your patient's neck for general symmetry and visible masses.[4] Note any obvious deformity, deviation, tugging, masses, surgical scars, gland enlargement, or visible lymph nodes. Examine any penetrating injuries to the neck closely for damage to the trachea or major blood vessels; handle gently to avoid dislodging a clot that has halted bleeding. Immediately cover any open wounds with an occlusive dressing to prevent air from entering a lacerated jugular vein during inspiration. Look for jugular vein distention while your patient is sitting upright and at a 45-degree incline.

Palpate the trachea for the midline position (Procedure 5-7a). Then gently palpate the carotid arteries, one at a time, and note the rate and quality of their pulses (Procedure 5-7b). Palpate the butterfly-shaped thyroid gland

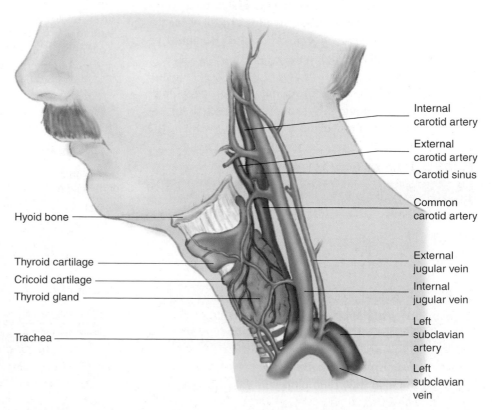

Hyoid bone

Thyroid cartilage
Cricoid cartilage
Thyroid gland

Trachea

Internal carotid artery
External carotid artery
Carotid sinus
Common carotid artery
External jugular vein
Internal jugular vein
Left subclavian artery
Left subclavian vein

FIGURE 5-34 The neck.

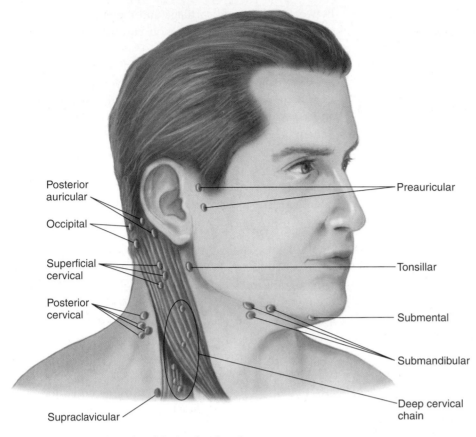

FIGURE 5-35 Lymph nodes of the head and neck.

nodes are palpable, and sometimes even visible. Note their size, shape, mobility, consistency, and tenderness. Tender, swollen, and mobile nodes suggest inflammation, usually from infection. Hard or fixed nodes suggest a malignancy. Inspect and palpate for subcutaneous emphysema, the presence of air just below the skin. This generally suggests a tear in the tracheobronchial tree or a pneumothorax.

Chest and Lungs

Anatomy and Physiology

The chest is a protective cage of bones, muscles, and cartilage (Figure 5-36).[11] The bony cage comprises the three bones of the sternum (manubrium, body, and xiphoid process), the 12 pairs of ribs and their cartilaginous attachments, and the spinal column. In most adults, the transverse

from behind your patient. Rest your thumbs on his trapezius muscles and place two fingers of each hand on the sides of the trachea just beneath the cricoid cartilage (Procedure 5-7c). Have your patient swallow and feel for the movement of the gland. If you can feel it, it should be small, smooth, and free of nodules.

Examining the lymph nodes requires a systematic approach (Table 5-7). Using the pads of your fingers, palpate the nodes by moving the skin over the underlying tissues in each area (Procedure 5-7d). When swollen, the

Pediatric Pearls

Evaluate the child's neck for stiffness, which—when associated with a fever—suggests meningitis. Evaluate for lymphadenopathy (enlarged lymph nodes) in the neck by assessing the nodes' size, warmth, tenderness, and mobility. Certain infectious diseases, such as mononucleosis, rubella, and mumps, are associated with lymphadenopathy. Nodes commonly feel enlarged as a result of recurrent upper respiratory infections.

Table 5-7 Lymph Node Examination

Node	Exam
Preauricular	Press on the tragus and "milk" anteriorly.
Postauricular	Palpate on or under the mastoid process.
Occipital	Palpate at the base of the skull lateral to thick bands of muscle.
Submental	Palpate at the base of the mandible under the chin.
Submaxillary	Palpate along the underside of the jawline.
Anterior cervical	Palpate anterior to the sternocleidomastoid muscle.
Posterior cervical	Palpate posterior to the sternocleidomastoid muscle.
Deep cervical	Encircle and palpate the sternocleidomastoid muscle.
Supraclavicular	Palpate just above the clavicle in the deep groove.

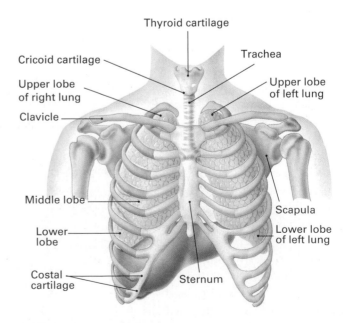

FIGURE 5-36 The thorax.

Procedure 5-7 Examining the Neck

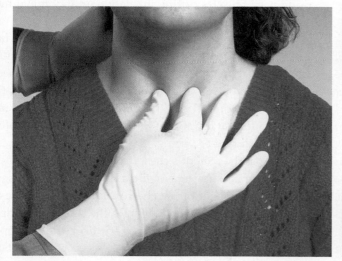

5-7a Assess the trachea for midline position.

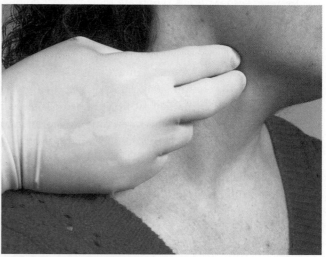

5-7b Palpate the carotid arteries, one at a time.

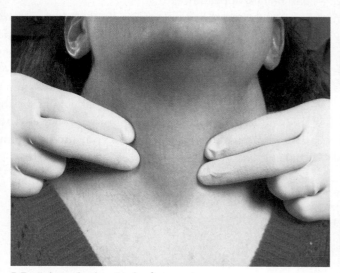

5-7c Palpate the thyroid gland.

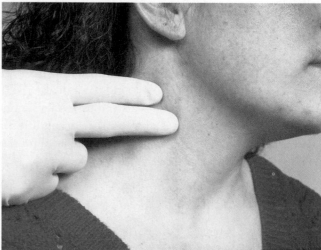

5-7d Palpate the lymph nodes.

(side-to-side) diameter exceeds the anterior–posterior (front-to-back) diameter.

The chest is divided into three cavities: the mediastinum, the right pleural cavity, and the left pleural cavity. The right chest contains three lung lobes (upper, middle, lower), whereas the left contains only two (upper, lower), to make room for the heart. The mediastinum contains the heart, the great vessels (vena cava, aorta, and pulmonary arteries and veins), the trachea, and the esophagus.

The chest wall can expand to create a vacuum that draws air into the lungs and helps return blood to the heart. The primary muscles of respiration are the diaphragm and external intercostals. During inhalation, the diaphragm contracts and moves downward and the external intercostals pull the chest wall upward and outward.

The lungs, attached to the inner chest wall by a membrane called the pleura, also expand.

The pleura consist of a parietal layer (lining the inner chest wall) and a visceral layer (covering the lungs) that glide over each other during breathing. A small amount of liquid between the layers helps create the vacuum for inhaling and acts as a lubricant. In cases of airway obstruction, a variety of accessory muscles in the neck and chest help lift the chest wall. Exhalation is primarily a passive process of muscle relaxation unless disease or injury forces the use of accessory muscles in the chest and abdomen to help expel air from the lungs.

A neurochemical process controls normal breathing. Specialized chemoreceptors monitor the blood for increases in carbon dioxide, decreases in oxygen, and changes in pH.

The brain sends signals to the primary respiratory muscles to begin inspiration. The phrenic nerve, arising from cervical nerves 3, 4, and 5, innervates the diaphragm, whereas the thoracic spinal nerves innervate their respective intercostal muscles.[5]

Assessment

To assess the chest and thorax, you will need a stethoscope with a bell and diaphragm, a marking pen, and a centimeter ruler.[11] Have your patient sit upright, if possible, and expose his entire chest. At the same time, try to maintain your female patient's dignity when assessing her thorax and lungs by keeping her breasts covered. Perform your exam in the standard sequence—inspect, palpate, percuss, auscultate—and compare the findings from side to side. Always try to visualize the underlying lobes of the lungs during your exam.

Observe your patient's breathing. Look for signs of acute respiratory distress. Count the respiratory rate and note the patient's breathing pattern. Obviously prolonged inhalation or exhalation indicates difficulty moving air in or out of the lungs. Do you hear sounds of an upper airway obstruction (inspiratory stridor) or a lower airway obstruction (expiratory wheezing, rhonchi)? Any gross abnormalities in the respiratory rate or pattern require rapid emergency intervention.

Inspect the anterior chest wall and assess its symmetry. Funnel chest (pectus excavatum) is a condition in which the lower portion of the sternum is depressed (Figure 5-37a). With a pigeon chest (pectus carinatum), the sternum curves outward (Figure 5-37b). Do both sides of your patient's chest wall rise in unison? Note whether he is using neck muscles during inhalation or abdominal muscles during exhalation.

If the patient's skin retracts in the area above his clavicles (supraclavicular), at the notch above his sternum (suprasternal), and between his ribs (intercostal), suspect a ventilation problem. If multiple ribs are fractured, creating a "floating segment" or "traumatic flail chest," you may find paradoxical (opposite) movement of that part of the chest wall during breathing.

Look at the patient's chest from the side. Normally, an adult's thorax is twice as wide as it is deep. That is, the transverse diameter of the chest wall is usually twice the anteroposterior diameter. In infants, the elderly, or patients with chronic pulmonary disease, however, the anteroposterior diameter is increased and may even be equal to the transverse diameter (Figure 5-37c), giving the patient a barrel-chest appearance.

Next, examine the posterior chest. Ask your patient to fold his arms across his chest and breathe normally during the exam. This moves his scapulae out of the way and allows you more access to his posterior lung fields. Inspect his posterior chest for deformities and symmetrical movement as he breathes. Some patients may exhibit thoracic kyphoscoliosis, an abnormal spinal curvature that deforms the chest and makes your lung exam more challenging.

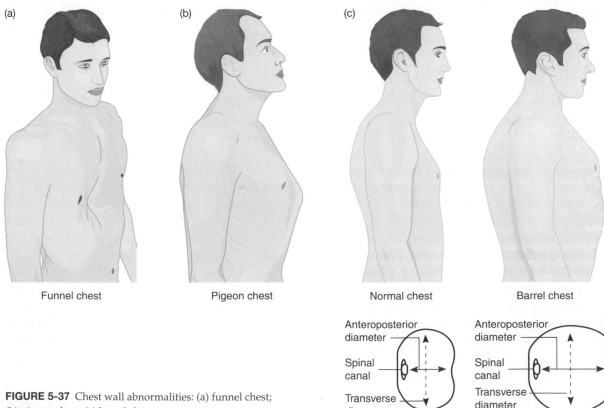

FIGURE 5-37 Chest wall abnormalities: (a) funnel chest; (b) pigeon chest; (c) barrel chest.

Inspect the intercostal spaces for retractions or bulging; both are abnormal. Retractions may appear when airflow is impeded during inspiration. Bulging may appear when airflow is impeded during exhalation. Respiratory movement should be smooth and effortless. When it is not, suspect underlying respiratory disease or structural impairment.

Palpate the rib cage for rigidity. Feel for tenderness, deformities, depressions, loose segments, asymmetry, and crepitus. Then evaluate for equal expansion. First, locate the level of the posterior 10th rib. To do this, find the lowest rib and simply move up two more ribs. An alternate method for locating the posterior 10th rib is to palpate the spinous processes. Ask your patient to touch his chin to his chest. The most prominent spinous process is the 7th cervical vertebra. Locate it and count down to T-10 in the midline.

Place your hands parallel to the 10th rib on your patient's back with your fingers spread. Lightly grasp his lateral rib cage with your spread hands (Procedure 5-8a). Ask him to inhale deeply. Normally, the distance between your thumbs will increase symmetrically by 3 to 5 centimeters during deep inspiration. If you detect decreased thoracic expansion or feel unilateral delay, suspect a disorder of the underlying lung, pleura, or diaphragm.

When your patient speaks, you can feel vibrations on his chest wall. This is known as *tactile fremitus*. Place the palm of your hand on your patient's chest wall and have him say "ninety-nine" or "one-on-one." As he does, palpate the posterior chest; feel the vibrations in different areas of the chest wall and compare symmetrical areas of the lungs (Procedure 5-8b). Identify and note any areas of increased, decreased, or absent vibrations. You will feel increased fremitus when sound transmission is enhanced through areas of consolidated lung tissue such as in a tumor, pneumonia, or pulmonary fibrosis. You will feel decreased or absent fremitus when sound transmission is diminished in a certain area, as may occur with a pleural effusion, emphysema, or pneumothorax.

Percuss your patient's posterior chest to determine whether the underlying tissues are air filled, fluid filled, or solid. Also percuss to determine the position and boundaries of the diaphragm and underlying organs. Percuss both sides of the chest symmetrically from the apex to the base at 5-centimeter intervals, avoiding bony areas such as the scapulae (Procedure 5-8c). Percuss at least twice in each area and compare both sides of the thorax. Identify and note any area of abnormal percussion. For example, a hyperresonant sound in the right chest may indicate a pneumothorax, whereas a dull sound in the same area may indicate a hemothorax. Assess the percussion sounds according to their quality, intensity, pitch, and duration. Practice percussing the chest so that you will become familiar with the normal resonance of the lungs and be able to identify abnormal sounds.

Next, assess for diaphragmatic excursion. Identify the level of the diaphragm during quiet breathing by percussing for dullness as the diaphragm moves during the respiratory cycle. Percuss at the lower rib margin on one side and note when dullness (muscle) replaces resonance (air). With a pen, mark the location of the diaphragm at the end of inhalation and at the end of exhalation. The distance between the marks is the diaphragmatic excursion. In the normal healthy adult at rest, the diaphragmatic excursion should be approximately 6 centimeters.

Measure diaphragmatic excursion on the opposite side, and compare the marks. If you find asymmetrical diaphragmatic levels, a paralyzed phrenic nerve may be the problem. Here, reevaluate your patient's respiratory depth for adequacy and provide the appropriate intervention as needed.

Auscultate your patient's chest for normal breath sounds, adventitious breath sounds, and voice sounds. Auscultate all lung fields and compare side to side. Evaluate the normal breath sounds produced by airflow through the upper and lower airways. These include tracheal, bronchial, bronchovesicular, and vesicular breath sounds (Table 5-8). Besides the normal breath sounds already mentioned, you also may hear adventitious sounds. These include crackles, wheezes, rhonchi, stridor, and pleural rubs.

Also known as *rales*, **crackles** are light crackling, popping, nonmusical sounds heard usually

CONTENT REVIEW

➤ Adventitious Breath Sounds
- Crackles
- Wheezes
- Rhonchi
- Stridor
- Pleural rubs

Table 5-8 Normal Breath Sounds

Sound	Description	Location	Duration
Tracheal	Very loud, harsh	Over the trachea	Nearly equal inspiratory and expiratory phases
Bronchial	Loud, high pitch, hollow	Over the manubrium	Prolonged expiratory phase
Bronchovesicular	Soft, breezy, lower pitch	Between the scapulae/2nd–3rd ICS lateral to the sternum	Approximately equal inspiratory and expiratory phases
Vesicular	Soft, swishy, lowest pitch	Lung periphery	Prolonged inspiratory phase

Procedure 5-8 Examining the Chest

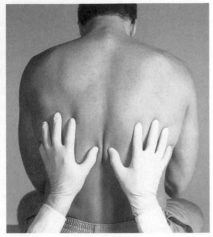

5-8a Palpate the posterior chest for excursion.

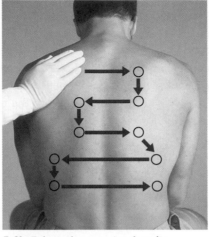

5-8b Palpate the posterior chest for tactile fremitus.

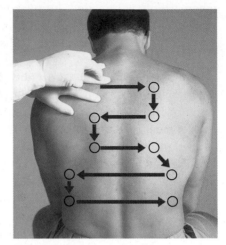

5-8c Percuss the posterior chest.

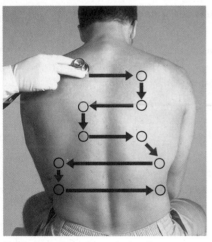

5-8d Auscultate the posterior chest.

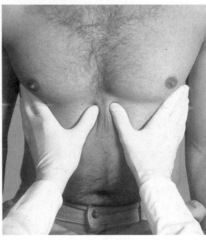

5-8e Palpate the anterior chest for excursion.

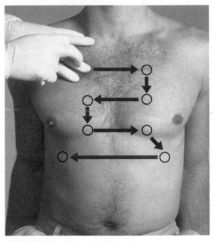

5-8f Percuss the anterior chest.

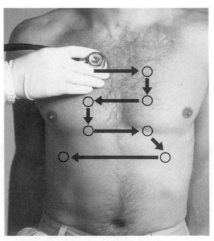

5-8g Auscultate the anterior chest.

during inspiration. They are produced by air passing through moisture in the bronchoalveolar system or from the abrupt opening of closed alveoli. Early inspiratory crackles, associated with chronic bronchitis and heart failure, begin shortly after inspiration starts, and they stop soon thereafter. These are coarse crackles—loud, low pitched, and long, similar to the sound of water boiling. They are often audible at the mouth.

Late inspiratory crackles, associated with congestive heart failure and interstitial lung diseases, begin in the first half of the inspiratory phase and continue into late inspiration. They are fine crackles—soft, high-pitched, and very brief, similar to the sound of Rice Krispies crackling. They commonly appear first at the base of the lungs and move upward as your patient's condition worsens. Usually, you can expect them to shift to dependent regions with changes in your patient's position. For example, if your heart failure patient is sitting up, expect to hear crackles first in the bases. If he is bedridden, expect to hear crackles first in the back.

Wheezes are continuous, high-pitched musical sounds similar to a whistle. They result when air moves through partially obstructed smaller airways. Their causes include asthma, bronchospasm, and foreign bodies. You may hear them without a stethoscope or by auscultating the chest during any or all phases of the respiratory cycle. They often originate in the small bronchioles and first appear at the end of exhalation. The closer to inspiration they appear, the worse your patient's condition.

Rhonchi are continuous sounds with a lower pitch and a snoring quality. They are caused by secretions in the larger airways, a common finding in bronchitis (diffuse) and pneumonia (localized). Rhonchi usually appear in early exhalation but may occur in early inspiration as well.

Stridor is a predominantly high-pitched inspiratory sound. It indicates a partial obstruction of the larynx or trachea.

Pleural friction rubs are the squeaking or grating sounds of the pleural linings rubbing together. They occur where the pleural layers are inflamed and have lost their lubrication. Pleural rubs are common in pneumonia and pleurisy (inflammation of the pleura). Because these sounds occur whenever your patient's chest wall moves, they appear during the entire respiratory cycle.

You may hear no breath sounds in some areas. This may result from effusion (fluid in the pleural space causing a decrease in functional lung tissue) or consolidation (infectious pus causing collapsed alveoli). In either case, note the area's size and intervene appropriately to ensure adequate ventilation and oxygenation of your patient.

Auscultate the posterior chest systematically. Have your patient fold his arms across his chest and breathe through his mouth more deeply and slowly than usual. Auscultate the same areas you percussed and compare the bilateral findings (Procedure 5-8d). Listen for at least one full breath at each location. Be alert for patient discomfort or hyperventilation. Note the pitch, intensity, and duration of each inspiratory and expiratory sound. If the sounds are decreased, suspect impaired airflow or poor sound transmission. If the sounds are absent, suspect no airflow. Note whether you hear sounds where you normally should. For example, when you auscultate over the peripheral lung fields, you should not hear tracheal, bronchial, or bronchovesicular breath sounds. Listen carefully and note what you hear, where you hear it, and when you hear it during the respiratory cycle. Also note whether the sounds change when your patient coughs or changes position.

If you hear abnormally located tracheal, bronchial, or bronchovesicular breath sounds, assess your patient's transmitted voice sounds. Ask him to repeat the words "ninety-nine" as you auscultate his chest wall. Normally you should hear muffled, indistinct sounds. Hearing the words clearly is an abnormal finding known as **bronchophony**. Bronchophony occurs when fluid (water, blood) or consolidated tissue (pus, tumor) replaces the normally air-filled lung. After you check your patient for bronchophony, assess him for **whispered pectoriloquy** and **egophony**. For pectoriloquy, ask your patient to whisper "ninety-nine" while you auscultate. As with bronchophony, the words will be clear and distinct if sound transmission through an area is abnormally enhanced. For egophony, ask him to repeat the long "e" sound while you auscultate. You should hear a muffled, long "e." If vocal resonance is abnormally increased, you will hear an "a" sound instead. This is known as "e to a egophony."

Your examination of the anterior chest will be similar to your examination of the posterior chest. Begin by having your patient lie supine with his arms relaxed but slightly abducted at his sides. Look for any gross deformities or asymmetrical movements. Does the chest wall rise symmetrically? Is there accessory muscle use? Look for abnormal retractions in the suprasternal, supraclavicular, and intercostal areas. Also check for callused elbows from tripoding (leaning with elbows on a table or chair arms), and finger clubbing—both common signs of chronic lung disease. Is the trachea midline or deviated? Does it tug during inhalation? In cases of tension pneumothorax, the trachea will deviate away from the affected side. In cases of pulmonary fibrosis and atelectasis, it will tug toward the affected side during inhalation.

Palpate the anterior chest for deformities and areas of tenderness. Check for chest expansion by placing your thumbs along the costal margins on both sides and gently grasping the lateral rib cage (Procedure 5-8e). Ask your patient to inhale deeply. Normally, your thumbs will separate symmetrically and the distance between them will increase from 3 to 5 centimeters. If you detect decreased thoracic expansion or feel unilateral delay, suspect a disorder of the underlying lung, pleura, or diaphragm.

Pediatric Pearls

The rib cage in infants and small children is elastic and flexible. Because it comprises more cartilage than bone at this age, rib fractures are rare. On the other hand, lung contusions are common, because the lung tissue is very fragile. Small children also have a mobile mediastinum with a greater tendency to develop a tension pneumothorax. The chest muscles are not well developed, so children are mostly diaphragm breathers until about age 7.

The chest muscles are considered accessory muscles in the young child; to evaluate his breathing, observe both the chest and abdomen for movement. A child in severe respiratory distress may exhibit a "seesaw" pattern in which his sternum

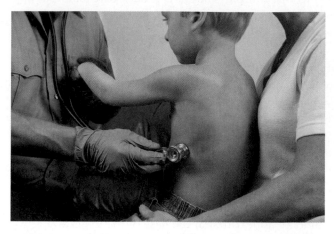

FIGURE 5-38 Place your stethoscope along your young patient's midaxillary line.

Table 5-9 Normal Pediatric Vital Signs

Age Group	Respiratory Rate	Heart Rate	Systolic BP
Newborn	30–60	100–180	60–90
Infant	30–60	100–160	87–105
Toddler	24–40	80–110	95–105
Preschooler	22–34	70–110	95–110
School Age	18–30	65–110	97–112
Adolescent	12–26	60–90	112–128

and abdomen rise and fall in opposition to each other. Count the respiratory rate without touching your patient, if possible. Assess the rate, quality, and depth of his respirations. Normal respiratory rates vary with age, but generally they decrease as the child grows older. Table 5-9 gives normal vital signs for the various pediatric age groups. Auscultate for breath sounds with the bell of your stethoscope at the midaxillary line (Figure 5-38). Use this location to avoid hearing transmitted breath sounds from the opposite lung fields.

As with the posterior chest, test for tactile fremitus, bronchophony, whispered pectoriloquy, and egophony if you detect abnormal breath sounds.

Percuss your patient's anterior chest to help determine whether the underlying tissues are air filled, fluid filled, or solid and to determine the position and boundaries of the diaphragm and underlying organs. Percuss each side of your patient's anterior chest from its apex to its base at 5-centimeter intervals at the midclavicular lines (Procedure 5-8f). Percuss at least twice in each area and compare both sides of the thorax. Identify and note any area of abnormal percussion. Remember that when percussing the right chest, you will hear dullness at the upper border of the liver. On the left side, you will hear the normal resonance of the lung change to tympany when you reach the stomach. You also will percuss an area of cardiac dullness from the third to the fifth intercostal spaces.

Finally, auscultate the anterior and lateral thorax systematically. Have your patient breathe through his mouth more deeply and slowly than usual. Auscultate the same areas you percussed and compare symmetrical areas (Procedure 5-8g). Listen for at least one full breath at each location. Be alert for patient discomfort or hyperventilation. As with posterior chest auscultation, note the pitch, intensity, and duration of each inspiratory and expiratory sound and whether you heard sounds where you should normally expect them. Listen for adventitious sounds. If you hear abnormally located tracheal, bronchial, or bronchovesicu-

lar breath sounds, assess for bronchophony, whispered pectoriloquy, and egophony.[6]

Many EMS calls involving children are for respiratory system complaints, and it is critical to adequately assess the child's respiratory system, including breath sounds. This can prove challenging when children are frightened, as they often are in the presence of strangers—especially when they are ill. Try to obtain their trust; consider having the child sit in his parent's lap.

It is often difficult to get a child to take a deep breath. Either he does not understand what you are asking, or he is afraid to comply. In these cases, some visual imagery often proves helpful. Engage the parent's assistance by pretending to hold a candle or birthday cake. Ask the child to blow, just as if he's blowing out a candle. Get the parent to do this once, and the child will often follow.

When the child prepares to "blow out the candle," listen to his chest. He will take a deep breath, and you can usually accurately auscultate the chest. Have him repeat the "candle blowing" until your auscultation is complete. As an alternative, use your fingers as the candles, folding them down as the child blows and repeating as many times as needed for adequate auscultation.

Another visualization technique is to ask the child if he's heard of the story "The Three Little Pigs." If so, have the child imitate the big bad wolf in the story and attempt to blow down the little pigs' house. When the child inhales to blow down the pigs' house, you can hear breath sounds well.

Always follow a standardized approach when assessing the chest: inspection, palpation, percussion (if indicated), and auscultation.

Heart and Blood Vessels
Anatomy and Physiology

Mentally picture the heart and great vessels as you inspect the chest (Figure 5-39).[5] The heart sits just behind the sternum between the third and sixth costal cartilages and rotated to the left. Its most anterior surface, therefore, is the right ventricle. The pulmonary artery, which carries deoxygenated blood to the lungs, leaves the right ventricle at the third costal cartilage, close to the sternum.

The left ventricle sits behind the right ventricle and a little to its left. It forms the left border of the heart and produces the apical impulse at the fifth intercostal space, near the midclavicular line. This is the point of maximal impulse (PMI), usually the same as the apical impulse, which occurs at the apex of the heart. The aorta curves upward from the left ventricle to the level of the sternal angle (second costal cartilage), arches backward, and then turns back downward. To the right of the aorta, the superior vena cava returns blood to the right atrium.

The heart is an electrical-mechanical pump. Its job is to begin the movement of blood through the circulatory system. Its effectiveness is measured by cardiac output. **Cardiac output** is the amount of blood the heart ejects each minute, measured in milliliters per minute. It is the product of the heart rate and the stroke volume. **Stroke volume** is the amount of blood the heart ejects in one beat. Changes in any of these components may severely affect cardiac output. For example, if your patient's heart rate falls to 30 beats per minute, or if a massive heart attack destroys 30 to 40 percent of his left ventricle, the cardiac output will greatly decrease.

Three factors determine stroke volume: preload, contractile force, and afterload. **Preload**, also known as end-diastolic pressure, is the amount of blood returned to the heart from the body. The greater the preload, the more the cardiac muscles will stretch, the harder they will contract, and the more blood the heart will eject (Starling's law). *Contractile force* refers to how forcefully the heart muscle contracts. It is regulated by the autonomic nervous system and the body's needs. **Afterload** refers to the resistance in the vessels that the heart must overcome to eject blood. It is determined mostly in the medium-sized arterioles.

With each contraction of your patient's heart, you should feel an arterial pulse. Blood pressure is a measurable estimate of the pressure in the circulatory system during **systole** and **diastole**. Arterial blood pressure is affected by the stroke volume (left ventricular effectiveness), the condition of the aorta and large arteries, the peripheral vascular resistance (condition of the arterioles), and the circulating blood volume. Changes in any of these components can severely affect your patient's blood pressure. For example, if your patient loses 30 to 40 percent of his blood volume or experiences massive vasodilation, his blood pressure will drop drastically.

Venous pressure, on the other hand, is much lower than arterial pressure. It will remain so unless something restricts blood flow through the heart. For example, in congestive heart failure, a weakened heart cannot effectively move all the blood it receives from the body or the lungs. The resulting backup eventually raises venous pressure. Cardiac tamponade and tension pneumothorax inhibit venous return, causing a dramatic rise in venous pressure. You can easily observe and measure increases in venous pressure in the external jugular veins.

Several changes occur with aging. Because most patients with cardiac complaints are older, an understanding of these changes is essential. Changes in chest wall diameter make it more difficult to find the apical pulse. Extra heart sounds are more common. Many older patients will have heart murmurs, especially affecting the aortic valve, which becomes stenotic over time. The aorta and large arteries stiffen from atherosclerosis, raising blood pressure. Older patients often develop mitral valve murmurs and regurgitation (backflow leakage into the left atrium during ventricular systole).

The peripheral arterial system delivers oxygenated blood to the tissues of the extremities (Figure 5-40). Where the arteries lie close to the skin, the pulse is

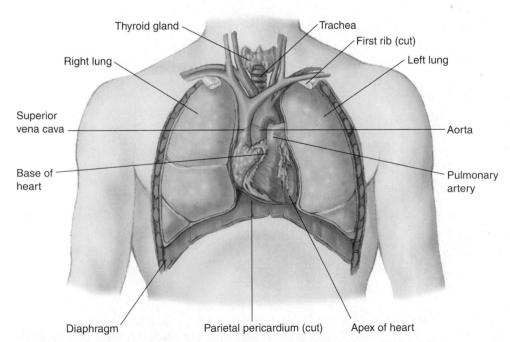

Thyroid gland — Trachea — First rib (cut) — Right lung — Left lung — Superior vena cava — Aorta — Base of heart — Pulmonary artery — Diaphragm — Parietal pericardium (cut) — Apex of heart

FIGURE 5-39 The heart and great vessels.

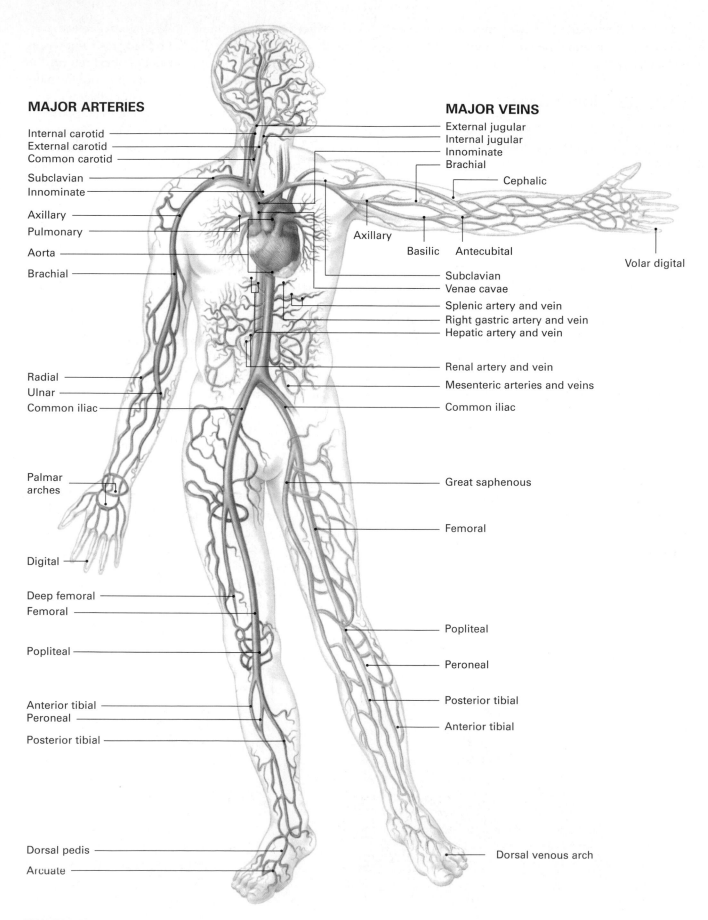

MAJOR ARTERIES

Internal carotid
External carotid
Common carotid

Subclavian
Innominate

Axillary
Pulmonary

Aorta

Brachial

Radial
Ulnar
Common iliac

Palmar
arches

Digital

Deep femoral
Femoral

Popliteal

Anterior tibial
Peroneal

Posterior tibial

Dorsal pedis

Arcuate

MAJOR VEINS

External jugular
Internal jugular
Innominate
Brachial

Cephalic

Axillary

Basilic   Antecubital

Volar digital

Subclavian
Venae cavae

Splenic artery and vein
Right gastric artery and vein
Hepatic artery and vein

Renal artery and vein
Mesenteric arteries and veins

Common iliac

Great saphenous

Femoral

Popliteal

Peroneal

Posterior tibial

Anterior tibial

Dorsal venous arch

FIGURE 5-40 The circulatory system.

palpable. The brachial artery runs along the medial humerus and delivers blood to the arm and hand. Palpate the brachial pulse just above the elbow and medial to the biceps tendon and muscle. The brachial artery splits into the radial and ulnar arteries that deliver blood to the forearm and hand. Palpate the radial artery just above the wrist on the thumb side; palpate the ulnar artery just above the wrist on the other side.

In the lower extremities, the femoral artery delivers blood to the legs and feet. Palpate the femoral artery just below the inguinal ligament midway between the anterior-superior iliac spine and the symphysis pubis. The femoral artery then branches into the popliteal artery, which passes behind the knee and is easily palpated there. Below the knee, the popliteal artery branches into the posterior tibial artery, which travels behind the tibia and can be felt just below the medial malleolus. The anterior branch can be felt as the dorsalis pedis pulse on top of the foot just lateral to the extensor tendon of the big toe.

The venous system comprises deep, superficial, and communicating veins that return blood to the heart. In the upper extremities, superficial veins are visible in the back of the hand, the inside of the arms, and in the antecubital fossa (crook of the elbow). These veins are used for venous access in the emergency setting. They eventually deliver their blood into the superior vena cava en route to the right atrium.

In the legs, the vast majority of venous return happens via deep veins. The superficial veins, however, also play an important role. The great saphenous vein originates in the foot and joins the deep vein system near the inguinal ligament. The small saphenous vein, which also begins in the foot, joins the deep system in the popliteal space behind the knee. The two saphenous systems and the deep system are connected in other places by communicating veins and anastomotic vessels. The veins of the lower extremities deliver their blood into the inferior vena cava en route to the heart. Venous flow occurs via muscular contractions that push the blood against gravity toward the heart and one-way valves that prohibit backflow.

The lymphatic system (Figure 5-41) is a network of vessels that drains fluid, called *lymph*, from the body tissues and delivers it to the subclavian vein. Lymph nodes in the neck, the axilla, and the groin help filter impurities en route to the heart. They are palpable when congested with infectious products.

The lymphatic system plays an important role in the body's immune system. It also plays an important role in our circulatory system.

When arterial blood flows into a capillary bed, hydrostatic pressure pushes fluid across the capillary membrane into the tissues. As the blood flows through the capillary bed, this pressure diminishes. Plasma proteins in the capillaries create an oncotic pressure gradient that draws fluid back into the bloodstream. On the venous side of the capillary bed, the oncotic pressure drawing fluid in is greater than the hydrostatic pressure pushing fluid out. The net effect is that fluid returns to the capillary for its return to the heart.

In a perfect system, whatever fluid enters the tissues should exit at the other end. In reality, some fluid usually

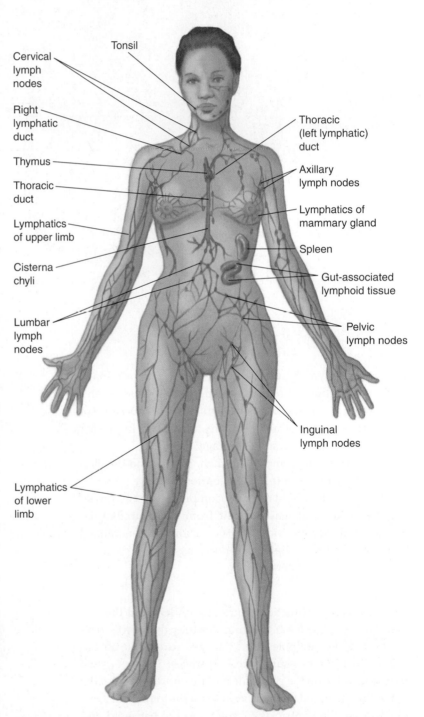

FIGURE 5-41 The lymphatic system.

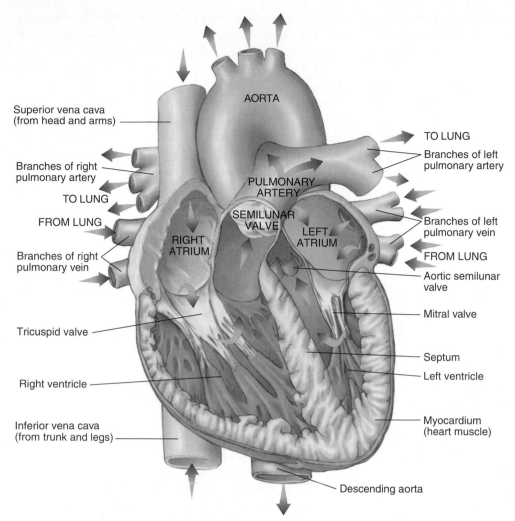

Labels (clockwise): AORTA · TO LUNG · Branches of left pulmonary artery · PULMONARY ARTERY · Branches of left pulmonary vein · FROM LUNG · Aortic semilunar valve · Mitral valve · Septum · Left ventricle · Myocardium (heart muscle) · Descending aorta · Inferior vena cava (from trunk and legs) · Right ventricle · Tricuspid valve · Branches of right pulmonary vein · FROM LUNG · TO LUNG · Branches of right pulmonary artery · Superior vena cava (from head and arms) · RIGHT ATRIUM · SEMILUNAR VALVE · LEFT ATRIUM

FIGURE 5-42 Anatomy of the heart and blood flow.

remains. The lymph system acts as an auxiliary drainage system, collecting the remaining fluid from the tissues and returning it to the heart. Tissue edema can occur because of an increase in hydrostatic pressure, a decrease in plasma proteins, or a lymph system blockage.

As we age, the arteries lengthen, stiffen, and develop atherosclerosis. A complete evaluation of your patient's circulatory system is an essential component of any physical exam. Many diseases result from poor circulation, either localized (specific artery occlusion) or generalized (cardiovascular collapse). Carefully assess your elderly patient's end-organ perfusion.[5]

Assessment

To assess cardiac function, you must understand the cardiac cycle (Figure 5-42).[4] During diastole, the heart's resting period, the ventricles relax. The pressure in the atria is greater than the pressure in the ventricles. This opens the tricuspid valve on the right side and the mitral valve on the left, allowing blood from the atria to fill the ventricles. During systole, the ventricles contract and the tricuspid and mitral valves close, preventing backflow into the atria. The

vibrations of these valves' closings generate the first heart sound—S1, or the "lub."

The increased pressure in the right ventricle opens the pulmonic semilunar valve, sending deoxygenated blood to the lungs. The increased pressure in the left ventricle opens the aortic semilunar valve, sending freshly oxygenated blood to the body. At the end of systole, as pressure in the ventricles falls, the pulmonic and aortic semilunar valves close tightly to prevent backflow. These vibrations generate the second heart sound—S2, or the "dub." This cycle repeats approximately 60 to 100 times per minute in the healthy adult at rest. Extra sounds known as *heart murmurs* result when valves do not fully open or close, causing turbulent flow that an experienced clinician can detect.

You must auscultate for heart sounds at the proper places on the chest wall (Figure 5-43). Always listen downstream. For example, because the tricuspid and mitral valves direct blood flow to the ventricles, which are toward your patient's feet, listen for S1 at the apex of the heart. This is found near the lower left

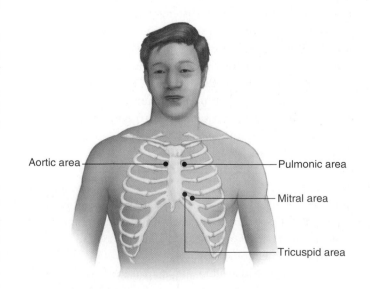

Labels: Aortic area · Pulmonic area · Mitral area · Tricuspid area

FIGURE 5-43 Sites for cardiac auscultation.

sternal border. Because the aortic and pulmonic valves direct blood flow to the lungs and aorta, which are toward your patient's head, listen for S2 at the base of the heart. This is found at the second intercostal space near the sternum.

Begin your cardiovascular assessment by inspecting for signs of arterial insufficiency or occlusion in your patient's trunk and extremities. Look for skin pallor and other signs of decreased perfusion. Assess the arterial pulses. Inspect the carotid arteries for visible pulsations just medial to the sternocleidomastoid muscles. Palpate the carotid arteries at the level of the cricoid cartilage to avoid pressing on the carotid sinus (Procedure 5-9a). Never palpate both carotids simultaneously; doing so may decrease cerebral blood flow.

Assess the carotid pulse for rate, rhythm, and quality. Does its quality vary? Do the variations correspond to respiration? For example, in pulsus paradoxus, the amplitude of the pulse diminishes with inspiration and increases with exhalation. Do you feel a vibration or humming (**thrills**) when you palpate the carotid artery? If so, auscultate the area with your stethoscope for **bruits**, the sounds of turbulent blood flow around a partial obstruction (Procedure 5-9b). The presence of a bruit suggests at least an 80 percent occlusion of the artery.

If you have not already taken your patient's blood pressure, do so now. Also check for jugular venous pressure, which approximates your patient's right atrial pressure. Position your patient supine, with his head elevated to about 45 degrees.

Adjust the head angle so the top of the jugular vein is generally in the middle of the neck. Measure the height of the venous column from the angle of Louis (i.e., second intercostal space, midsternum). Add 5 centimeters to this measurement, which determines the measurement from the chest wall to the right atrium. Examine the external jugular veins for equality of distention. Abnormal bilateral distention indicates fluid volume overload or that something such as congestive heart failure or cardiac tamponade is blocking venous return to the heart. Unilateral distention suggests a localized problem.[12] To determine whether jugular venous distention (JVD) is the result of CHF or fluid overload, place your right hand on the patient's midabdomen and apply steady pressure to indent the abdomen about 4 to 5 cm. When you do this, the blood column in the neck veins will immediately rise. The initial rise usually results when the patient performs a Valsalva maneuver (a forced exhalation against a closed glottis). If the veins remain elevated after the patient has resumed normal breathing (within 10 to 15 seconds), this finding (referred to as the *abdominojugular reflex*) is indicative of congestive heart failure.[13]

With your patient's head still raised to about 45 degrees, inspect and palpate the chest for the point of maximal impulse (PMI), or apical impulse (Procedure 5-9c).

When examining a woman with large breasts, gently displace the left breast upward and laterally, if needed, or ask her to do this for you. First, look for a pulsation at the cardiac apex, normally at the fifth intercostal space just medial to the midclavicular line. This pulsation represents the PMI. It helps you locate the left ventricle's apex. If you cannot see the pulsation, ask your patient to exhale and stop breathing for a few seconds. Lateral displacement of the PMI indicates an enlarged right ventricle.

The PMI may be displaced upward and to the left in pregnant women. If your patient is obese or has a very muscular chest wall or a barrel chest, you may not detect the PMI. Percussion may help if you have difficulty palpating the PMI. Start lateral and work your way toward the midline (Procedure 5-9d). When you hear a change from resonance (lung) to dull (heart), you have located the PMI.

Using the diaphragm of your stethoscope, auscultate your patient's anterior chest for normal heart sounds and for abnormal or extra heart sounds (Procedure 5-9e). Listen for the high-pitched sounds of S1 at the fifth intercostal space at the left sternal border (tricuspid valve) and at the PMI (mitral valve) using the diaphragm of your stethoscope. Listen for the high-pitched sounds of S2 at the second intercostal space at the right sternal border (aortic valve) and second intercostal space at the left sternal border (pulmonic valve). For a comprehensive auscultation of heart sounds, you should also listen at the third and fourth intercostal spaces. Although nothing is specifically behind those spaces, you may hear something there that you will not hear in the other places if the heart is not anatomically perfect.

Because the mitral and aortic valves (left side) close slightly before the tricuspid and pulmonic valves (right side), you may hear two sets of sounds instead of one. This is known as *splitting*. A split S1 sounds like "la-lub," a split S2 like "da-dub." Instead of "lub-dub" you will hear "la-lub—da-dub." Splitting of S2 during inspiration is normal in healthy children and young adults. Expiratory or persistent splitting suggests an abnormality.

You also may hear extra or abnormal heart sounds, depending on your patient's age and condition. A third heart sound, S3, is sometimes called the *ventricular gallop*. It is the "dee" of "lub-dub-dee" and has the same cadence as the word "Kentucky." This extra heart sound develops from vibrations that result when blood fills a dilated ventricle. Commonly heard in children and young adults, an S3 is usually considered pathological in patients over age 30. It generally develops with ventricular failure and ventricular volume overload and disappears when the problem is resolved. S3 is a low-pitched sound heard in early to mid-diastole. Listen for S3 at the apex using the bell of your stethoscope with your patient lying on his left side.

Atrial gallop is the fourth heart sound, S4. It is the "dee" of "dee-lub-dub" and has the same cadence as the word

Procedure 5-9 Assessing the Cardiovascular System

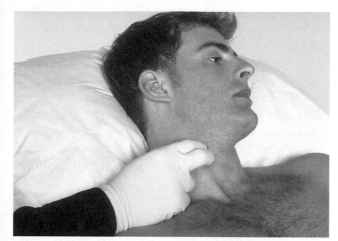

5-9a Assess the carotid pulse.

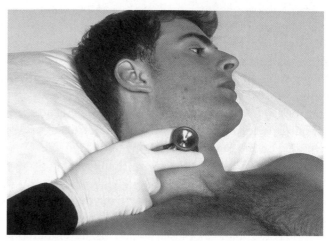

5-9b Auscultate for bruits.

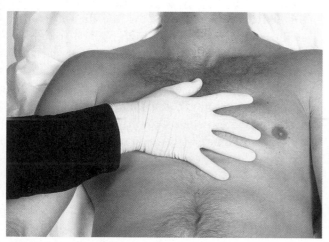

5-9c Palpate for the point of maximal impulse (PMI).

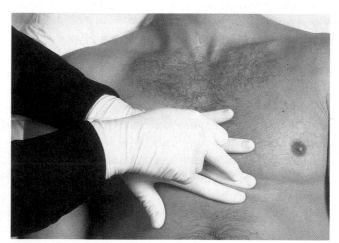

5-9d Percuss for the PMI.

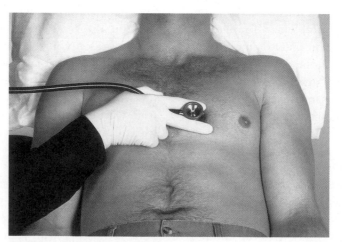

5-9e Auscultate for heart sounds.

"Tennessee." An S4 develops from vibrations produced in late diastole when atrial contraction forces blood into a ventricle that has decreased compliance or that resists filling and causes volume overload. It usually disappears when the problem is resolved. Listen for the low-pitched S4 at the apex using the bell of your stethoscope with your patient lying on his left side.

Experienced cardiologists can also detect clicks, snaps, friction rubs, and murmurs. An *ejection click* results from a stiff or stuck valve. An *opening snap* results when a stenotic mitral or tricuspid valve's leaflets recoil abruptly after ventricular diastole. A *pericardial friction rub* occurs when inflammation causes the heart's visceral and parietal surfaces to rub together at each heartbeat. A *murmur* is a rumbling or vibrating noise that results from turbulent blood flow through the heart valves, a large artery, or a septal defect.

To assess your patient's peripheral vascular system, inspect both arms from the fingertips to the shoulders. Note their size and symmetry. Observe swelling, venous congestion, the color of the skin and nail beds, and the skin texture. Yellow or brittle nails or poor color in the fingertips indicates chronic arterial insufficiency. Palpate the peripheral arteries to evaluate pulsation (Procedures 5-10a and 5-10b) and capillary refill and to assess skin temperature. To palpate a peripheral pulse, lightly place your finger pads over the artery's pulse point. Increase the pressure slowly until you feel a maximum pulsation. Note the rate, regularity, equality, and quality of the pulses. Count the number of beats in 1 minute. Then determine whether the pulse is regular, regularly irregular, or irregularly irregular.

Finally, assess the quality of the pulse by noting its amplitude and contour; rate its quality from 0 to 3+, as shown in Table 5-10. Determine whether it is absent, normal, weak, or bounding, and note any *thrills*, humming vibrations that feel similar to the throat of a purring cat. Thrills suggest a cardiac murmur or vascular narrowing. Expect the pulse of a normal adult to range between 60 and 100 beats per minute with a regular rhythm and normal amplitude.

Compare peripheral pulses bilaterally. If you detect a weak or absent pulse in one extremity, suspect an arterial occlusion proximal to the pulse point. Also compare distal and proximal pulses for equality. If you cannot palpate a distal artery, move proximally to another artery. For example, if you cannot palpate the radial artery, move to the brachial artery in the antecubital area. While you are at the elbow, you can also assess the epitrochlear lymph nodes; they will be palpable only if inflamed.

Next, assess the feet and legs. Have your patient lie down and ask him to remove his socks. Inspect the legs from the feet to the groin. Note their size and symmetry. Evaluate the presence of swelling, venous congestion,

Table 5-10 Assessing a Peripheral Pulse

Score	Description
0	Absent pulse
1+	Weak or thready
2+	Normal
3+	Bounding

the color of the skin and nail beds, and the skin texture. Note any venous enlargement. Evaluate scars, pigmentation, rashes, and ulcers. Palpate and compare the femoral pulses (Procedure 5-10c). Note the rate, regularity, equality, and quality of the pulses. Palpate the popliteal pulse behind the knee (Procedure 5-10d), the dorsalis pedis pulse on top of the foot (Procedure 5-10e), and the posterior tibial pulse just behind the medial malleolus (Procedure 5-10f).

Feel the temperature of the legs, feet, and toes with the back of your fingers and compare both sides. Unilateral coldness indicates an arterial occlusion. Bilateral coldness is due to an environmental problem, bilateral occlusion (saddle embolus), or a general circulatory problem (shock). Palpate the superficial inguinal lymph nodes for enlargement and tenderness.

Observe the legs for **edema**, the presence of an abnormal amount of fluid in the tissues. Compare one leg and foot with the other. Note their relative size and symmetry. Are veins, tendons, and bones easily visible under the skin? Edema will usually obscure these structures. Palpate for pitting edema by pressing firmly with your thumb for 5 seconds over the top of the foot, behind each medial ankle, and over the shins (Procedure 5-10g). Pitting is a depression left by the pressure of your thumb. Normally there should be no depression. If edema is present, evaluate the degree of pitting, which can range from slight to marked (Figure 5-44). You can grade the depth of the pitting according to the appropriate scale in Table 5-11. Expect the pit to disappear within 10 seconds after you release the pressure.

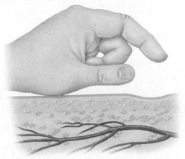
+1 Slight pitting edema

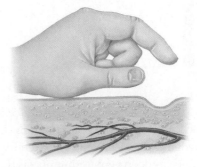
+4 Deep pitting edema

FIGURE 5-44 Assessing for edema.

Procedure 5-10 Assessing the Peripheral Vascular System

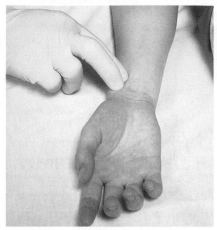

5-10a Palpate the radial artery.

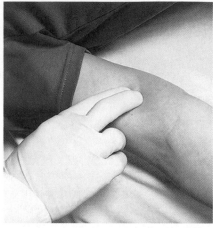

5-10b Palpate the brachial artery.

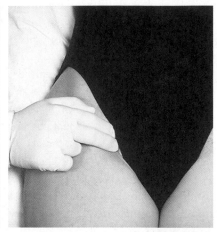

5-10c Palpate and compare the femoral arteries.

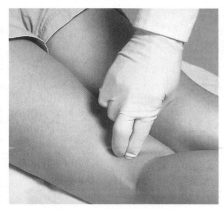

5-10d Palpate the popliteal pulse.

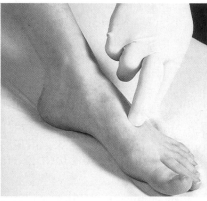

5-10e Palpate the dorsalis pedis pulse.

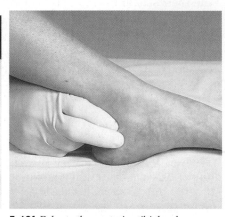

5-10f Palpate the posterior tibial pulse.

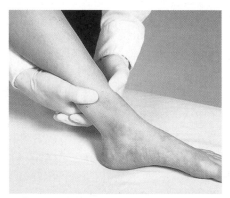

5-10g Palpate for edema.

Bilateral edema suggests a central circulatory problem, such as congestive heart failure or renal failure; unilateral edema suggests a lower extremity circulation abnormality, such as deep venous thrombosis (DVT) or venous occlusion. Note the extent of the edema. How far up the leg does it spread? The higher the edema, the more severe the problem.

During your assessment, look for visible venous distention. An associated swollen, painful leg suggests a DVT. Palpate the femoral vein just medial to the femoral artery. If you detect a tender femoral vein, flex the knee and palpate the calf for tenderness, another classic sign of DVT. Is there a local redness or warmth? Feel for a

Table 5-11 Pitting Edema Scale

Score	Description
1+	One-quarter inch (0.6 cm) or less
2+	One-quarter to one-half inch (0.6–1.2 cm)
3+	One-half to one inch (1.2–2.5 cm)
4+	One inch (2.5 cm) or more

Assessment Pearls

When you encounter a patient with a penetrating injury to an extremity, such as a gunshot or knife wound, you should always be concerned about the presence of a vascular injury. Ideally, you want to be able to palpate pulses distal to the injury. However, in certain situations (e.g., cold weather, entrapment), this can be difficult. In patients with suspected peripheral vascular disease, the oximeter probe can be placed distally to detect any perfusion. Placing the oximeter probe distal to the injury will help determine the presence and quality of perfusion and can also allow you to monitor perfusion during treatment and transport.

To accomplish this, take the probe from your pulse oximeter and apply it to the toes or fingers of the extremity in question. If peripheral perfusion is present, you should get a reading. Move the probe from toe to toe (or finger to finger) and note any difference. For example, if your patient's pulse oximetry readings drop off when you move the probe from the third to the fourth and fifth fingers, your index of suspicion about an ulnar artery injury should be raised.

Likewise, when you encounter a patient with a knee or elbow dislocation, you should always worry about vascular compromise.

cordlike vessel. Evaluate the skin for discoloration, ulcers, and unusual thickness. Finally, ask your patient to stand. Evaluate his legs for varicose veins and, if present, palpate them for signs of thrombophlebitis (redness, swelling, pain, and tenderness).

Pediatric Pearls

Unless the child has a congenital defect, his heart will be strong and healthy. His heart rate will vary with age, but generally it will decrease as he gets older. If the child is alert and uncooperative, measure his pulse rate by listening to the heart. Place your stethoscope between the sternum and nipple on your patient's left side. Children have thin chest walls, so you will usually be able to observe the apical impulse of the heart. Remember that tachycardia or bradycardia can be a response to hypoxia in infants and young children. Bradycardia is the initial response to this condition in the newborn; without aggressive intervention, cardiopulmonary arrest will soon follow. Blood pressure will vary in children, but generally it will rise as they grow older. Children respond to hypovolemia by increasing cardiac function.

Abdomen
Anatomy and Physiology

The key to evaluating the abdomen is visualizing the organs in the region you are examining. The abdominal cavity is divided into four quadrants: the right upper (RUQ), right lower (RLQ), left upper (LUQ), and left lower (LLQ). Their dividing lines intersect at the umbilicus (Figure 5-45). Age changes in the abdomen include increased fat storage around the midsection and hips and weakened abdominal musculature. The result is the "beer belly" appearance. Decreased sensation may diminish the normal signs and symptoms of serious disease. The classic signs and symptoms of abdominal diseases are often missing in the elderly.

Major organs of the digestive, urinary, reproductive, cardiovascular, and lymphatic systems lie in the abdomen. The peritoneum, a protective membrane, covers most of them.

DIGESTIVE SYSTEM Food travels down the esophagus to the stomach (in the LUQ) (Figure 5-46).[5] It then passes into the first section of the small intestine, the duodenum, where digestive enzymes from the pancreas (just behind the stomach) and gallbladder (just behind the liver in the RUQ) help digestion. Food then begins its journey through the remainder of the long small intestine (the jejunum and ileum), where the mesentery veins absorb nutrients from the food. Blood travels from the mesentery veins to the liver (RUQ) for processing and detoxification before it returns to the right heart. The appendix lies at the point where the small intestine turns into the large intestine (RLQ).

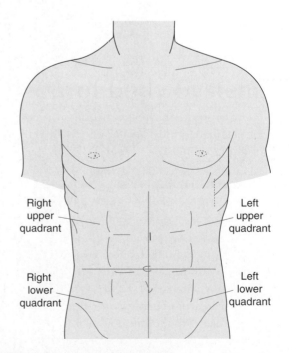

FIGURE 5-45 The abdominal quadrants.

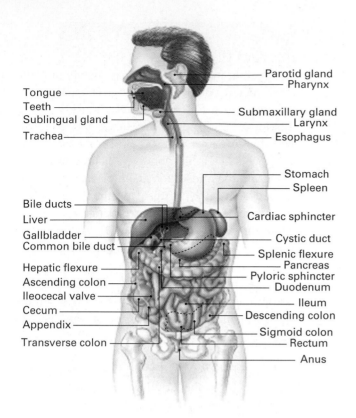

Tongue
Teeth
Sublingual gland
Trachea

Parotid gland
Pharynx
Submaxillary gland
Larynx
Esophagus

Bile ducts
Liver
Gallbladder
Common bile duct
Hepatic flexure
Ascending colon
Ileocecal valve
Cecum
Appendix
Transverse colon

Stomach
Spleen
Cardiac sphincter
Cystic duct
Splenic flexure
Pancreas
Pyloric sphincter
Duodenum
Ileum
Descending colon
Sigmoid colon
Rectum
Anus

FIGURE 5-46 The digestive system.

The large intestine, or colon, has three distinct sections: the ascending colon (RLQ to RUQ), the transverse colon (RUQ to LUQ), and the descending colon (LUQ to LLQ). The large intestine is responsible for absorbing water from the feces and returning it to the general circulation. The remaining waste continues through the sigmoid colon (LLQ), rectum (midline), and anus.

URINARY SYSTEM The kidneys are pear-shaped solid organs embedded in fat in the retroperitoneal space (RUQ, LUQ) (Figure 5-47).[5] They receive blood from the renal arteries, which branch off the abdominal aorta. The kidneys filter blood and excrete impurities, acids, and electrolytes from the blood before returning it to the general circulation. The waste product is called urine. Ureters bring the urine to the bladder, just behind the pubic bone in the midline. The urethra connects the urinary bladder to the outside.

FEMALE REPRODUCTIVE SYSTEM The ovaries (RLQ, LLQ) are walnut-sized organs that manufacture and produce the ova for fertilization (Figure 5-48). The fallopian tubes transport the ova toward the uterus (midline just above the urinary bladder). Fertilization occurs in the tubes. The fertilized ovum travels and implants in the uterus. The cervix is the opening to the uterus. The vagina is the birth canal.[5]

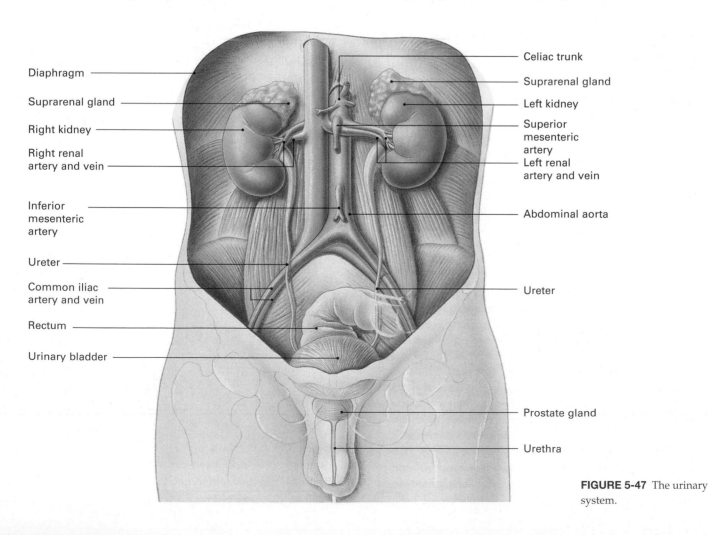

Diaphragm
Suprarenal gland
Right kidney
Right renal
artery and vein
Inferior
mesenteric
artery
Ureter
Common iliac
artery and vein
Rectum
Urinary bladder

Celiac trunk
Suprarenal gland
Left kidney
Superior
mesenteric
artery
Left renal
artery and vein
Abdominal aorta
Ureter
Prostate gland
Urethra

FIGURE 5-47 The urinary system.

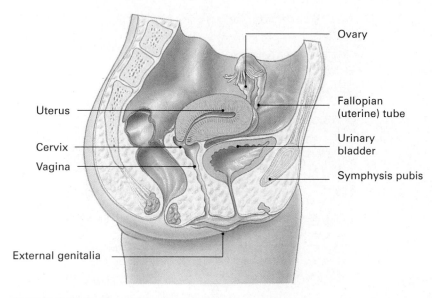

FIGURE 5-48 The female reproductive system.

MALE REPRODUCTIVE SYSTEM The testes are located in the scrotal sac and produce reproductive sperm (Figure 5-49). The sperm collect in a small reservoir called the *epididymis*, which can become inflamed. During sex, the sperm travel via the vas deferens (RLQ, LLQ) through an opening in the inguinal ligament known as the *inguinal canal*. The testicular blood supply also runs through this opening, an anatomic weak point that is the site of male hernias. The vas deferens moves the sperm toward the prostate gland, where they mix with seminal fluid and are ejected via the penile urethra.[5]

CARDIOVASCULAR SYSTEM The large abdominal aorta delivers blood from the heart to all organs of the

abdominal cavity (Figure 5-50). Palpate the aorta just to the left of the umbilicus. The inferior vena cava delivers blood that is deoxygenated and high in carbon dioxide from the abdominal organs and lower extremities to the heart. The mesenteric arteries and veins and portal circulation systems deliver blood to and from the intestines and back to the heart for general distribution.

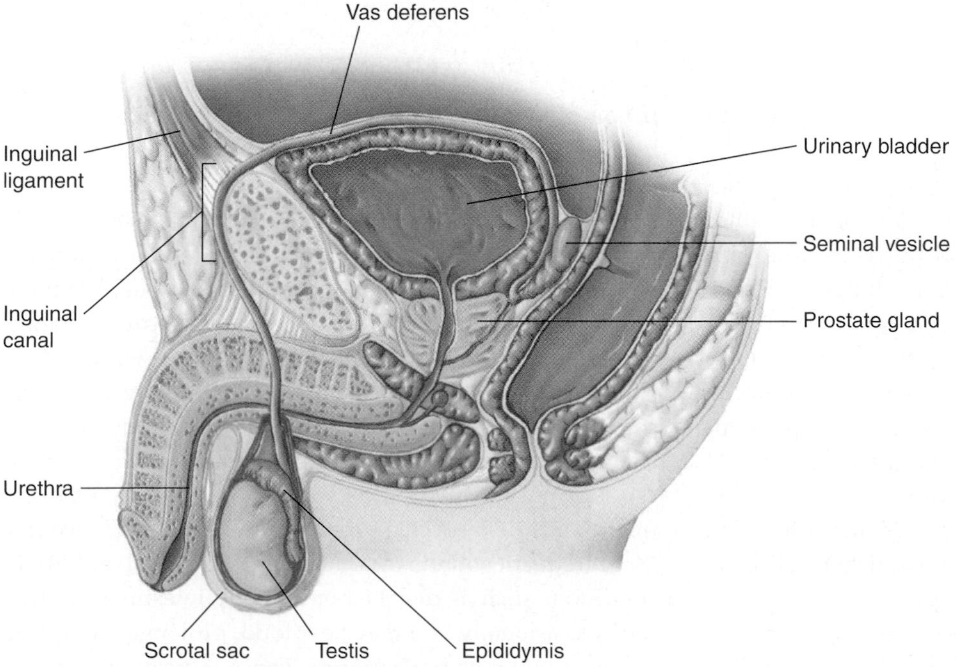

LYMPHATIC SYSTEM The spleen (LUQ) is the major organ of the lymphatic system. The vast network of lymph vessels helps drain excessive fluid and return it to the heart and aids the immune and infection control systems.

Assessment

To examine the abdomen, you need good lighting, a relaxed patient, and exposure from above the xiphoid process to the symphysis pubis.[5] Make sure that your patient does not have a full bladder. Make him comfortable in the supine position with one pillow under the head and another under the knees. Have him place his hands at his sides. This helps relax his abdominal muscles, making the examination easier for you and more comfortable for him.

Ask your patient to point out any areas of pain or tenderness. Examine these areas last. Use warm hands and a warm stethoscope and keep your fingernails short. If your hands are cold, palpate your patient through his clothes until your hands warm up. Begin your exam slowly and avoid any quick, unexpected movements.

Monitor your patient's facial expressions for pain and discomfort. During the exam, distract him with conversation or questions. Use inspection, auscultation, percussion, and palpation to perform the exam. Always auscultate before percussing or palpating, because these manipulations may alter your patient's bowel motility and resulting bowel sounds.

When you examine the abdomen, you assess the gastrointestinal organs and other nearby organs and structures. Inspect the skin of the abdomen and flanks for scars, dilated veins, stretch marks, rashes, lesions, and pigmentation changes. Look for discoloration over the umbilicus (**Cullen's sign**) or over the flanks

FIGURE 5-49 The male reproductive system.

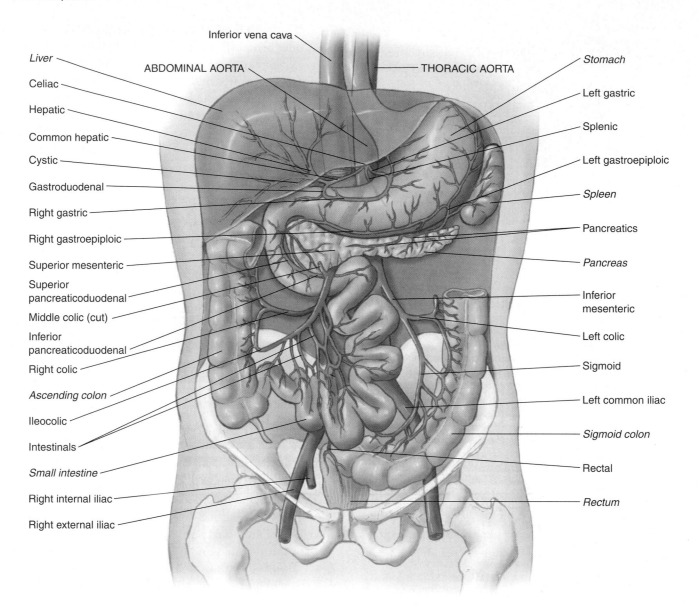

Inferior vena cava

Liver

ABDOMINAL AORTA

THORACIC AORTA

Stomach

Celiac

Left gastric

Hepatic

Splenic

Common hepatic

Left gastroepiploic

Cystic

Spleen

Gastroduodenal

Pancreatics

Right gastric

Pancreas

Right gastroepiploic

Superior mesenteric

Inferior mesenteric

Superior pancreaticoduodenal

Left colic

Middle colic (cut)

Sigmoid

Inferior pancreaticoduodenal

Left common iliac

Right colic

Sigmoid colon

Ascending colon

Ileocolic

Rectal

Intestinals

Small intestine

Rectum

Right internal iliac

Right external iliac

FIGURE 5-50 The abdominal arteries.

(**Grey Turner's sign**); these are late signs suggesting intraabdominal bleeding.

Assess the size and shape of your patient's abdomen to determine whether it is scaphoid (concave), flat, round, or distended. Ask the patient whether this is its usual size and shape. Note its symmetry. Check for bulges, hernias, or distended flanks. **Ascites** appear as bulges in the flanks and across the abdomen and indicate edema usually caused by severe liver disease, congestive heart failure, or advanced renal failure. A distended bladder or pregnant uterus can cause a suprapubic bulge. Bulges in the inguinal or femoral areas suggest a hernia.

Look at your patient's umbilicus. Note its location and contour and observe for any signs of herniation or inflammation. Check for any visible pulsation, peristalsis (the wavelike motion of organs moving their contents through the digestive tract), or masses. You may see the normal pulsation of the aorta just lateral to the umbilicus.

If you notice a bounding or exaggerated pulsation, suspect an aortic aneurysm. Visible peristalsis may indicate a bowel obstruction.

Next, auscultate for bowel sounds and other sounds such as bruits throughout the abdomen. To auscultate for bowel sounds, first warm your stethoscope's diaphragm in your hand, because a cold diaphragm might cause abdominal tension. Gently place the diaphragm on your patient's abdomen and proceed systematically, listening for bowel sounds in each quadrant. Note the location, frequency, and character of these sounds.

Normal bowel sounds consist of a variety of high-pitched gurgles and clicks that occur every 5 to 15 seconds. More frequent sounds indicate increased bowel motility in conditions such as diarrhea or an early intestinal obstruction. Occasionally you may hear loud, prolonged, gurgling sounds known as **borborygmi**. These indicate hyperperistalsis. Decreased or absent sounds suggest a paralytic

Procedure 5-11 Examining the Abdomen

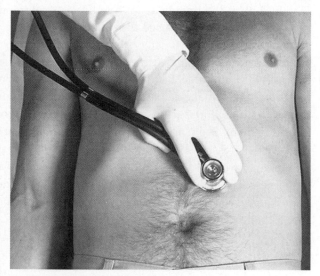

5-11a Auscultate for renal bruits.

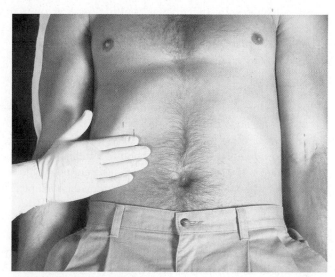

5-11b Light abdominal palpation.

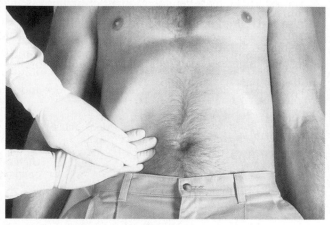

5-11c Deep abdominal palpation.

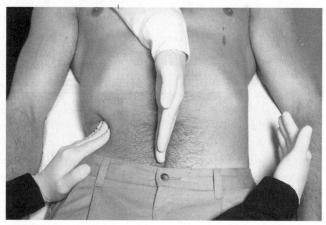

5-11d Test for ascites.

ileus or peritonitis. Listen for at least 2 minutes for bowel sounds if the abdomen is silent.

Bruits are swishing sounds that indicate turbulent blood flow. To confirm bruits, use the bell of your stethoscope and listen in areas over abdominal blood vessels such as the aorta and renal arteries (Procedure 5-11a). If you hear a bruit, suspect an arterial disorder such as an abdominal aortic aneurysm or renal artery stenosis.

Percussing the abdomen produces different sounds based on the underlying tissues. These sounds help you detect excessive gas and solid or fluid-filled masses. They also help you determine the size and position of solid organs, such as the liver and spleen. Percuss the abdomen in the same sequence you used for auscultation. Note the distribution of tympany and dullness. Expect to hear tympany in most of the abdomen; expect dullness over the solid abdominal organs, such as the liver and spleen.

Palpate the abdomen last to detect tenderness, muscular rigidity, and superficial organs and masses. Before you begin palpation, ask your patient whether he has any pain or tenderness. If he does, ask him to point to the area with one finger. Palpate that area last, using gentle pressure with a single finger. Ask him to cough and tell you if and where he experiences any pain. If coughing causes pain, suspect peritoneal inflammation.

Ask your patient to take slow, deep breaths with his mouth open, and have him flex his knees to relax his abdominal muscles. Perform light palpation by moving your hand slowly and just lifting it off the skin (Procedure 5-11b). Palpate all areas in the same sequence you used for auscultation and percussion. Watch your patient's face for signs of discomfort. Identify any masses and note their size, location, contour, tenderness, pulsations, and mobility. Abdominal pain on light palpation suggests

Assessment Pearls

Some of your patients will be, frankly, ticklish. Tickling is a tingling, tactile sensation, considered both pleasant and unpleasant, which results in laughter, smiling, and involuntary twitching movements of the head, limbs, and torso. This reaction is probably a remnant of the mammalian scratch-touch reflex. (Ever scratched a dog's stomach and watched as it rhythmically moved a leg?)

Most patients are ticklish when it comes to their abdomen. To help in the assessment of a ticklish patient, have him put his hand on his abdomen and place your hand on top of his. (A person can't tickle himself.) Continue your physical exam as best you can, using the patient's hand as a buffer. Eventually, the patient will relax and allow you to use your own hand for the exam without a ticklish response. You can then complete a comprehensive examination.

peritoneal irritation or inflammation. If you feel rigidity or guarding while palpating, determine whether it is voluntary (patient anticipates the pain or is not relaxed) or involuntary (peritoneal inflammation).

Next, palpate the abdomen deeply to detect large masses or tenderness. Use one hand on top of another and push down slowly (Procedure 5-11c). Many clinicians assess for rebound tenderness by pushing down slowly and then releasing their hands from the tender area quickly. If the peritoneum is inflamed, your patient will experience pain when you let go. Having your patient simply cough will accomplish the same thing without causing him excessive pain. Another method is to simply hold your hand 1 centimeter above your patient's abdomen at rest. Then ask him to push his abdomen out to touch your hand. Limitation by pain suggests peritoneal irritation.

If you note a protruding abdomen with bulging flanks and dull percussion sounds in dependent areas, you might perform two tests for ascites. First, assess for areas of tympany and dullness while your patient is supine. Then ask him to lie on one side. Percuss again, noting once more any areas of tympany and dullness. If your patient has ascites, the area of dullness will shift down to the dependent side and the area of tympany will shift up.

To test for fluid wave, ask an assistant to press the edge of his hand firmly down the midline of your patient's abdomen (Procedure 5-11d). With your fingertips, tap one flank and feel for the impulse's transmission to the other flank through excess fluid. If you detect the impulse easily, suspect ascites.

Pediatric Pearls

A child's liver and spleen are proportionally larger and more vascular than an adult's. Thus, they extend beyond the rib cage and are more exposed. Likewise, the child's immature abdominal muscles provide less protection than an adult's. Inspect the abdomen first for movement. Normally, only respiratory movements should be visible; peristalsis is not normally observable.

Next, assess contour. The abdomen normally bulges by the end of inspiration. Note any asymmetry. Inspect the groin area for inguinal hernias, common in male children. Finally, look at the umbilicus for any hernias, common in children under 3 years of age. Percuss and auscultate the abdomen as in the adult.

Before you begin palpating the abdomen, make sure the child is comfortable. Bend his knees to relax the abdominal muscles and make palpation easier. Your hands should be warm. If the child is ticklish, cover his hands with yours as you palpate. Begin with light palpation and gradually increase the pressure. Palpate all four quadrants. Deep palpation is performed next. You are feeling for masses and tenderness. The child's facial expression is a better guide to pain than his words, because he may interpret your pressure as pain.

Female Genitalia

Anatomy and Physiology

The external female genitalia consist of highly vascular tissues that protect the entrance to the birth canal (Figure 5-51). The mons pubis is the hair-covered fat pad that covers the pubic symphysis. The labia majora and labia minora are rounded folds of tissue that protect the opening to the vagina. Extensions of the labia form the prepuce and clitoris.

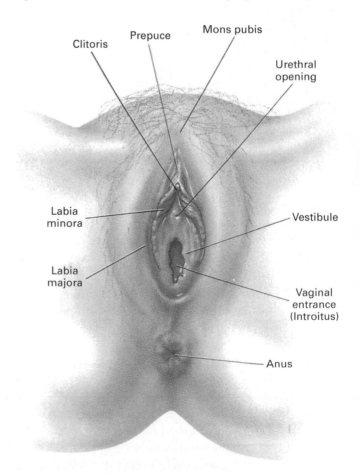

FIGURE 5-51 The external female genitalia.

The vagina is the receptacle for the penis during sexual intercourse. The urethral opening lies between the clitoris and the vagina. The perineum refers to the tissue between the vagina and the anus.

The external genital organs begin to mature and take adult proportions during adolescence. Puberty also marks the appearance of breast buds, pubic hair, and the first period (menarche). The age in which sexual development occurs varies among individuals. As women grow older, ovarian function diminishes, menstrual periods cease, and pubic hair becomes gray and sparse. The labia and clitoris become smaller; the vagina narrows and shortens and its lining (the mucosa) becomes thin, pale, and dry. The ovaries and uterus decrease in size.

Assessment

Except in cases of trauma or abuse, you rarely would be expected to examine the female genitalia. Before examining the external female genitalia, make sure that the room is warm and quiet and that your patient's bladder is empty. Be sure to maintain privacy during this examination. To reduce any anxiety or embarrassment your patient may feel, explain what you are doing during the exam. Expose her body areas only as necessary, be sensitive to her feelings, and project a professional demeanor. Place a pillow under her head and shoulders to help relax her abdominal muscles.

Begin your assessment by inspecting your patient's external genitalia. Look at the mons pubis, labia, and perineum for abnormalities such as inflammation, swelling, or lesions. These abnormalities may signal a sebaceous cyst or a sexually transmitted disease, such as syphilis or a herpes simplex virus infection. Check the bases of the pubic hair for signs of lice, such as excoriation or small, itchy, red maculopapules.

Retract the outer labia and inspect the inner labia and urethral meatus (opening). Assess for vaginal discharge. The normal discharge is clear or cloudy and has little or no odor. A white, curdlike discharge with no odor or a yeasty, sweet odor may suggest a fungal infection (candidiasis). A yellow, green, or gray discharge with a foul or fishy odor may suggest a bacterial infection (gonorrhea or *Gardnerella*).

Examining the external female genitalia can be an embarrassing, uncomfortable experience, especially for male clinicians. Remember, it is probably twice as awkward for your patient. It is customary for male clinicians to have a female partner present during the examination.

Male Genitalia

Anatomy and Physiology

The external male genitalia consist of the penis and scrotum. The penis is the male organ for copulation. It houses the urethra and specialized erectile tissue (Figure 5-52). The scrotum contains the testes. The glans, a conical structure at the end of the penis, is covered by a fold of skin called the foreskin, or prepuce. The foreskin may have been surgically removed by circumcision.

The genital organs begin to mature and take adult proportions during adolescence. Puberty also marks a noticeable increase in the size of the testes. As in the female, the actual age in which sexual development occurs will vary widely. As men grow older, the penis decreases in size and the testes hang lower in the scrotum. The pubic hair becomes gray and sparse.

Assessment

Except for trauma, you rarely would be expected to inspect the male genitalia. Before examining the male genitalia,

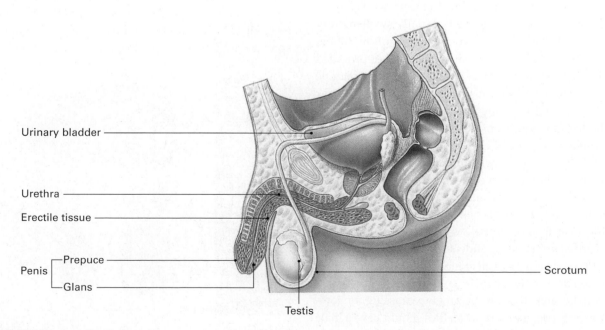

FIGURE 5-52 Male reproductive anatomy.

make sure that the room is warm and quiet and that your patient's bladder is empty. Be sure to maintain privacy during this examination. To reduce any anxiety or embarrassment your patient may feel, explain what you are doing during the exam. Expose his body areas only as necessary, be sensitive to his feelings, and project a professional demeanor.

Begin your assessment by inspecting your patient's penis and scrotum. Note any inflammation and inspect the skin around the base of the penis for abnormalities, such as lesions that may be caused by sexually transmitted diseases. Also check the bases of the pubic hair for signs of lice, such as excoriation or small, itchy, red maculopapules.

Next, inspect the glans for signs of degeneration or other abnormalities. If the foreskin is present, ask your patient to retract it. Assess any discharge from the urethral meatus. Normally, no discharge is present. A profuse, yellow discharge may be a sign of gonorrhea. A scant, clear or white discharge may suggest a nongonococcal urethritis.

Inspect the anterior surface of the scrotum and note its contour. Then, lift the scrotum to inspect its posterior surface and note any swelling or lumps. Always check the testicles in male patients with abdominal pain. Many cases of male abdominal pain are actually the result of problems in the testicles—especially in children. During development, the testicles are in the abdomen and (usually) descend into the scrotum before birth. Thus, pain from the testicles can often be interpreted as abdominal pain because of the innervation of the testicles.

Testicular torsion (twisting of the testicle on the spermatic cord) is the most common pediatric genitourinary emergency. The testicles hang freely in the scrotum and, in certain situations, can twist. (The right testicle usually twists counterclockwise and the left usually twists clockwise.) When this occurs, blood flow to the testicle is cut off, causing pain. The torsed testicle is usually swollen, very tender to touch, and rides higher in the scrotum. Often, associated vomiting is present. If surgery is not provided to relieve the torsion within 6 hours, the testicle may be lost. Expect acute epididymitis or testicular torsion if your patient has scrotal swelling and lower abdominal pain. Testicular torsion requires immediate intervention.

Priapism is a painful and prolonged erection of the penis. In the trauma patient, it may indicate cervical spine injury with autonomic nervous system dysfunction. Nontraumatic causes are many and include sickle cell disease and other blood disorders, as well as drug overdose, including overdose of erectile dysfunction medications such as vardenafil (Levitra), sildenafil (Viagra) and tadalafil (Cialis). Priapism is a medical emergency requiring prompt intervention by a urologist or emergency physician.

Again, because this can be an embarrassing, uncomfortable experience, female paramedics should have a male partner present during this type of examination.

Anus

Anatomy and Physiology

The rectum and anus mark the most distal end of the gastrointestinal system (Figure 5-53). The anal canal is approximately 2.5 to 4.0 cm long and is kept closed by the internal and external anorectal sphincters. The internal ring has smooth muscle that the autonomic nervous system controls. When the rectum fills with feces, the internal sphincter relaxes, resulting in the urge to defecate. Because the external sphincter has striated muscle, defecation is under voluntary control.

The lower half of the anal canal contains sensory fibers, whereas the upper half is somewhat insensitive. Hence, many problems of the lower anus cause pain, but those in the upper region do not. The lower anus is also rich in venous circulation, promoting internal and external hemorrhoids.

Assessment

Examining the anus is normally not a prehospital assessment practice. Unless your patient presents with rectal bleeding, there will be no reason for you to examine this area. Because routine internal rectal and prostate examinations are beyond the scope of this course, this section will focus on the external anal exam. As always, your aim is gentleness, a calm demeanor, and talking to your patient about what you are doing.

Before examining the anus, make sure the room is warm and quiet. Be sure to maintain privacy during this examination. To reduce any anxiety or embarrassment your patient may feel, explain what you are doing during the exam. Drape your patient appropriately and expose his body areas only as necessary; be sensitive to his feelings and project a professional demeanor. Place your patient on his left side with his legs flexed and his buttocks near the edge of the examination table. Glove your hands and spread the buttocks apart. Inspect the sacrococcygeal and

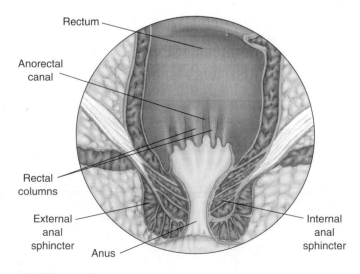

FIGURE 5-53 The anus.

perianal areas for lumps, ulcers, inflammations, rashes, or excoriation. Palpate any abnormal areas carefully and note any tenderness or inflammation. If appropriate, obtain a fecal sample and test it for occult blood. Simply smear a small sample onto a special test slide and add a couple of drops of developer onto the sample. If it turns blue, there is blood in the stool.

Musculoskeletal System

Anatomy and Physiology

The musculoskeletal system consists of at least 206 bones and their associated muscles, tendons, ligaments, and cartilage.[5] Its main functions are to give form to the body and to allow for movement. Skeletal muscle is attached to bone by tendons (Figure 5-54). The proximal attachment is the *origin*, and the distal attachment is the *insertion*. When a muscle contracts, the distal attachment usually moves toward the origin. Movement of one bone on another occurs at a joint. In an elaborate system, the muscles and tendons act like ropes, the bones like levers, and the joints like fulcrums to make movement possible.

Each joint's structure, along with the number and size of the surrounding ligaments, determines its range of motion. Hinge joints, such as the fingers and elbows, allow only flexion and extension (Figure 5-55). Ball-and-socket joints, such as the shoulder and hip, allow rotation and a wide range of motion. Saddle joints, such as those in the thumbs, permit movement in several planes. Condyloid joints, such as the wrist, are similar to ball-and-socket joints but do not allow rotation. Gliding joints, such as those in the hands and feet, permit a movement in which one bone slides across another. Pivot joints, as in the first two cervical vertebrae, allow a turning motion.

The bones within a joint do not touch each other (Figure 5-56). Instead, their articulating surfaces are covered with cartilage. A synovial membrane at the outer margins of the cartilage creates a synovial cavity into which it secretes synovium, a viscous lubricating fluid. A joint capsule surrounds and protects the synovial capsule. In turn, strong ligaments surround the joint capsule and extend to the articulating bones. In some joints, such as those in the spinal column, cartilaginous disks instead of synovial cavities separate the bones. These disks cushion the vertebrae and absorb shocks.

Bursae—fluid-filled, disk-shaped sacs—lie between the skin and the convex surface of a bone where friction may occur. They appear where tendons or muscles might rub against a bone or ligament or another muscle or tendon, such as in the knee and shoulder.

The musculoskeletal system's most obvious physical change with age is the gradual shortening in height. This occurs because the intervertebral disks become thinner and may even collapse. As a result, your patient's limbs may appear longer than they should in proportion to his trunk. The other visible change is in posture. The anteroposterior diameter of the chest increases owing to kyphosis (abnormal curvature of the spine), particularly in women. In addition, skeletal muscles decrease in size and strength, and the ligaments lose some of their pliability. As a result, the range of motion decreases. Osteoporosis also contributes to this loss of mobility.

Assessment

An examination of the musculoskeletal system must include a detailed assessment of function and structure. Inspect and palpate your patient's joints, their structure, their range of motion, and the surrounding tissues.[11] Begin your assessment with a general observation of posture, build, and muscular development. Watch the way your patient's body parts move, and observe their resting positions.

Begin the exam with your patient sitting to evaluate his head, neck, shoulders, and upper extremities. Then have him stand to assess his chest, back, and ilium; ask him to walk, so you can assess his gait. Finally, ask him to lie down, so you can examine his hips, knees, ankles, and feet.

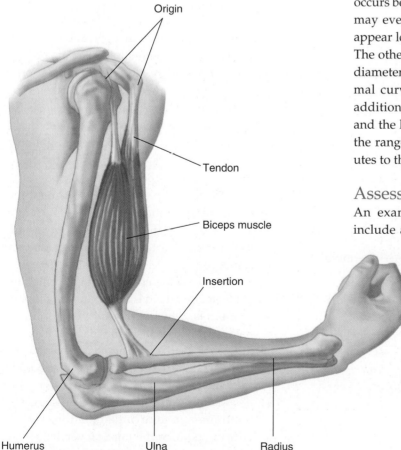

FIGURE 5-54 Interaction of bone, muscle, and tendon.

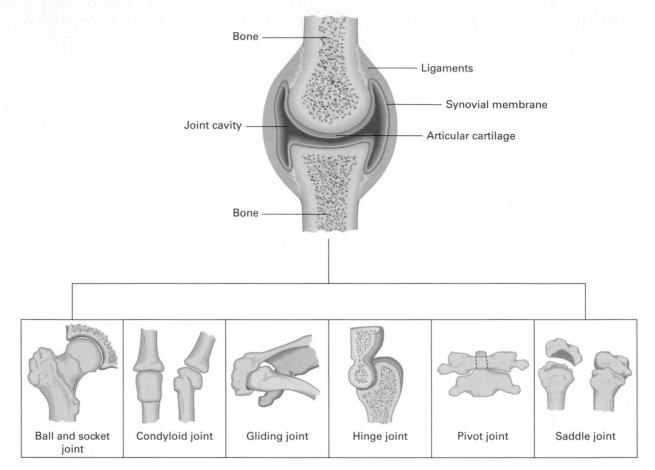

FIGURE 5-55 Types of joints.

Inspect for swelling in or around joints, changes in the surrounding tissue, redness of the overlying skin, deformities, and symmetry of impairment. Swelling may be caused by trauma to the area or by excess synovial fluid in the joint space or tissues surrounding the joint. Tissue changes may include muscle atrophy, skin changes, and subcutaneous nodules resulting from rheumatoid arthritis or rheumatic fever. Skin redness may suggest inflammation or arthritis. Deformities may be produced by restricted range of motion, misalignment of the articulating bones, dislocation (complete separation of bone ends), or subluxation (partial dislocation). Symmetrical impairment is usually associated with a disorder such as rheumatoid arthritis.

Inspect and palpate each body part, then test its range of motion and muscle strength, as explained in the "Motor System" section later in this chapter. Examine each joint and compare joints on opposite sides for equal size, shape, color, and strength. Swelling in a joint usually involves the synovial membrane or a bursa, which will feel spongy on deep palpation within the joint space. It also may involve the surrounding structures, such as ligaments, cartilage, tendons, or the bones themselves.

Redness of the overlying skin suggests a nontraumatic joint inflammation, such as arthritis, gout, or rheumatic fever. Palpate for tenderness in and around the joint. Try to identify the specific structure that is tender,

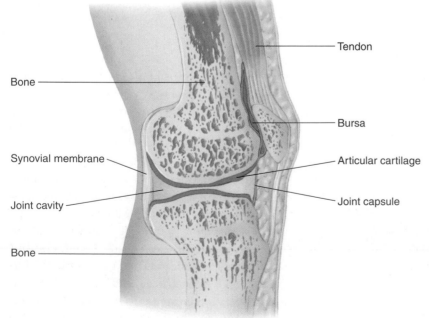

FIGURE 5-56 A synovial joint.

such as a ligament or tendon. Some common causes of a tender joint include arthritis, tendonitis, bursitis, or osteomyelitis. With the back of your hand, feel over the tender area for increased temperature, which suggests arthritis.

After you have inspected and palpated each body part with your patient at rest, assess range of motion. Test each joint for passive range of motion, range of motion against gravity, and range of motion against resistance. First, test the joint's passive range of motion by moving it in the directions that it normally allows. For example, test the elbow—a hinge joint—for flexion and extension. Note any resistance and whether the range of motion is within normal limits. Test the range of motion against gravity by asking your patient to perform the same movements by himself. Again, note the range of motion and any difficulties. Finally, test the range of motion against resistance. Have your patient perform the same movements while you apply resistance.

Passive and active ranges should be equal. A discrepancy indicates either a muscle weakness or a joint problem. If your patient has difficulty with passive and active tests, suspect a joint problem. If he has difficulty only with active tests, suspect a weakened muscle or nerve disorder. A decreased range of motion could indicate arthritis or injury, whereas an increased range of motion suggests a loosening of the structures that support the joint.

Listen for **crepitus**, the crunching sounds of unlubricated parts rubbing against each other, while you manipulate the joint. Crepitus may indicate an inflamed joint or osteoarthritis. An obvious traumatic deformity could indicate a sprained ligament, a bone fracture, or a dislocation. In these cases, modify your manipulation and range-of-motion exam accordingly. Nontraumatic deformities are caused by arthritis or the misalignment of bones. Avoid manipulating a painful joint.

The extremities are the arms and legs. A complete examination of your patient's extremities will include wrists and hands, elbows, shoulders, ankles and feet, knees, and hips.

WRISTS AND HANDS   The radius and ulna articulate with the carpal bones at the wrist, or *radiocarpal joint* (Figure 5-57). The carpals articulate with the metacarpals. The metacarpals articulate with the proximal phalanges at the metacarpophalangeal (MCP) joint. The proximal phalanges articulate with the middle phalanges at the proximal interphalangeal (PIP) joint. The middle phalanges articulate with the distal phalanges at the distal interphalangeal (DIP) joint. Movement at the wrist includes flexion, extension, radial deviation, and ulnar deviation. Movement at the

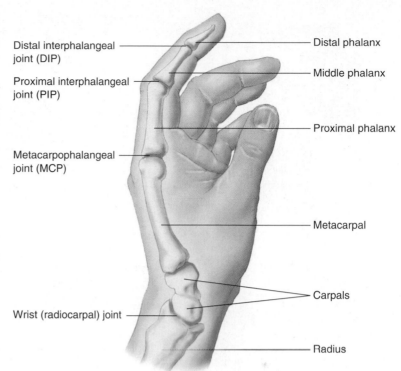

FIGURE 5-57 Bones and joints of the hand and wrist.

MCP, PIP, and DIP joints includes flexion and extension. The MCP joints also allow abduction (spreading the fingers out) and adduction (bringing them back together). The major flexor muscles are the flexor carpi radialis and flexor carpi ulnaris (Figure 5-58). The major extensor muscles are the extensor carpi radialis longus, extensor carpi radialis brevis, and extensor carpi ulnaris.

Begin by inspecting your patient's hands and wrists. Next, palpate them by feeling the medial and lateral aspects of the DIP joints and then the PIP joints with your thumb and forefinger (Procedure 5-12a). Note any swelling, sponginess, bony enlargement, or tenderness. Then, palpate the tops and bottoms of these joints in the same manner. Ask your patient to flex his hand slightly so you can examine each MCP. Compress the MCP joints by squeezing the hand from side to side between your thumbs and fingers and note any swelling, tenderness, or sponginess (Procedure 5-12b). Finally, palpate each wrist joint with your thumbs and note any swelling, sponginess, or tenderness (Procedure 5-12c). If your patient has had swelling of both his wrists or his finger joints for several weeks, suspect an inflammatory condition such as rheumatoid arthritis.

To assess range of motion, ask your patient to make a fist with each hand and then to open his fist and extend and spread his fingers. He should be able to make a tight fist and spread his fingers smoothly and easily. Next, ask him to flex and then extend his wrist. Normal flexion is 90 degrees, extension 70 degrees (Procedure 5-12d). Check for radial and ulnar deviation by asking your patient to flex

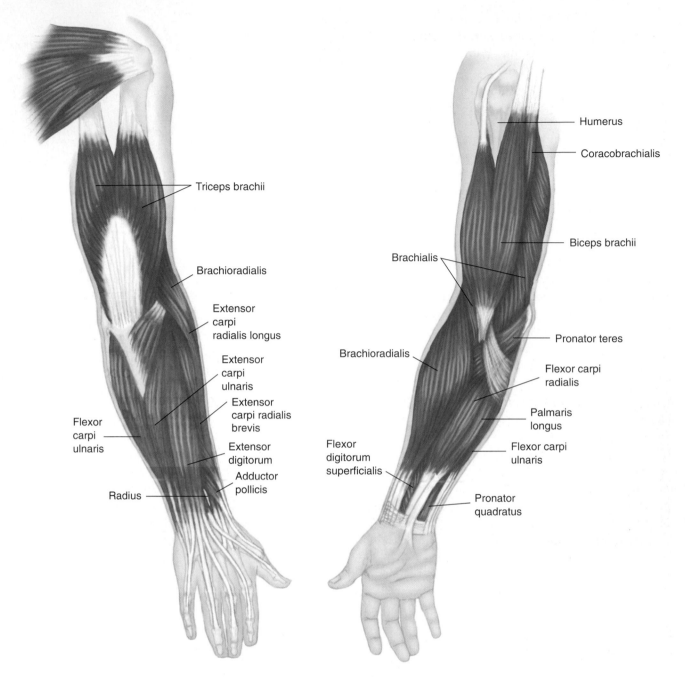

Triceps brachii

Brachioradialis

Extensor carpi radialis longus

Extensor carpi ulnaris

Extensor carpi radialis brevis

Flexor carpi ulnaris

Extensor digitorum

Adductor pollicis

Radius

Humerus

Coracobrachialis

Biceps brachii

Brachialis

Pronator teres

Brachioradialis

Flexor carpi radialis

Palmaris longus

Flexor digitorum superficialis

Flexor carpi ulnaris

Pronator quadratus

FIGURE 5-58 Muscles of the arm.

his wrist and move his hands medially and laterally. Normal radial movement is 20 degrees, ulnar movement 45 degrees (Procedure 5-12e).

If your patient complains of hand pain and numbness, especially at night, suspect carpal tunnel syndrome, the painful inflammation of the median nerve. To detect additional signs of this disorder, hold your patient's wrists in acute flexion for 60 seconds (Procedure 5-12f). In carpal tunnel syndrome, he will develop numbness or tingling in the areas innervated by the median nerve—the palmar surface of his thumb, index, and middle fingers, and part of his ring

finger. Throughout these maneuvers, watch for deformities, redness, swelling, nodules, or muscular atrophy.

ELBOWS The lateral and medial epicondyles (large rounded edges) of the distal humerus, the olecranon process of the proximal ulna, and the proximal radius constitute the elbow joint (Figure 5-59). Between the olecranon process and skin lies a bursa. The ulnar nerve (the "funny bone" nerve) extends through the groove between the olecranon process and the medial epicondyle. The elbow is a hinge joint, allowing flexion and extension. The major flexor muscles

Procedure 5-12 Examining the Wrist and Hand

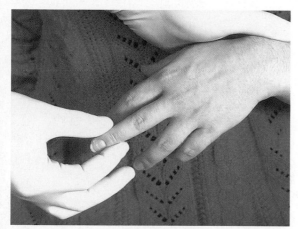

5-12a Palpate the DIP and PIP joints.

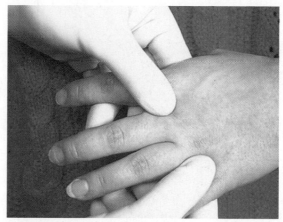

5-12b Palpate the MCP joints.

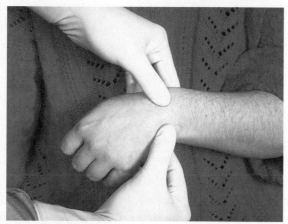

5-12c Palpate the wrist.

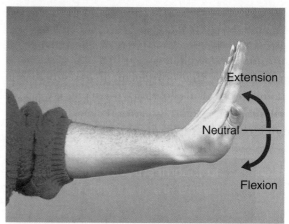

Extension

Neutral

Flexion

5-12d Assess wrist flexion and extension.

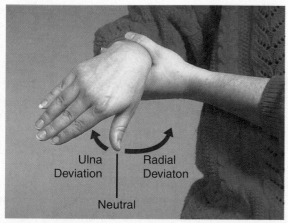

Ulna Deviaton

Radial Deviaton

Neutral

5-12e Assess radial and ulnar deviation.

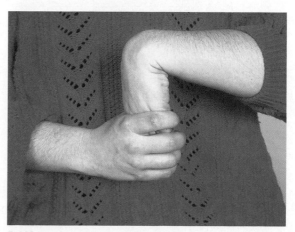

5-12f Test for carpal tunnel syndrome.

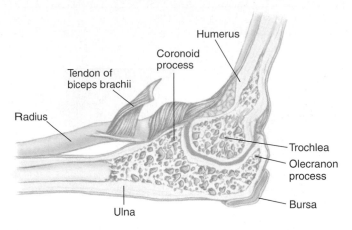

FIGURE 5-59 The elbow.

are the biceps (Figure 5-60). The major extensor muscles are the triceps (Figure 5-61). Just below the elbow, the relationship of the radius and ulna to the pronator and supinator muscles allows the forearm to supinate (turn palm up) and pronate (turn palm down) (Figure 5-62).

To examine the elbow, support your patient's forearm with your hand so that his elbow is flexed about 70 degrees (Procedure 5-13a). Inspect the elbow joint and note any deformities, swelling, or nodules. Palpate the joint struc-

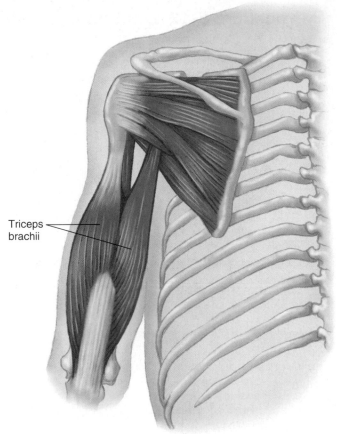

Posterior

FIGURE 5-61 Elbow extensors.

tures for tenderness, swelling, or thickening. Press on the medial and lateral epicondyles (Procedure 5-13b). Inflammation of either the medial epicondyle (tennis elbow) or of the lateral epicondyle (golfer's elbow) suggests tendonitis at those muscle insertion sites. To assess range of motion, ask your patient to flex and extend his elbow (Procedure 5-13c). Normally he will flex his elbow up to 160 degrees and return it to the neutral position. Then ask him to keep his elbows flexed and his arms at his sides. Now, have him turn his palms up and then down. Normally, both supination and pronation are 90 degrees (Procedure 5-13d).

SHOULDERS The shoulder girdle consists of articulations between the clavicle and the scapula and between the scapula and the head of the humerus (Figure 5-63). The sternoclavicular joint, which joins the clavicle and the manubrium, is the only bony link between the upper extremity and the axial skeleton. Movement at this joint is largely passive and occurs as a result of active movements of the scapula. The distal clavicle articulates with the acromion, or acromion process, of the scapula at the acromioclavicular (AC) joint. The clavicle acts as a strut, keeping the upper limbs away from the thorax and permitting a greater range of motion. The AC joint also helps provide stability

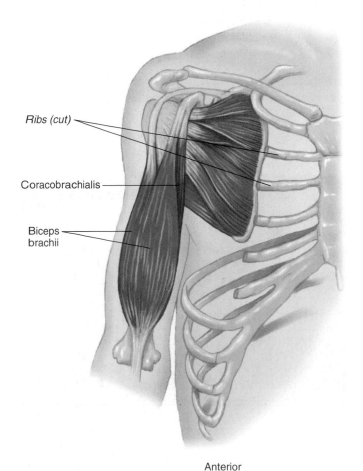

Anterior

FIGURE 5-60 Elbow flexors.

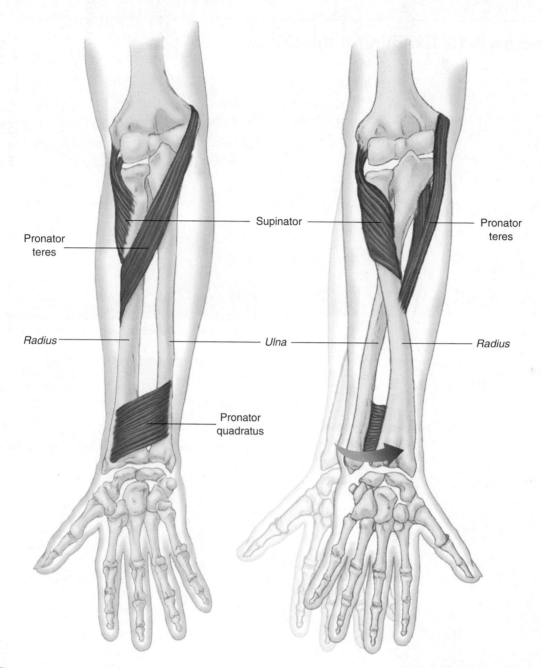

FIGURE 5-62 Pronator–supinator muscles.

to the upper limbs, reducing the need for muscle energy to keep the shoulders in their proper alignment.

The glenohumeral joint is a ball-and-socket joint that allows flexion, extension, internal and external rotation, abduction, and adduction. It has the greatest range of motion of any joint in the body and as a result is the most frequent site for dislocation. The head of the humerus (ball) fits into the glenoid cavity (socket) of the scapula. The proximal humerus has two rounded protrusions called the greater and lesser tubercles. The biceps tendon runs through the bicipital groove between the greater and lesser tubercles and is easily palpable on the lateral surface of the shoulder.

The glenohumeral joint is encapsulated and reinforced by the tendons and four muscles that make up the rotator cuff and by the large deltoid muscle (Figure 5-64 and Fig-

ure 5-65). The muscles of the rotator cuff include the supraspinatus, the infraspinatus, the teres minor, and the subscapularis muscles.

To assess range of motion, ask your patient to raise both arms forward and then straight overhead (flexion) (Procedure 5-14b). Expect to see forward flexion of 180 degrees. Next, ask him to extend both arms behind his back (extension). Normal extension is 50 degrees. Have him raise both arms overhead from the side (abduction) (Procedure 5-14c). Normal abduction is 180 degrees. Then, ask him to lower his arms and swing them as far as he can across his body (adduction). Normal shoulder adduction is 75 degrees. Finally, have him abduct his shoulders to 90 degrees, pronate, and flex his elbows 90 degrees to the front of his body.

Procedure 5-13 Examining the Elbow

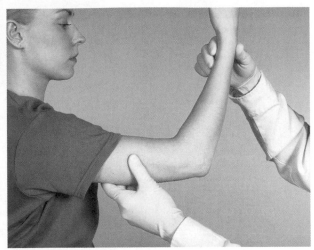

5-13a Inspect the elbow.

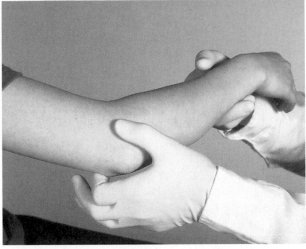

5-13b Palpate the lateral and medial epicondyles.

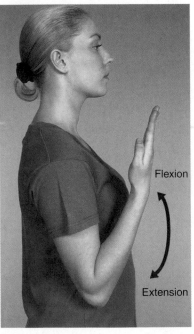

5-13c Assess elbow flexion and extension.

Flexion

Extension

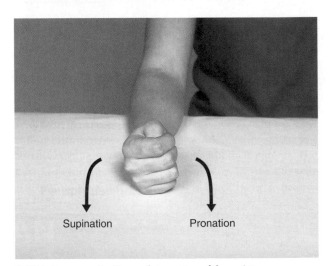

5-13d Assess supination and pronation of the wrist.

Supination   Pronation

Assessment Pearls

Dugas Sign. It is sometimes difficult to determine whether a patient has a dislocated shoulder. A shoulder may dislocate during the injury and reduce (go back into normal position) when the patient relaxes. To test for shoulder dislocation, consider testing for the Dugas sign. Have the patient place the hand of the affected side on the opposite shoulder and then have him bring his elbow to his chest. If he cannot bring his elbow to his chest (Dugas sign), the shoulder is likely dislocated. To assess your patient's shoulders, look at them from the front and then look at the scapulae from the back. Inspect the

entire shoulder girdle for swelling, deformities, or muscular atrophy. Before you palpate, ask your patient if he has any pain in his shoulders. If so, have him point to it with one finger; palpate this area last. Palpate the shoulders with your fingertips, moving along the clavicles out toward the humerus (Procedure 5-14a). Palpate the sternoclavicular joint, AC joint, subacromial region, and the bicipital groove for tenderness (biceps tendonitis) or swelling (bursitis). Palpate over the greater tubercle of the humerus as you abduct the arm at the shoulder. Then palpate the scapulae.

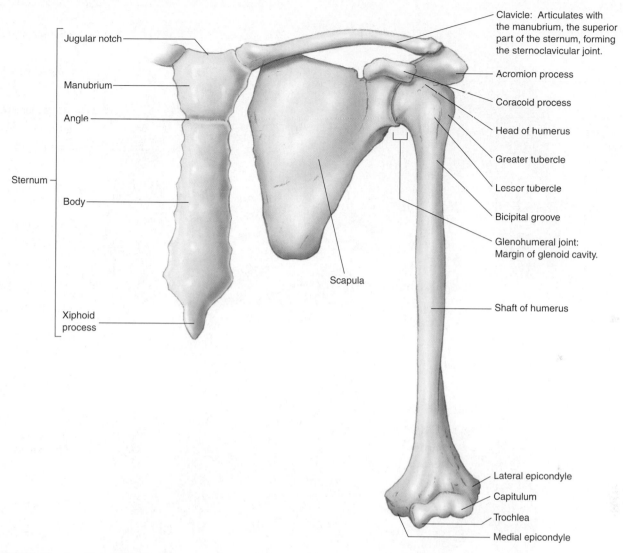

Jugular notch

Manubrium

Angle

Sternum

Body

Xiphoid process

Clavicle: Articulates with the manubrium, the superior part of the sternum, forming the sternoclavicular joint.

Acromion process

Coracoid process

Head of humerus

Greater tubercle

Lesser tubercle

Bicipital groove

Glenohumeral joint: Margin of glenoid cavity.

Scapula

Shaft of humerus

Lateral epicondyle

Capitulum

Trochlea

Medial epicondyle

FIGURE 5-63 The shoulder girdle.

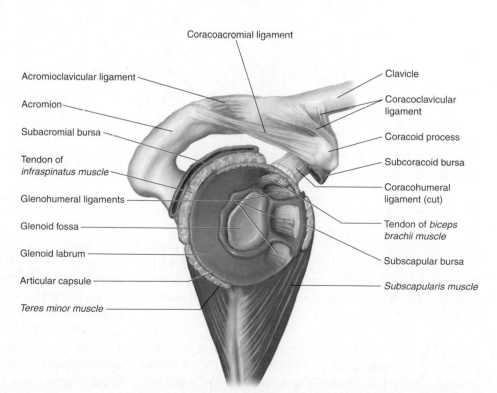

Coracoacromial ligament

Acromioclavicular ligament

Acromion

Subacromial bursa

Tendon of *infraspinatus muscle*

Glenohumeral ligaments

Glenoid fossa

Glenoid labrum

Articular capsule

Teres minor muscle

Clavicle

Coracoclavicular ligament

Coracoid process

Subcoracoid bursa

Coracohumeral ligament (cut)

Tendon of *biceps brachii muscle*

Subscapular bursa

Subscapularis muscle

FIGURE 5-64 Shoulder girdle ligaments.

(a)

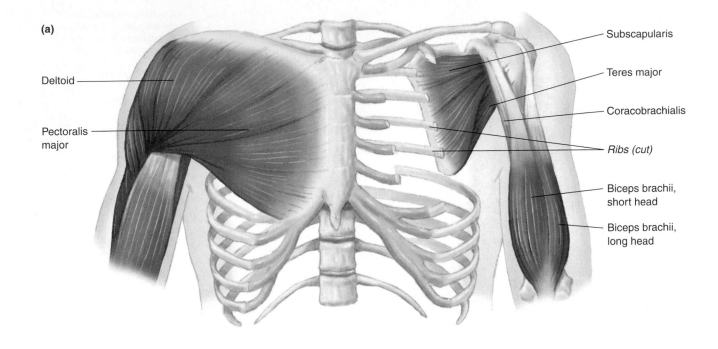

Deltoid

Pectoralis major

Subscapularis

Teres major

Coracobrachialis

Ribs (cut)

Biceps brachii, short head

Biceps brachii, long head

(b)

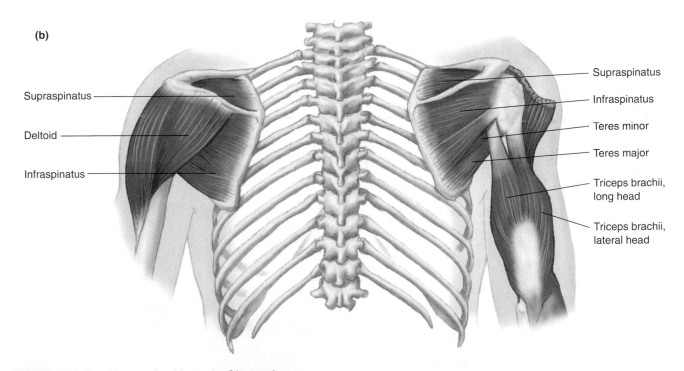

Supraspinatus

Deltoid

Infraspinatus

Supraspinatus

Infraspinatus

Teres minor

Teres major

Triceps brachii, long head

Triceps brachii, lateral head

FIGURE 5-65 Shoulder muscles: (a) anterior (b) posterior.

Ask the patient to rotate his shoulders to the "goal post" position (external rotation) (Procedure 5-14d). Normal external rotation is 90 degrees. Finally, ask him to place both hands behind the small of his back (internal rotation). Normal internal rotation is 90 degrees. During these motions, cup your hands over your patient's shoulders and note any crepitus.

ANKLES AND FEET The foot is composed of 7 tarsal bones, 5 metatarsal bones, and 14 phalanges (Figure 5-66). The talus, the calcaneus (heel), and the other tarsals articu-

late in a system of joints that allows inversion (lifting the inside of the foot) and eversion (lifting the outside of the foot). The most distal tarsals articulate with the metatarsals, which articulate with the proximal phalanges at the metatarsophalangeal joints.

At the ankle joint, the distal tibia (medial malleolus) and the distal fibula (lateral malleolus) articulate with the talus (Figure 5-67). Ligaments stretching from each malleolus to the foot itself hold the ankle joint together. The strong Achilles tendon, which inserts on the calcaneus (heel), also helps maintain the ankle's integrity. Movement in the ankle

Procedure 5-14 Examining the Shoulder

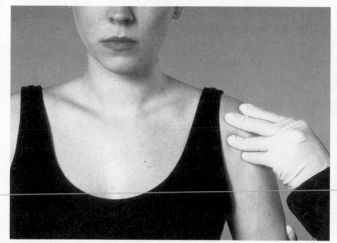

5-14a Palpate the shoulder with your fingertips.

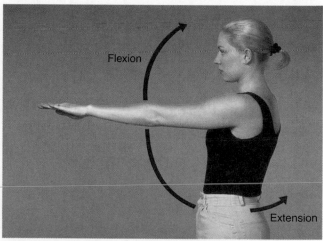

5-14b Assess shoulder flexion and extension.

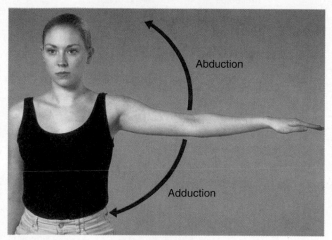

5-14c Assess shoulder abduction and adduction.

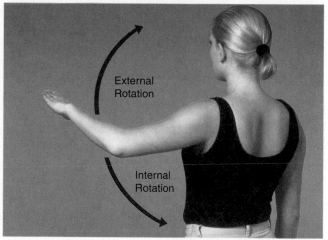

5-14d Assess internal and external shoulder rotation.

is limited to dorsiflexion (raising the foot) and plantar flexion (lowering the foot). The major dorsiflexor muscle is the tibialis anterior (Figure 5-68). The major plantar flexor is the gastrocnemius (calf muscle) (Figure 5-69).

Inspect the foot and ankle for obvious deformities, nodules, swelling, calluses, or corns. Palpate the anterior aspect of each ankle joint with your thumbs and note any sponginess, swelling, or tenderness (Procedure 5-15a). Feel along the Achilles tendon for tenderness or nodules. Exert pressure between your thumbs and fingers on each metatarsophalangeal joint (Procedure 5-15b). Acute inflammation of these joints suggests gout. Tenderness is an early sign of rheumatoid arthritis.

To test range of motion, ask your patient to bring his foot upward (dorsiflexion) (Procedure 5-15c). Normal dorsiflexion is 20 degrees. Then have him point it downward (plantar flexion). Normal plantar flexion is 45 degrees. Next, while stabilizing the ankle with one hand, grasp the heel with the other hand and invert the foot, then evert it (Procedure 5-15d). Normal inversion is 30 degrees, normal eversion 20 degrees. These four movements test the ankle joint's stability.

A sprained ankle will cause your patient pain when the injured ligament is stretched or torn. Because the lateral ligaments are smaller and weaker than the medial ligaments, lateral sprains are more common, causing severe pain on inversion and plantar flexion. In arthritis, pain and tenderness will accompany movement in any direction. Finally, flex and extend the toes (Procedure 5-15e). Expect a great range of motion in these joints, especially the big toes.

KNEES The knee joint involves the distal femur, the proximal tibia, and the patella (Figure 5-70). The distal femur and the proximal tibia meet at this joint and are cushioned by the lateral meniscus and the medial meniscus, which form a cartilaginous surface for pain-free movement. The

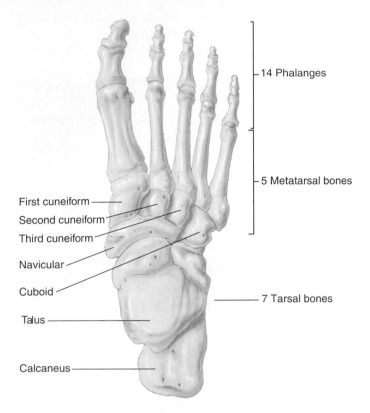

First cuneiform
Second cuneiform
Third cuneiform
Navicular
Cuboid
Talus
Calcaneus

14 Phalanges
5 Metatarsal bones
7 Tarsal bones

FIGURE 5-66 Bones of the foot.

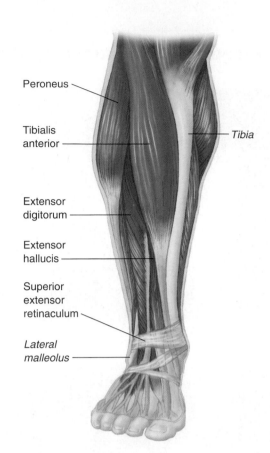

Peroneus
Tibialis anterior
Extensor digitorum
Extensor hallucis
Superior extensor retinaculum
Lateral malleolus
Tibia

FIGURE 5-68 The dorsiflexors.

joint capsule contains synovial fluid. Several ligaments surround the knee joint and help maintain its integrity. The medial and lateral collateral ligaments provide side-to-side stability and are easily palpable. The anterior and posterior cruciate ligaments, which give the knee front-to-back stability, lie deep within the joint capsule and are not palpable.

The knee is a modified hinge joint, allowing flexion and extension, with some rotation during flexion. The major flexors are a group of three muscles (biceps femoris, semimembranosus, and semitendinosus) known as the hamstrings (Figure 5-71). The major extensors are a group of four muscles (vastus lateralis, vastus intermedius, vastus medialis, and rectus femoris) known as the quadriceps (Figure 5-72). The femur can rotate on the tibia slightly. The

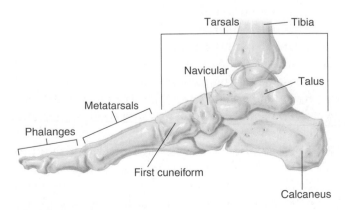

Tarsals — Tibia
Navicular
Talus
Metatarsals
Phalanges
First cuneiform
Calcaneus

FIGURE 5-67 The foot and ankle.

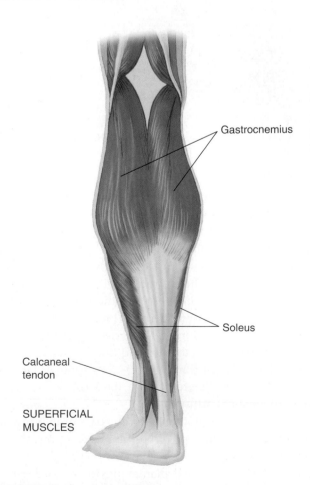

Gastrocnemius
Soleus
Calcaneal tendon

SUPERFICIAL MUSCLES

FIGURE 5-69 The plantar flexors.

Procedure 5-15 Examining the Ankle and Foot

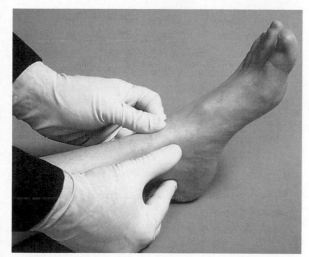

5-15a Palpate the ankle and foot.

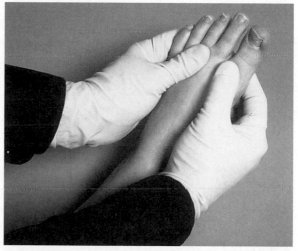

5-15b Palpate the metatarsophalangeal joints.

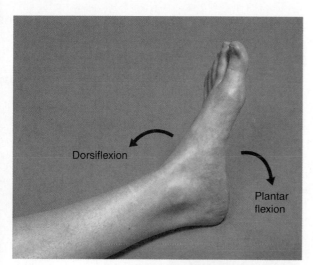

5-15c Assess dorsiflexion and plantar flexion.

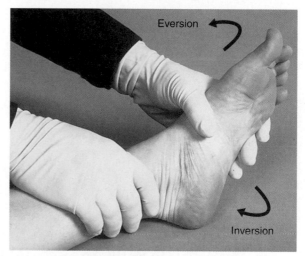

5-15d Assess inversion and eversion of the foot.

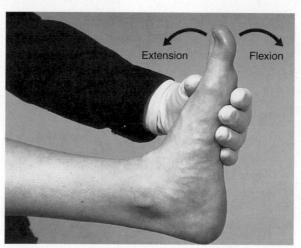

5-15e Test flexion and extension of the toes.

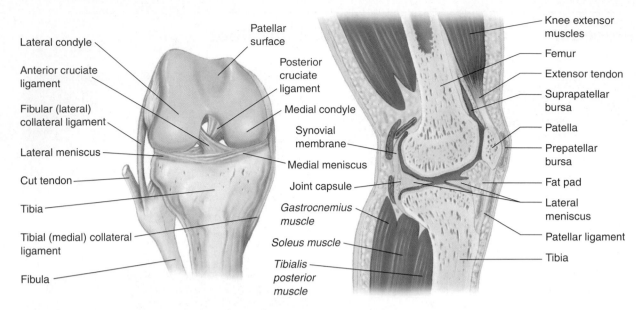

FIGURE 5-70 The knee.

Lateral condyle
Anterior cruciate ligament
Fibular (lateral) collateral ligament
Lateral meniscus
Cut tendon
Tibia
Tibial (medial) collateral ligament
Fibula

Patellar surface
Posterior cruciate ligament
Medial condyle
Synovial membrane
Medial meniscus
Joint capsule
Gastrocnemius muscle
Soleus muscle
Tibialis posterior muscle

Knee extensor muscles
Femur
Extensor tendon
Suprapatellar bursa
Patella
Prepatellar bursa
Fat pad
Lateral meniscus
Patellar ligament
Tibia

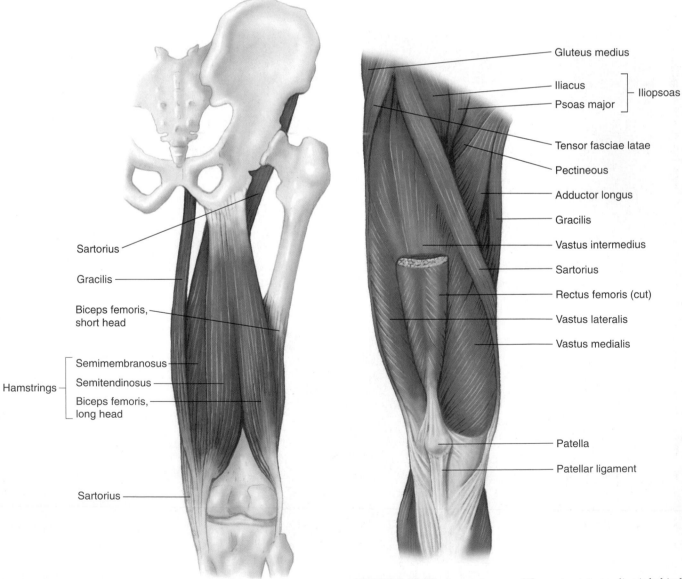

Sartorius
Gracilis
Biceps femoris, short head
Hamstrings
Semimembranosus
Semitendinosus
Biceps femoris, long head
Sartorius

Gluteus medius
Iliacus
Psoas major
Iliopsoas
Tensor fasciae latae
Pectineous
Adductor longus
Gracilis
Vastus intermedius
Sartorius
Rectus femoris (cut)
Vastus lateralis
Vastus medialis
Patella
Patellar ligament

FIGURE 5-71 The knee flexors.

FIGURE 5-72 The knee extensors. (The vastus intermedius is behind the rectus femoris.)

Procedure 5-16 Examining the Knee

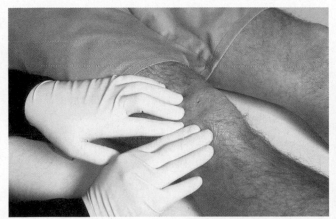

5-16a Palpate the knee.

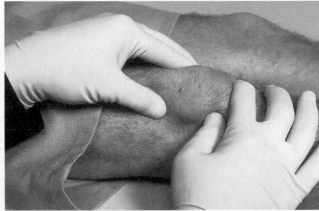

5-16b Palpate the patella.

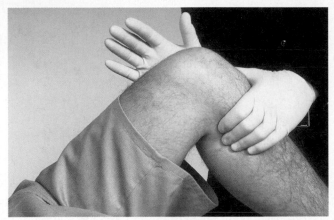

5-16c Test the collateral ligaments of the knee.

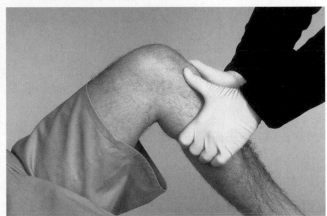

5-16d Test the cruciate ligaments of the knee.

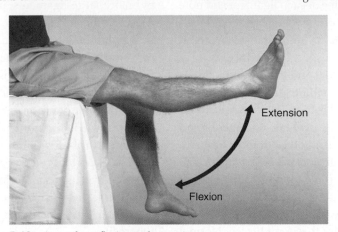

Extension

Flexion

5-16e Assess knee flexion and extension.

patella lies deep in the middle of the quadriceps tendon, which inserts on the tibial tuberosity below the knee. Concave areas at each side of the patella and below it contain synovial fluid.

Inspect your patient's knees for alignment and deformities. Look for the concave areas that usually appear on each side of the patella and just above it. The absence of these concavities indicates swelling in the knee or the surround-ing structures. If swelling is present, milk the medial aspect of the knee firmly upward two or three times to displace the fluid. Then press the knee just behind the lateral margin of the patella and watch for a return of fluid (a positive sign for effusion) (Procedure 5-16a). Feel for any thickening or swelling around the patella; these suggest synovial thickening or effusion. Compress the patella and move it against the femur (Procedure 5-16b). Note any pain or tenderness.

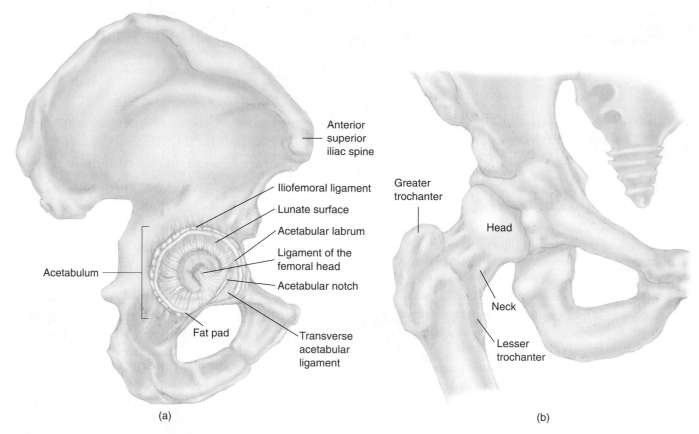

Anterior superior iliac spine

Iliofemoral ligament

Lunate surface

Acetabular labrum

Ligament of the femoral head

Acetabular notch

Acetabulum

Fat pad

Transverse acetabular ligament

Greater trochanter

Head

Neck

Lesser trochanter

(a)

(b)

FIGURE 5-73 The hip joint: (a) lateral view (b) anterior view.

To test for range of motion, have your patient flex his knee to 90 degrees. Press your thumbs into the joint and palpate along the tibial margins from the patellar tendon laterally. Palpate along the course of each ligament and note any points of tenderness. If your patient has tenderness, expect damage to the meniscus or to lateral ligaments. If you feel irregular bony ridges, suspect osteoarthritis.

Test for stability of the medial and collateral ligaments by moving the knee joint from side to side with the knee flexed to 30 degrees (Procedure 5-16c). There should be little movement if the joint is stable. Evaluate the anterior and posterior cruciate ligaments by using the "drawer" test. Try to move the knee joint anterior and posterior, much like opening and closing a drawer (Procedure 5-16d). Again, if the ligaments are strong, there should be little movement.

Have your patient sit at the edge of the exam table with his lower legs dangling. Ask him to extend his leg. Normal extension is 90 degrees (Procedure 5-16e). Ask him to lie down on his stomach and try to touch his foot to his back. Normal flexion is 135 degrees. With your patient standing, inspect the posterior surface of his legs, especially the popliteal region behind his knees. Note any deformity or abnormalities, such as bowlegs, knock-knees, or flexion contracture—the inability to fully extend the knee.

HIPS The hip joint involves the head of the proximal femur (ball) and the acetabulum (socket) of the ischium

(Figure 5-73). Although the hip is a ball-and-socket joint like the shoulder, the two are very different. Whereas the shoulder has a wide range of motion, the hip joint is restricted by many large ligaments, a bony ridge in the pelvis, and capsular fibers. Hip flexion, the most important movement, occurs via the iliopsoas muscle group (Figure 5-74). Other movements, although much more limited in range than the shoulder, include extension, abduction, adduction, and internal and external rotation.

A number of muscle groups control these movements. One of these is the gluteus, a series of adductor muscles and lateral rotators (Figure 5-75). Three bursae in the hip play an important role in pain-free movement. The iliopectineal bursa sits just anterior to the hip joint. The trochanteric bursa lies just to the side and behind the greater trochanter. The ischiogluteal bursa resides under the ischial tuberosity.

Inspect the hips for deformities, symmetry, and swelling. Palpate for tenderness all around the joint, including the three bursae and greater trochanter of the femur (Procedure 5-17a). Test the hip's range of motion with your patient supine. Ask him to raise his knee to his chest and pull it firmly against his abdomen. Observe the degree of flexion at the knee and hip (normally 120 degrees) (Procedure 5-17b).

Flex the hip at 90 degrees and stabilize the thigh with one hand while you grasp the ankle with the other. Swing

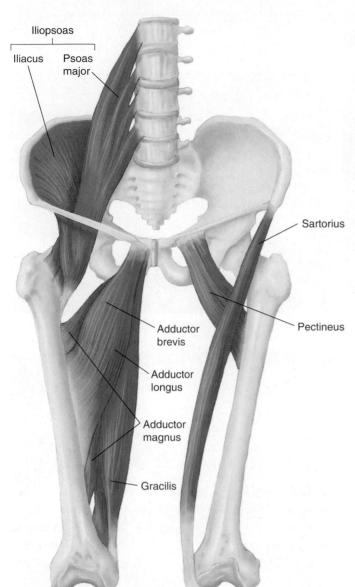

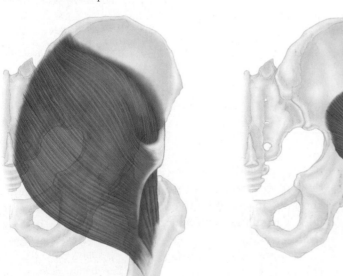

FIGURE 5-74 The hip flexors.

Assessment Pearls

Evaluating for a Hip Fracture. The presence of an occult hip fracture can be difficult to discern in older patients—especially those who are demented or bedridden. Often, the patient has a history of falling out of bed or falling in the shower. Because the patient is nonambulatory, it is difficult to determine whether a fracture exists. One trick is to auscultate for the fracture.

This test is performed by percussing the patella and simultaneously auscultating with the bell of a stethoscope over the symphysis pubis. The percussion note is then compared with the opposite (contralateral) side in a similar fashion. A positive test is one that results in a diminished percussion note on the side where pain is felt. A negative test is defined as one in which no difference in percussion note is obtained. This test was first described in 1846 and remains valid today. Diagnostic X-rays, of course, will still be needed.

the lower leg medially to evaluate external rotation and laterally to evaluate internal rotation (Procedure 5-17c). Normal external rotation is 40 degrees, and normal internal rotation is 45 degrees. Arthritis restricts internal rotation.

To test for hip abduction, have your patient extend his legs. Then, while you stabilize the anterior superior iliac spine with one hand, abduct the other leg until you feel the iliac spine move. This marks the degree of hip abduction, which is normally 45 degrees (Procedure 5-17d). If your patient complains of hip pain or if the range of motion is limited, palpate the three bursae for swelling (bursitis) and tenderness.

SPINE The spine comprises the cervical, thoracic, lumbar, sacral, and coccygeal vertebrae (Figure 5-76). Cartilaginous disks separate the vertebrae from one another, except for those in the sacrum and coccyx, which fuse in

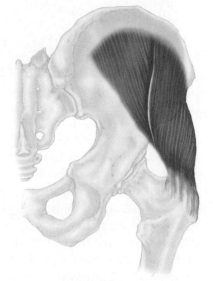

Gluteus maximus

Gluteus minimus

Gluteus medius

FIGURE 5-75 The gluteus muscles.

Procedure 5-17 Examining the Hip

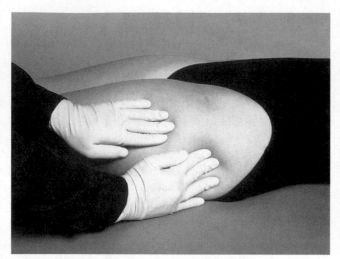

5-17a Palpate the hip.

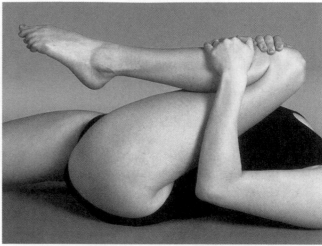

5-17b Assess hip flexion with the knee flexed.

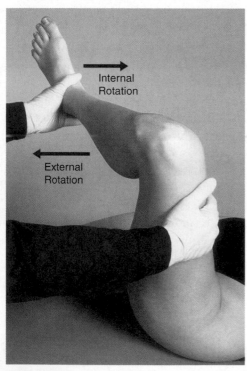

Internal
Rotation

External
Rotation

5-17c Assess external and internal rotation of the hip.

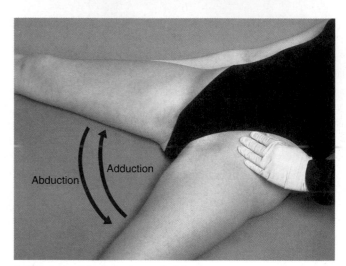

Abduction Adduction

5-17d Assess hip abduction and adduction.

adulthood. The vertebrae form a series of gliding joints that permit a variety of movements.

The cervical vertebrae are the most mobile. C1 and C2 share a special structural relationship. C1, also known as the *atlas*, because it supports the head much as the mythical Atlas supported the world, allows flexion and extension between itself and the skull. This enables us to look up and down. C2, also known as the *axis*, has a fingerlike projection called the *odontoid process*. The atlas sits atop the odontoid process and rotates around it. The cervical spine (C2 through C7) permits flexion, extension, lateral bending, and rotation in a fairly wide range of motion in all directions.

The thoracic vertebrae (T1 through T12) articulate with the 12 sets of ribs that protect the vital organs of the chest. The lumbar

CONTENT REVIEW

➤ Vertebrae from Head to Tail
  • Cervical (C1–C7)
  • Thoracic (T1–T12)
  • Lumbar (L1–L5)
  • Sacral (S1–S5, fused in adulthood)
  • Coccygeal

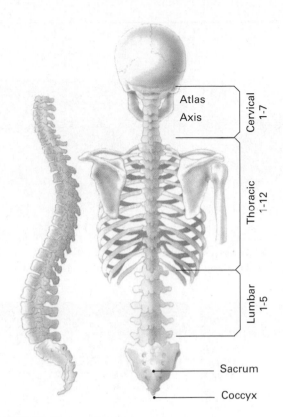

FIGURE 5-76 The spinal column.

vertebrae (L1 through L5) are the most massive because they bear most of the body's weight when it is standing erect. Similar to the cervical vertebrae, they are not well protected and are the site of frequent back problems. They, too, allow flexion, extension, lateral bending, and rotation.

The spinal cord runs through a foramen (opening) in the center of each vertebra. Nerve roots for both sensory and motor nerves leave the spinal cord bilaterally at each level and innervate the various body regions (Figure 5-77). Damage to the cord or nerve roots can render those regions numb and immobile. Ligaments, tendons, muscles, and various other connective tissues hold the vertebrae in

place. When these supporting structures are injured, the risk of damage to the spinal column, and ultimately to the spinal cord, becomes a priority concern.

To assess your patient's spine, first inspect his head and neck for deformities, abnormal posture, and asymmetrical skin folds. The head should be erect and the spine straight. Ask your patient to bend forward slightly while you visually identify the spinous processes, the paravertebral muscles, the scapulae, the iliac crests, and the posterior iliac spines (usually marked by dimples). Draw imaginary horizontal lines across the shoulders and iliac crests. Then, draw an imaginary vertical line from T1 to the space between the buttocks (gluteal cleft). Any deviations suggest a variety of pathologies.

Next, observe your patient from the side. Evaluate the curves of the cervical, thoracic, and lumbar spine and note any irregularities. Common abnormalities of the spine include lordosis, scoliosis, and kyphosis (Table 5-12). Using the pads of your fingers, palpate the spinous processes for tenderness (Procedure 5-18a). Feel the supporting structures for muscle tone, symmetry, size, and tenderness or spasms. If your patient exhibits tenderness of the spinous processes and paravertebral muscles, suspect a herniated intervertebral disk, most commonly found between L4 and S1.

Test the range of motion. First, test for flexion by asking your patient to touch his chin to his chest (Procedure 5-18b). Flexion is normally 45 degrees. Next, ask him to bend his head backward. This tests extension, which normally is up to 55 degrees. Test for rotation by asking your patient to touch his chin to each shoulder (Procedure 5-18c). Normal rotation is 70 degrees on each side. Finally, ask him to touch his ears to his shoulders without raising his shoulders. This assesses lateral bending, which normally is 40 degrees on each side (Procedure 5-18d).

Test for flexion of the lower spine with your patient standing. Ask him to bend and touch his toes (Procedure 5-18e). Note the smoothness and symmetry of movement, the range of motion, and the curves in the lumbar region. Normal flexion ranges from 75 degrees to 90 degrees. If the lumbar area remains concave or appears asymmetrical during this exam, your patient may have a muscle spasm. Next, stabilize your patient's pelvis with your hands and have him bend sideways; normal lateral bending is 35 degrees on each side (Procedure 5-18f). To assess

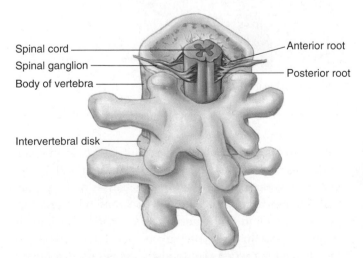

FIGURE 5-77 The vertebrae.

Table 5-12 Spinal Curvatures

Condition	Description
Normal	Concave in cervical and lumbar regions, convex in thorax
Lordosis	Exaggerated lumbar concavity (swayback)
Kyphosis	Exaggerated thoracic convexity (hunchback)
Scoliosis	Lateral curvature

Procedure 5-18 Assessing the Spine

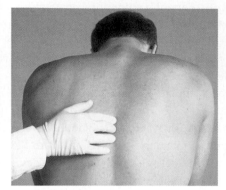

5-18a Palpate the spine.

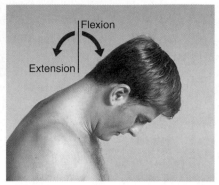

5-18b Test flexion and extension of the head and neck.

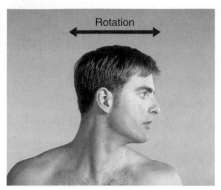

5-18c Test rotation of the head and neck.

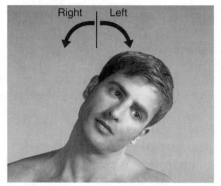

5-18d Test lateral bending of the head and neck.

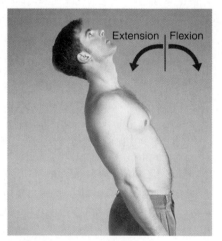

5-18e Assess flexion of the lower spine.

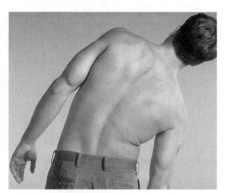

5-18f Assess lateral bending of the lower spine.

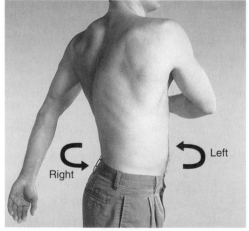

5-18g Assess spinal extension.

5-18h Assess spinal rotation.

hyperextension, ask him to bend backward toward you; normal hyperextension is 30 degrees (Procedure 5-18g). Finally, test spinal rotation by asking your patient to twist his shoulders one way, then the other. Normally, they will rotate 30 degrees to each side (Procedure 5-18h).

If your patient complains of lower back pain radiating down the back of one leg, assess it by having him lie supine on the table. Ask him to raise his straightened leg until he feels pain. Note the angle of elevation at which the pain occurs, as well as the quality and distribution of the pain. Dorsiflex your patient's foot. If this causes a sharp pain that radiates from your patient's back down his leg, suspect compression of the nerve roots of the lower lumbar region. Repeat this test with the other leg. Increased pain in the affected leg when the opposite leg is raised confirms the finding.

Neurologic System

A comprehensive physical exam includes a thorough evaluation of your patient's mental status and thought processes.[5] On the scene of an emergency, you would limit your mental exam to level of consciousness and basic orientation questions such as "What is your name?" "Where are you right now?" "What day is it today?" If you are conducting a full physical exam or evaluating someone with altered mentation, some or all of the following techniques will be useful.

When you conduct a neurologic exam, you are attempting to answer two vital questions. First, are the findings symmetrical or unilateral? Second, if the signs are

Assessment Pearls

Lower back or neck pain are common reasons that people summon EMS or go to the emergency department. Most back pain is musculoskeletal in origin and resolves with conservative treatment. However, herniation of a spinal disk can be quite painful and refractory to treatment. How can you differentiate musculoskeletal back pain from diskogenic back pain? It's not always easy, but here are a few pointers.

When you are obtaining the history from the patient, listen for indications that the pain is worse on one side compared with the other. Diskogenic pain tends to be worse in one leg compared with the other.

Other clues to diskogenic pain include worsening of the pain when the patient coughs or bears down while having a bowel movement. Both of these cause an increase in the intrathecal pressure (i.e., the pressure within the spinal canal) and thus push on the herniated disk, which then pushes on the spinal nerve root, exacerbating the pain.

Numbness in one leg, especially along a spinal nerve dermatome, is usually the result of diskogenic disease. Bilateral numbness is usually not. The exception would be bilateral numbness on the inside of the thighs (i.e., saddle anesthesia), which is indicative of cauda equina syndrome and a neurosurgical emergency. (*Cauda equina syndrome* is compression of the nerve roots in the lower spinal cord, which causes paralysis and loss of bowel and bladder control. Patients have altered sensation between the legs, over the buttocks, and on the inner thighs, the back of the legs [saddle area], and the feet.)

On your physical exam, loss of muscle strength or loss of a deep tendon reflex on one side is indicative of diskogenic disease. Have a patient without recent trauma lie supine and raise both of his feet off the stretcher for about 30 seconds. If he can do this, diskogenic disease is unlikely. If he cannot do this, the weak side is the side where the spinal nerve root is compressed. Another test is the straight-leg lifting test. With the patient supine, pick up a leg, keeping it straight. If this causes pain before the leg can be completely raised, suspect diskogenic disease.

Pediatric Pearls

Evaluate pulses, sensation, movement, and warmth in all four extremities. Check for capillary refill and feel for peripheral pulses. Evaluate the skin, which reveals important clues in children. Its color, turgor, moisture, and temperature are key indicators of the cardiovascular system's condition. Unlike the adult's, the child's capillary refill time accurately reflects his peripheral perfusion status.

When examining the musculoskeletal system, remember the growth and posture at different stages of the child's development. For example, a toddler walks with a broad base for support and is likely to appear bowlegged. A teenager with poor posture may suffer from a skeletal problem, such as scoliosis.

Palpate the upper and lower extremities for swelling, tenderness, and contractions. Next, have the child demonstrate the range of motion of his joints while you feel for smoothness of movement. Examine all joints.

unilateral, is the site of origin in the central nervous system (brain and spinal cord) or in the peripheral nervous system (everything else)? You will conduct many parts of the neurologic exam while you assess other anatomic areas and systems. For example, you can examine the cranial nerves while evaluating the head and face. You can note any weaknesses or abnormal neurologic findings while evaluating the arms and legs during the musculoskeletal exam.

A nervous system exam covers five areas: mental status and speech, the cranial nerves, the motor system, the sensory system, and the reflexes. Because we covered mental status earlier in this chapter, we focus here on the cranial nerves, the motor system, the sensory system, and deep tendon reflexes. Again, this section covers the entire spectrum of a comprehensive neurologic exam. The chief complaint, the clinical condition of your patient, and time constraints will determine which parts you will actually use.

Cranial Nerves

The 12 pairs of cranial nerves originate from the base of the brain and provide sensory and motor innervation, mostly to the head and face (Figure 5-78). Each pair bears the name of its function and carries either sensory fibers or motor fibers, or both. Table 5-13 lists the cranial nerves' names, their specific functions, and the areas they innervate.

Most likely, you will conduct parts of the cranial nerve exam when you assess other areas, such as the eyes, ears, throat, and musculoskeletal system. The following is the cranial nerve exam in its entirety.

CN-I Test your patient's olfactory nerve by having him close his eyes and compress one nostril while you present him with a variety of common, nonirritating odors (Procedure 5-19a). Repeat the test with each nostril. Ask the

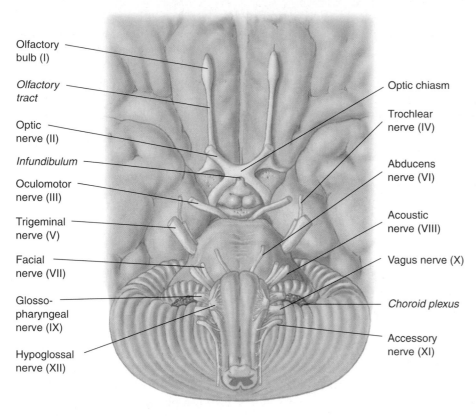

Olfactory bulb (I)

Olfactory tract

Optic nerve (II)

Infundibulum

Oculomotor nerve (III)

Trigeminal nerve (V)

Facial nerve (VII)

Glosso-pharyngeal nerve (IX)

Hypoglossal nerve (XII)

Optic chiasm

Trochlear nerve (IV)

Abducens nerve (VI)

Acoustic nerve (VIII)

Vagus nerve (X)

Choroid plexus

Accessory nerve (XI)

FIGURE 5-78 The cranial nerves.

patient to identify the odor. Most people will do so easily. If your patient cannot, several causes are possible. Bilateral loss of smell suggests head trauma, nasal stuffiness, smoking, cocaine use, or a congenital defect. A unilateral loss of smell without nasal disease suggests a frontal lobe lesion.

CN-II Test the optic nerve with the visual acuity and visual field tests described earlier in this chapter in the "Assessment" section on the eyes.

CN-III Test the oculomotor nerve with the optic nerve when you perform pupil reaction tests. Inspect the size and shape of your patient's pupils and compare one side with the other. A slight inequality may be normal. Usually the pupil is midpoint. Constricted or dilated pupils may result from medications, drug abuse, glaucoma, and neurologic disease.

Darken the room, if possible, to test for pupillary reaction. Ask your patient to look straight ahead. Shine a bright light obliquely into one of his pupils. Watch for direct reaction (pupillary constriction in the same eye) and for consensual reaction (pupillary constriction in the opposite eye). Repeat this test on the other side. Now assess for the near-response, asking your patient to follow your finger as you move it in toward the bridge of his nose. Watch for his pupils to constrict and his eyes to converge.

CN-III, IV, VI Test the oculomotor, trochlear, and abducens nerves by evaluating your patient's extraocular movements

Table 5-13 Cranial Nerves

Cranial Nerve	Function	Innervation
I—Olfactory	Sensory	Smell
II—Optic	Sensory	Sight
III—Oculomotor	Motor	Pupil constriction; superior rectus, inferior rectus, inferior oblique muscles
IV—Trochlear	Motor	Superior oblique muscles
V—Trigeminal	Sensory Motor	Ophthalmic (forehead), maxillary (cheek), and mandibular (chin) regions Chewing muscles
VI—Abducens	Motor	Lateral rectus muscle
VII—Facial	Sensory Motor	Tongue Facial muscles
VIII—Acoustic	Sensory	Hearing, balance
IX—Glossopharyngeal	Sensory Motor	Posterior pharynx, taste to anterior tongue Posterior pharynx
X—Vagus	Sensory Motor	Taste to posterior tongue Posterior palate and pharynx
XI—Accessory	Motor	Trapezius, sternocleidomastoids
XII—Hypoglossal	Motor	Tongue

Procedure 5-19 Assessing the Cranial Nerves

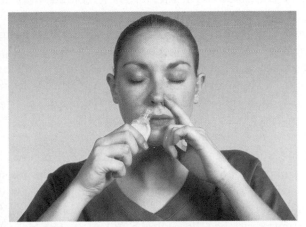

5-19a Test the olfactory nerve by having your patient identify common odors.

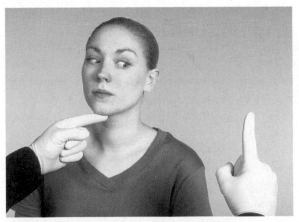

5-19b Test the oculomotor, trochlear, and abducens nerves by evaluating your patient's extraocular movements.

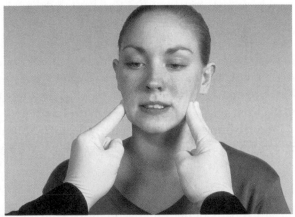

5-19c Test motor function of the trigeminal nerve by palpating the temporal and masseter muscles.

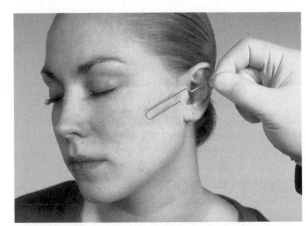

5-19d Test sensory function of the trigeminal nerve with sharp and dull objects.

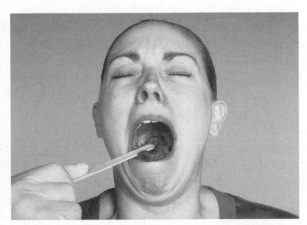

5-19e Test the glossopharyngeal and vagus nerves with a tongue blade.

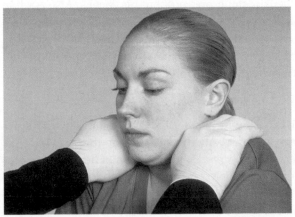

5-19f Test the spinal accessory nerve by having your patient shrug her shoulders against resistance.

(EOMs). Ask him to follow your finger with only his eyes as you move your finger through the six cardinal positions of gaze (Procedure 5-19b). Make a wide "H" in the air with your finger. Observe for conjugate (together) movements of your patient's eyes in each direction. Normally, your patient can follow your finger with no strabismus (deviation) or nystagmus (involuntary movements). Inability to move in any direction can be the result of a problem with a cranial nerve, an ocular muscle, or an eye orbit that may be fractured and impinging on the muscle or nerve. Finally, look for ptosis (a droopy eyelid) that may be the result of CN-III palsy or myasthenia gravis.

CN-V Test function of the trigeminal nerve by asking your patient to clench his teeth while you palpate the temporal and masseter muscles (Procedure 5-19c). Note the strength of the muscle contraction. Unilateral weakness or the inability to contract suggests a trigeminal nerve lesion. Bilateral dysfunction suggests motor neuron involvement.

To test for sensory function in the three main divisions of the trigeminal nerve, first ask your patient to close his eyes. Using something sharp and something dull, lightly scrape the objects across the forehead, cheek, and chin on both sides and ask your patient to distinguish the sensations (Procedure 5-19d). The two ends of a paper clip work well for this procedure; straighten one end and use its tip as the sharp object. Unilateral loss of sensation suggests a trigeminal nerve lesion. Finally, test the corneal reflex. Ask your patient to look up and away as you touch his cornea lightly with some fine cotton fibers. He should blink. Repeat this test on the other eye.

CN-VII First, assess your patient's face at rest and during conversation. Note any asymmetry, eyelid drooping, or abnormal movements, such as tics. Test the facial nerve by having your patient assume a variety of facial expressions. Ask him to raise his eyebrows, frown, show his upper and lower teeth or smile, and puff out his cheeks. Also ask him to close his eyes tightly so that you cannot open them; then to test muscle strength, try to open them.

Bell's palsy is an inflammation of CN-VII. Your patient will present with unilateral facial drooping from paralysis of this nerve.

CN-VIII Ask your patient to occlude one ear with a finger. Then whisper something softly into the other ear. Ask him to repeat what you said. Any loss of hearing warrants further testing to detect air and bone conduction problems. Test the acoustic nerve for the senses of hearing and balance. Ask your patient to stand erect and close his eyes. Evaluate his balance and then ask him to open his eyes. If he does not become dizzy and opens his eyes to your command, the eighth nerve is functioning appropriately.

CN-IX, X Test the glossopharyngeal and vagus nerves together. Listen to your patient's voice. Hoarseness suggests a vocal cord problem; a nasal quality suggests a palate problem. Ask your patient to swallow; note any difficulties. Ask him to open his mouth and say "aaahhh"; watch for the soft palate and uvula to rise symmetrically. The posterior pharynx should move medially. If the vagus nerve is paralyzed, the soft palate and uvula will deviate toward the side of the lesion. Test the gag reflex with a tongue blade on the posterior tongue (Procedure 5-19e). Absence of a gag reflex suggests a lesion in one of these nerves.

CN-XI Inspect the upper portions of your patient's trapezius muscles and sternocleidomastoid muscles for symmetry at rest. To test his trapezius muscles, place your hands on his shoulders and ask him to raise his shoulders against resistance (Procedure 5-19f). Now, test his sternocleidomastoid muscles. Place your hands along his face and ask him to turn his head to each side as you apply resistance. Note any bilateral or unilateral weaknesses. A supine patient with bilateral weakness of the sternocleidomastoids will have trouble lifting his head.

CN-XII First, evaluate your patient's speech articulation. Then ask him to stick out his tongue; watch for a midline projection. A CN-XII lesion will make the tongue deviate away from the affected side. Have your patient move his tongue from side to side as you watch for symmetry.

You may conduct a cranial nerve exam according to this sequence. More likely, you will develop your own efficient system of testing these nerves.

Motor System

Thirty-one pairs of nerves arise from the spinal foramina on both sides of the spinal column (Figure 5-79). The anterior root of the peripheral nerves carries the motor, or efferent, nerve fibers from the brain and spinal cord through three pathways: the pyramidal, extrapyramidal, and cerebellar systems. The pyramidal tract, which begins in the motor cortex of the brain, mediates voluntary movements. Its fibers travel down the brainstem, where they crisscross to innervate the opposite sides of the body. These tracts guide voluntary skeletal muscle movement and allow for fine motor movements by stimulating some muscles and inhibiting others. The motor system's net effect is coordinated, skilled movements.

When this system is damaged, function is lost below the level of the injury, and movements become weak or paralyzed. Inhibition is lost, so muscle tone is increased and deep tendon reflexes are exaggerated. If the damage occurs above the crossover point in the brainstem, then the effects will be seen on the opposite (contralateral) side of the body. If the damage is below the crossover point, the damage will be on the same (ipsilateral) side. For example,

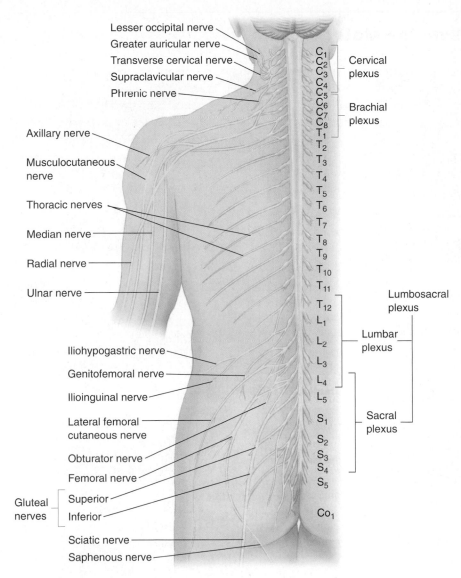

Lesser occipital nerve
Greater auricular nerve
Transverse cervical nerve
Supraclavicular nerve
Phrenic nerve

Axillary nerve

Musculocutaneous nerve

Thoracic nerves

Median nerve

Radial nerve

Ulnar nerve

Iliohypogastric nerve
Genitofemoral nerve
Ilioinguinal nerve
Lateral femoral cutaneous nerve
Obturator nerve
Femoral nerve

Gluteal nerves — Superior / Inferior

Sciatic nerve
Saphenous nerve

C_1 C_2 C_3 C_4 Cervical plexus
C_5 C_6 C_7 C_8 T_1 Brachial plexus
T_2 T_3 T_4 T_5 T_6 T_7 T_8 T_9 T_{10} T_{11} T_{12} L_1 L_2 L_3 L_4 L_5 S_1 S_2 S_3 S_4 S_5 Co_1

Lumbosacral plexus

Lumbar plexus

Sacral plexus

FIGURE 5-79 The peripheral nerves.

ASSESSMENT Inspect your patient's general body structure, muscle development, positioning, and coordination. What is his position at rest? Is he erect or does he slump to one side, suggesting unilateral paralysis or weakness? Note any obvious asymmetries, deformities, or involuntary movements. Are there tremors, tics, or fasciculations (twitches)? If so, note their location, rate, quality, rhythm, amplitude, and relation to your patient's posture, activity, fatigue, emotion, and other factors. For example, if your patient's hand begins to shake only when you ask him to perform a task with it, such as writing his name or lifting a spoon, this suggests a postural tremor. Conversely, a tremor at rest that may disappear with voluntary movement suggests Parkinson's disease. To assess involuntary movement, observe your patient throughout the exam.

To determine your patient's muscle bulk, observe the size and contour of his muscles. Look for atrophy, a decrease in bulk and strength; hypertrophy, an increase in bulk and strength; or pseudo-hypertrophy, an increase in bulk and decrease in strength, as in muscular dystrophy. Flattened or concave contours, especially with fasciculations, may result from lower motor neuron disease. Some degree of muscle atrophy may be a normal part of the aging process or may result from the effects of diabetes on the peripheral nervous system. Look for signs of general muscle atrophy by checking for flattening of the thenar (thumb) muscle and for furrowing between the metacarpals. Unilateral muscle atrophy in the hands suggests median or ulnar nerve paralysis.

To assess muscle tone, feel the muscle's resistance to passive stretching in the extremities. Ask your patient to relax one of his arms. Then put the arm, wrists, hands, and elbows through a moderate range-of-motion exam (Procedure 5-20a). Repeat the exam in the lower extremities. If you detect decreased resistance, shake the hand loosely back and forth. It should move freely, but it should not be floppy (flaccid). Increased resistance may be caused by tension. Does the resistance persist throughout the motion (lead-pipe rigidity) or does it vary? If the resistance increases at the extreme limits of the movement, it is called *spasticity*. A ratchetlike jerkiness in the resistance is known as "cog-wheel rigidity," a common finding in a patient faking his symptoms or trying to

if your patient suffers a stroke on the left motor strip controlling the hands, then the motor deficiencies will appear in the right hand. If your patient has swelling of the spinal cord from an injury that impinges on the left motor nucleus, the motor deficiencies will appear on the left side of his body.

The extrapyramidal tract controls body movements and maintains muscle tone through motor fibers and pathways outside the pyramidal system. Because the extrapyramidal tract is mostly inhibitory, damage to this system causes increased muscle tone, abnormal gait and posture, and involuntary movements. This is commonly seen in patients who have adverse reactions to drugs in the phenothiazine class. They appear flushed and stiff, with motor control problems. The cerebellar system coordinates muscular activity and helps to maintain equilibrium and posture through its motor fibers. Cerebellar damage causes abnormal changes in gait, coordination, and equilibrium.

Procedure 5-20 Assessing the Motor System

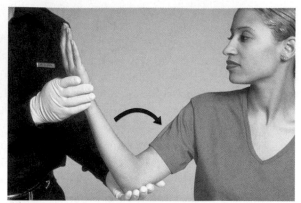

5-20a Assess the elbow's range of motion.

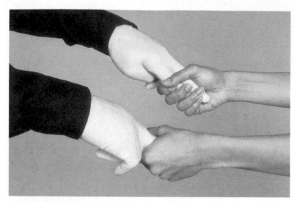

5-20b Test your patient's grip.

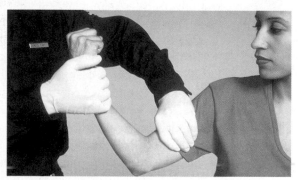

5-20c Test arm strength.

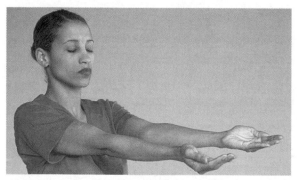

5-20d Test for pronator drift.

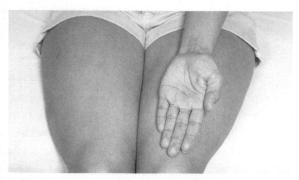

5-20e Test for coordination with rapid alternating movements.

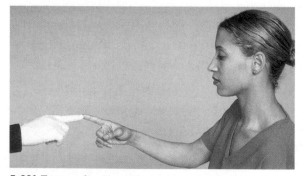

5-20f Test coordination with point-to-point testing.

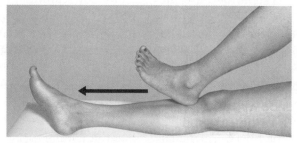

5-20g Assess coordination with heel-to-shin testing.

Table 5-14 Muscle Tone

Finding	Description
Spasticity	Increased tone when passive movement applied, especially at the end of range. Common in stroke.
Rigidity	Increased rigidity throughout movement (lead-pipe). Common in Parkinson's disease and extrapyramidal reactions. Cog-wheel motion is a patient-applied resistance.
Flaccidity	Loss of muscle tone causing limb to be loose. Common in stroke, spinal cord lesion, and Guillain-Barré syndrome.
Paratonia	Sudden changes in tone with passive movement. Can be increased or decreased resistance. Common in dementia.

Table 5-16 Muscle Strength Scale

Score	Description
5	Active movement against full resistance with no fatigue
4	Active movement against some resistance and gravity
3	Active movement against gravity
2	Active movement with gravity eliminated
1	Barely palpable muscle contraction with no movement
0	No visible or palpable muscle contraction

resist your examination. Table 5-14 describes some common muscle tone findings.

Now, focus on your patient's muscle strength. First, assess the strength of his grip. Test both grips simultaneously and compare them. Cross your middle finger over the top of your index finger to prevent your fingers from being hurt, then ask your patient to squeeze them as hard as possible (Procedure 5-20b). Normally, you will have difficulty removing your fingers from your patient's grip. Continue testing all the muscle groups listed in Table 5-15.

While assessing muscle strength, remember that each patient's age, gender, size, and muscular training will affect your exam results. When comparing sides, your patient's dominant side will be stronger. Test for muscle strength by having your patient move actively against your resistance (Procedure 5-20c). If the muscle is too weak

to perform against resistance, have your patient try the movement against gravity or with gravity eliminated (you support the limb). Grade muscle strength on a scale from 0 to 5 (Table 5-16).

To assess your patient's position sense and coordination, first observe his gait. Ask him to walk across the room, turn, and come back. Normally, he will be able to maintain his balance, swing his arms at his side, and turn easily. If his gait is ataxic—uncoordinated, reeling, or unstable—suspect cerebellar disease, loss of position sense, or intoxication. Next, ask him to walk heel-to-toe in a straight line. This "tandem walking" may reveal an ataxia not previously seen.

Ask your patient to walk first on his toes, then on his heels. This will assess plantar flexion and dorsiflexion of the ankle, as well as balance. Next, ask him to hop in place on each foot in turn. Difficulty hopping may result from leg muscle weakness, lack of position sense, or cerebellar dysfunction. Ask him to do a shallow knee bend on each leg in turn. Difficulty doing this suggests muscle weakness in the pelvic girdle and legs. If your patient is old and unable to hop or do knee bends, have him rise from a sitting position without arm support, or step up onto a stool.

Next perform the Romberg test. Ask your patient to stand with his feet together and eyes open. Now have him close his eyes for 20 to 30 seconds. Observe his ability to remain upright with minimal swaying and no support. Losing his balance indicates a positive Romberg test, caused by ataxia from a loss of position sense. An inability to maintain balance with eyes open and feet together represents a cerebellar ataxia.

Check your patient for pronator drift. Ask him to stand with his arms straight out in front of him with his palms up and his eyes closed (Procedure 5-20d). Ask him to maintain this position for 20 to 30 seconds. Normally, your patient can do this easily. If one forearm pronates, suspect a mild hemiparesis. If it drifts sideways or upward, suspect a loss of position sense.

To assess your patient's coordination, test for rapid alternating movements. These maneuvers can be difficult to describe, so you should always demonstrate them to your patient. Ask him to repeat them as rapidly as possible

Table 5-15 Muscle Strength Tests

Muscles	Nerves	Test
Biceps	C5, C6	Flexion of the elbow
Triceps	C6, C7, C8	Extension of the elbow
Wrist extensors	C6, C7, C8, radial nerve	Extension of the wrist
Fingers	C8, T1, ulnar nerve	Finger abduction
Thumb	C8, T1, median nerve	Thumb opposition
Iliopsoas	L2, L3, L4	Hip flexion
Hip extensor	S1	Hip extension
Hip abductors	L4, L5, S1	Hip abduction
Hip adductors	L2, L3, L4	Hip adduction
Quadriceps	L2, L3, L4	Knee extension
Hamstrings	L4, L5, S1, S2	Knee flexion
Feet	L4, L5	Dorsiflexion
Calf muscles	S1	Plantar flexion

while you observe for speed, rhythm, and smoothness. He should repeat all movements with both sides of the body. Keep in mind that his dominant hand usually will perform better than his nondominant hand. If his movements are slow, irregular, and clumsy, suspect cerebellar or extrapyramidal tract disease or upper motor neuron weakness.

First, have your patient tap the distal joint of his thumb with the tip of his index finger as rapidly as possible. Then ask him to place his hand, palm up, on his thigh, quickly turn it over palm down, and return it to palm up (Procedure 5-20e). Have him repeat this movement as quickly as possible for 15 seconds; evaluate both hands. Next, have him perform point-to-point testing. Ask him to alternate touching your index finger and his nose several times while you observe for accuracy and smoothness (Procedure 5-20f). Note any tremors or difficulty performing this task, indicating cerebellar disease; evaluate both hands.

Assess for point-to-point testing in your patient's legs. Ask him to touch his heel to the opposite knee, then run it down his shin to his big toe (Procedure 5-20g). Note the smoothness and accuracy of his actions. Repeat the test with the other leg. To test your patient's position sense, have him close his eyes and repeat this test for both legs. Abnormalities suggest cerebellar disease.

Sensory System

The posterior root of the peripheral nerves carries the sensory, or afferent, nerve fibers to the spinal cord and brain along two pathways. The spinothalamic tracts conduct the sensations of pain, temperature, and crude touch. The posterior column of the spinal cord conducts the sensations of position, vibration, and fine touch. Areas of the skin innervated by these afferent fibers are known as *dermatomes*. A dermatome chart is a road map depicting bands of skin innervated by sensory nerve fibers at each particular spinal level (Figure 5-80). By learning some basic landmarks, you can begin to identify approximate areas of spinal cord lesions according to the absence of skin sensation.

Assessment Pearls

Assessing peripheral sensory function is important for the trauma patient with possible spinal cord injury (or for the back-pain patient with reported sensory loss). Formerly, it was common practice to use a sharp object, such as the pin of a reflex hammer or a sterile needle, to test for sensory function. However, testing with a sterile needle will often result in bleeding, thus potentially exposing EMS personnel to bloodborne diseases. Instead, pick up a bunch of individually wrapped toothpicks (available at restaurant supply stores). When needed, open the wrapper, take out the toothpick, and break it in half. You can use the sharp end to test for sharp sensation and the dull end to test for dull sensation. Take both parts of the broken toothpick, separate them, and test for two-point discrimination. When through, drop the toothpick into the trash.

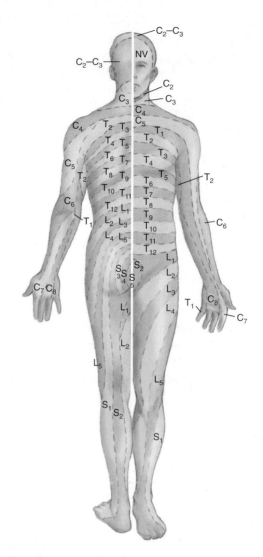

FIGURE 5-80 Dermatome chart. Knowing basic landmarks enables you to locate spinal cord lesions.

Pediatric Pearls

Check muscle strength in all muscle groups by asking the child to prevent you from moving a part of his body. A child's bones are more likely to break at the ends, where growth takes place. Until the child reaches adolescence, when these areas become as strong as the rest of the bone, injuries that occur near the joints are more likely to damage the bone than the ligaments or tendons. Assess the child's muscle coordination by having him stand and then hop on one foot. Repeat this for the other foot. Children usually enjoy this aspect of the physical examination. You can also have the child skip or jump.

You can test for cerebellar function with several games that children usually enjoy. First, as you move your finger, ask the child to touch his nose and then your finger. Consistent past-pointing should arouse your suspicion. An alternate test is to have the child pat his knees alternately with the palms and backs of his hands. Check for sensation over the child's face, trunk, arms, and leg. Check for hot and cold sensation by alternately touching the skin with warm and cold test tubes. Ask the child to close his eyes and tell you which he feels. Be sure to test for reflexes on both sides of the body, just as with an adult. If the child has difficulty relaxing, test the parent's reflexes to show that it does not hurt.

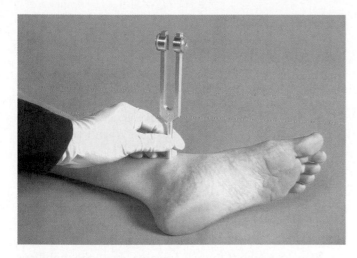

FIGURE 5-81 Test vibration sense with a tuning fork.

Table 5-17 Reflex Scale

Grade	Description
0	No response
+	Diminished, below normal
++	Average, normal
+++	Brisker than normal
++++	Hyperactive, associated with clonus

To assess the sensory system, test for pain, light touch, temperature, position, vibration, and discriminative sensations. Remember to compare distal areas with proximal areas, to compare symmetrical areas bilaterally, and to scatter the stimuli to assess most of the dermatomes. Ask your patient to close his eyes for each of these tests. To test for pain sensation, touch your patient's skin with a sharp object and ask him to tell you whether it is sharp or dull. Compare areas as you move along the different regions, intermittently substituting a dull object for the sharp one. To test for light touch, softly touch him with a fine piece of cotton. Ask him to tell you whenever he feels the cotton. An abnormality suggests a peripheral neuropathy.

Test for temperature sensation by touching your patient's skin with a vial filled with either hot or cold liquid. Then test for position sense by pulling one of his toes upward and asking him to tell you whether it is up or down. Test for vibration sense by placing the stem of a vibrating tuning fork against a bony prominence (Figure 5-81). Finally, test for discriminative sensation by putting a familiar object, such as a key, in your patient's hand and asking him to identify it.

Reflexes

The sensory pathways manage conscious sensation and participate in the reflex arc. The reflex arc connects some sensory impulses directly to motor neurons, triggering immediate responses to noxious stimuli, such as touching your hand to a flame. Deep tendon reflexes are a similar involuntary response to direct muscular stretch. Striking a slightly flexed tendon with a reflex hammer sends an impulse to the spinal cord, where a reflex arc occurs (Figure 5-82). This immediately sends a motor response back to the tendon, which begins the muscle contraction.

When you perform a nervous system exam, also test your patient's superficial and deep tendon reflexes. Always compare one side to the other. Grade the reflexes on a scale of 0 to 41 (Table 5-17) and record your findings on a stick figure (Figure 5-83). A hyperactive response suggests

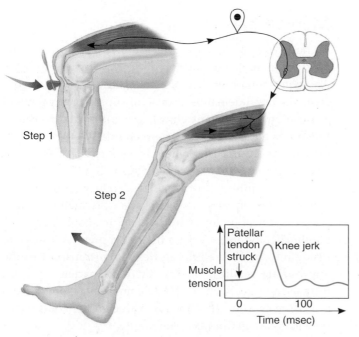

FIGURE 5-82 A reflex arc depicts muscle tension over time.

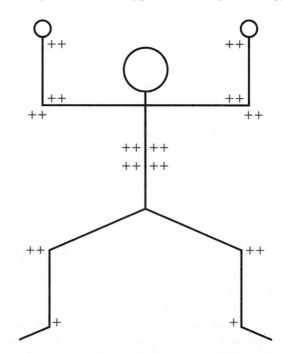

FIGURE 5-83 Reflex figures show grades on a scale of 0 to 4+.

upper motor neuron disease. A diminished response or no response suggests damage to the lower motor neurons or spinal cord.

Deep tendon reflexes can be tested at several places on the body. Use the pointed end of a reflex hammer for striking small areas and use the flat end for striking larger areas. First, ask your patient to relax. Then properly position the limb you are testing. Quickly strike the tendon using wrist motion only.

BICEPS   Support your patient's arm in the slightly flexed position with your thumb directly over the distal biceps tendon in the antecubital space (Procedure 5-21a). Strike your thumbnail with the point of the reflex hammer and watch for contraction of the biceps muscle and the resulting flexion of the elbow. This tests for spinal nerves C5 and C6.

TRICEPS   Flex your patient's arm at a right angle. With the point of your reflex hammer, strike the triceps tendon along the posterior aspect of the distal humerus (Procedure 5-21b). Watch for triceps contraction and the resulting elbow extension. This tests spinal nerves C6, C7, and C8.

BRACHIORADIALIS   Support your patient's arm with the forearm slightly pronated (Procedure 5-21c). Strike his radius about 2 inches above his wrist. Watch for contraction of the brachioradialis and the resulting flexion and supination of the forearm. This tests cervical nerves C5 and C6.

QUADRICEPS   Have your patient sit with his leg hanging off the end of the exam table. Tap the tendon just below the patella and watch for the quadriceps to contract and extend the knee (Procedure 5-21d). This tests lumbar nerves L2, L3, and L4.

ACHILLES TENDON   With your patient sitting, dorsiflex the foot at the ankle and strike the Achilles tendon (Procedure 5-21e). Watch for the calf muscles to contract and cause plantar flexion of the foot. This tests sacral nerves S1 and S2.

PLANTAR   Test the superficial abdominal reflexes and plantar response. These are initiated by stimulating the skin instead of muscle. Assess the plantar reflex by stroking the lateral aspect of the sole from the heel to the ball of your patient's foot, curving medially across the ball (Procedure 5-21f). Begin with the lightest stimulus that will elicit a response. If you detect no response, be more firm. Watch for plantar flexion of the toes. Note whether the big toe dorsiflexes while the other toes fan out. Known as a positive **Babinski's response**, this indicates a central nervous system lesion.

Test the abdominal reflex by lightly stroking each side of the abdomen above and below the umbilicus with an irregular object such as a reflex hammer, a broken cotton

Assessment Pearls

For various reasons, it is difficult to test for deep tendon reflexes (DTRs) in some patients. To enhance DTRs, use a technique referred to as *augmentation*. Have the patient isometrically tense muscles not directly involved in the reflex being tested. For example, if testing patellar DTRs, have the patient grab the fingers of his opposite hand, clench his fists, and try to pull both hands apart with fingers interlocked. When testing upper-extremity DTRs, have the patient clench his jaw or contract his quadriceps. These procedures will augment DTRs and provide a more accurate reading.

swab, or a split tongue blade (Procedure 5-21g). Note the contraction of the abdominal muscles and how the umbilicus deviates to the stimulus. The area above the umbilicus is innervated by thoracic nerves T8, T9, and T10. The area below the umbilicus is innervated by thoracic nerves T10, T11, and T12. The absence of abdominal reflexes can suggest either a central or peripheral nervous system disorder.

Reassessment

En route to the hospital, conduct an ongoing series of reassessments to detect trends, determine changes in your patient's condition, and assess the effectiveness of your interventions. Patient condition can change suddenly. You must steadfastly reassess mental status, airway patency, breathing adequacy, circulation, and any deterioration in areas already compromised. Conduct your reassessment every 15 minutes for stable patients and every 5 minutes for unstable patients. Compare your findings to the baseline findings and note any trends.

Mental Status

Recheck your patient's mental status by performing the AVPU exam frequently during transport (Procedure 5-22a). Any deterioration in mental status is cause for great concern. The brain demands a constant supply of oxygen and glucose and a constant elimination of waste products. When it is deprived of either—even briefly—expect rapid mental status changes. A falling level of response indicates either a direct or an indirect brain pathology.

For example, following a head injury, your patient who was alert and oriented at the scene gradually becomes sleepy and eventually unarousable. You should suspect a life-threatening increase in intracranial pressure (pressure inside the enclosed skull) and expedite transport to the appropriate medical facility. Or your patient with an intraabdominal hemorrhage becomes increasingly less arousable as a result of the decreased oxygenated blood flow to the brain (indirect pathology).

Sometimes patients improve following your interventions. After you administer 50 percent dextrose to your

Procedure 5-21 Testing the Reflexes

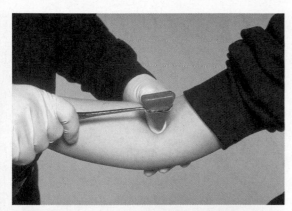

5-21a Test the biceps reflex (cervical nerves C5 and C6).

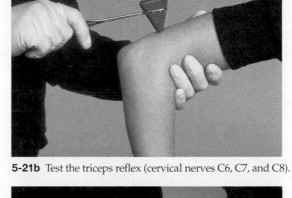

5-21b Test the triceps reflex (cervical nerves C6, C7, and C8).

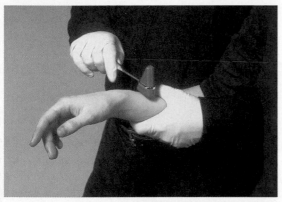

5-21c Test the brachioradialis reflex (cervical nerves C5 and C6).

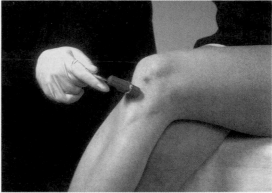

5-21d Test the quadriceps reflex (lumbar nerves L2, L3, and L4).

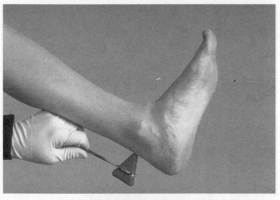

5-21e Test the Achilles reflex (sacral nerves S1 and S2).

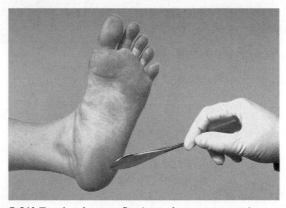

5-21f Test the plantar reflex (central nervous system).

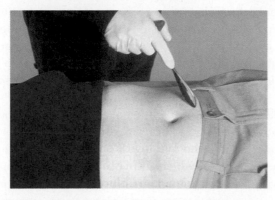

5-21g Test abdominal reflexes (thoracic nerves T8, T9, T10, T11, and T12).

Procedure 5-22 Reassessment

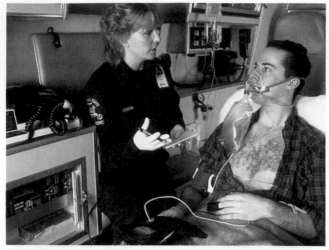

5-22a Reevaluate the ABCs.

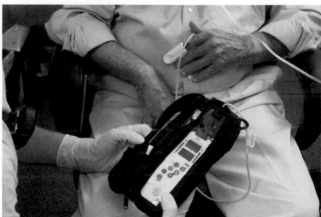

5-22b Take all vital signs again.

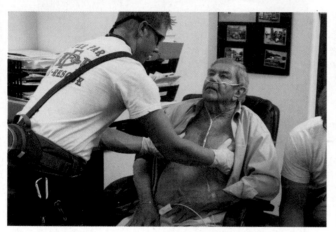

5-22c Perform your focused assessment again.

5-22d Evaluate your interventions' effects.

hypoglycemic diabetic patient, for instance, he becomes alert and begins talking.

Airway Patency

The patency of your patient's airway can change instantly. Bleeding, vomiting, and even secretions can suddenly obstruct the upper airway. Be prepared to suction your patient quickly. Respiratory burns and anaphylaxis can cause life-threatening swelling in a matter of minutes. Croup and epiglottitis also can quickly deteriorate into total upper airway occlusion.

Endotracheal intubation is the best way to secure the airway in patients with no gag reflex. However, endotracheal tubes can become dislodged easily during transport. Recheck for tube placement frequently during transport and every time you move your patient onto a backboard, onto the stretcher, or onto the hospital gurney.

The price of proper airway management is eternal vigilance and a pessimistic outlook—anything that can go wrong will go wrong. Be prepared for the worst.

Breathing Rate and Quality

A change in respiratory rate or quality might indicate improvement or deterioration. A sudden increase in rate or respiratory effort suggests deterioration. For example, if your patient suddenly begins to gasp for air, has retractions, and uses his accessory neck muscles, he has a serious problem.

Sometimes the signs are not so obvious. Subtle increases in respiratory rate can suggest a developing problem. A decrease in rate and effort could mean that your treatments are effective and your patient is improving. For example, after you administer an albuterol treatment, your patient breathes easier and his lung sounds improve. In infants and young children, however, a decrease in rate and effort may mean that your patient is exhausted and requires aggressive intervention. If, while assisting ventilation with a bag-valve mask, your partner suddenly complains that squeezing the bag is becoming more difficult, consider the possibility that a tension pneumothorax is developing or that bronchospasm or laryngospasm may be occurring. Airway and breathing management requires constant reevaluation.

Pulse Rate and Quality

Check central and peripheral pulses and compare the findings with earlier measurements. A rising pulse rate could indicate shock, hypoxia, or cardiac dysrhythmia. A falling rate could mean the terminal stage of shock or a rise in intracranial pressure. A sudden change in rate or regularity may suggest a cardiac dysrhythmia. The loss of peripheral pulses could mean decompensating shock.

Skin Condition

Similar to mental status, the skin quickly reflects the body's hemodynamic status. Reevaluate your patient's skin color, temperature, and condition. Cyanosis suggests decreased oxygenation. Lip cyanosis indicates central hypoxia (overall oxygen status), whereas peripheral cyanosis indicates decreased oxygen to the tissues.

Pallor and coolness suggest decreased circulation to the skin, as seen in shock. If your patient suddenly develops hives after you administer a medication, suspect an allergic reaction. A localized redness and warmth could indicate bleeding under the skin or vasodilation. Cyanosis and coolness in a lower extremity suggest a peripheral vascular problem, such as an arterial occlusion. A deep venous thrombosis will result in redness, swelling, and warmth in the lower leg.

Transport Priorities

Sometimes stable patients suddenly deteriorate en route to the hospital. For example, the formerly conscious and alert head injury patient now responds only to pain. Or your stable cardiac patient suddenly develops a life-threatening dysrhythmia. Or your patient suddenly cannot breathe because his simple pneumothorax has developed into a tension pneumothorax. In these cases, while you provide lifesaving treatments, change your transport decision to a higher priority. By the same token, if your unstable patient becomes stable, you may wish to downgrade your priority transport decision and decrease the danger and liability of driving with lights and siren on.

Vital Signs

Reassessing vital signs reveals trends clearly (Procedure 5-22b). A rising pulse rate combined with a falling blood pressure indicates shock. A decreasing pulse rate combined with a rising blood pressure, associated with an irregular respiratory pattern, suggests a rise in intracranial pressure. Any change in heart rate could indicate a cardiac dysrhythmia. A narrowing pulse pressure with a weakening pulse indicates cardiac tamponade, a tension pneumothorax, or hypovolemic shock. Reevaluate your critical patient's vital signs every 5 minutes and look for changes.

Focused Assessment

Elicit your patient's chief complaint again to determine whether the problem still exists or whether other problems have arisen. Often, following trauma, your patient will develop more complaints en route to the hospital, as the excitement of the incident begins to wear off. Patients often focus on their major injuries and might not even be aware of other problems. Repeat your focused assessment as your patient's chief complaint dictates (Procedure 5-22c).

Effects of Interventions

Evaluate the effects of any interventions (Procedure 5-22d). Did the albuterol treatment help open the lower airways? Did the oxygen and nitroglycerin relieve the chest pain? What are the effects of the fluid challenge on your patient's breathing? Did your intervention help or harm your patient? Is he getting better or worse? Know the expected therapeutic benefits of your interventions and then evaluate whether they worked. For example, you administer amiodarone to convert hemodynamically stable ventricular tachycardia. Following administration, observe your patient's electrocardiogram for changes while noting any harmful side effects such as nausea, vomiting, or seizures.

Management Plans

Evaluate whether your care is working. If it is not, consider another management plan. Develop the courage to admit when your plan is not working and the flexibility to change your course of action. For example, your patient, an elderly man with a history of congestive heart failure (CHF) and chronic obstructive pulmonary disease (COPD), presents with severe difficulty breathing and audible wheezing. You suspect he is having an exacerbation of his COPD, administer two nebulizer treatments, and begin transporting. En route, however, he is not improving, and now you also can hear crackles bilaterally. At this point, you suspect he is in CHF and change your management to administering nitroglycerin and continuous positive airway pressure (CPAP).

Patients often present with multiple complaints, symptoms, and histories. Formulating a definitive diagnosis is difficult without the hospital's labs, X-rays, and other assessment tools. Your ability to reassess your patient, reevaluate your field diagnosis, and alter your management plan will optimize patient care.

Summary

A comprehensive knowledge of anatomy and physiology is crucial in being able to perform a thorough secondary assessment. This knowledge will help you understand what should be normal and where to find and palpate specific organs and structures.

A thorough secondary assessment includes assessing and evaluating the entire patient, head to toe. As we have discussed, this is not always necessary, but it depends on the situation you are in. You should develop a consistent approach to assessment that will allow you the flexibility to deviate and adjust the assessment as necessary. By using a common approach, you are much less likely to overlook anything—and it could become a legal defense, if necessary.

Inspection, palpation, percussion, and auscultation are essential skills for all paramedics. Before a paramedic can begin to treat a patient, he must be able to determine the injury or illness and its extent through a combination of the primary assessment and secondary assessment. Time spent perfecting your assessment skills will prove to be invaluable throughout your career.

You Make the Call

You are on standby at the local raceway for a historic car race. About halfway through the final lap, you see a small roadster lose control on a sharp turn. You watch, as the vehicle appears to roll over twice before coming to rest on the driver side door. As you approach the scene and position the ambulance, you see that race safety personnel are quickly extricating the driver from the car. The patient is awake and has a patent airway, adequate respirations, and a rapid radial pulse. Following local protocols, you position the patient on your gurney and load him into your ambulance. As your paramedic partner starts an IV, you begin your secondary physical assessment.

1. A thorough physical exam involves auscultation, inspection, palpation, and percussion. Beginning with the head, list specifically what you will assess for in each area of the body. Identify the exam technique you will use. For example, you may assess the chest for the presence of a flail segment by palpation.

See Suggested Responses at the back of this book.

Review Questions

1. You are caring for a middle-aged male patient with abdominal pain. During your physical exam, which of the following should you do when palpating his abdomen?

   a. Always perform deep palpation first.

   b. Observe your patient's face during the procedure.

   c. Use the heel of one hand to perform deep palpation.

   d. Always palpate the painful area first.

2. You are assessing a patient with a history of COPD who has wrecked his car. He is complaining of chest pain and dyspnea. During your percussion of his chest, you note a hollow and vibrating resonance. This indicates the presence of _____

   a. air.   c. pleural fluid.

   b. blood.   d. pus.

3. Korotkoff sounds, which are generated by the cardiovascular system and heard with a stethoscope, represent _____

   a. the AV valves closing.

   b. the semilunar valves closing.

   c. blood hitting the arterial walls.

   d. a blockage in the carotid arteries.

4. You are managing a patient whose last three sets of vitals have yielded a pulse pressure of 32, 48, and 56 mmHg, respectively. This trend most likely represents _____

   a. increasing intracranial pressure.

   b. pericardial tamponade.

   c. tension pneumothorax.

   d. decompensated shock.

5. While you are transitioning your patient from a lying position to the wheeled cot, you help him stand for a brief moment. During this period, the pulse rate displayed on the finger pulse oximeter jumps 24 beats/minute in the standing position. What should you suspect?

    a. Congestive heart failure

    b. Volume depletion

    c. Severe hypertension

    d. Coronary artery disease

6. Which is the most reliable location for obtaining an accurate pulse rate on an infant?

    a. Apical

    b. Carotid

    c. Radial

    d. Brachial

7. During your secondary assessment, you note that the patient's alveolar breath sounds are now absent, and the pulse oximeter, which was registering 97%, now reads 90%. The patient has been responsive only to deep painful stimuli during the entire transport time, and her heart rate is slowly starting to rise. What should you do next, given these findings?

    a. Initiate positive pressure ventilation.

    b. Start a second IV and administer a fluid bolus.

    c. Divert transport to the closest certified stroke center.

    d. Immediately intubate the trachea.

8. Bilateral periorbital ecchymosis and/or mastoid process discoloration are classic signs of _____

    a. increased intracranial pressure.

    b. basilar skull fracture.

    c. orbital injury.

    d. TMJ dislocation.

9. Placing the tip of your finger into the depression just anterior to the tragus and asking your patient to open his mouth is the procedure for assessing his

    _____

    a. gag reflex.

    b. cranial nerve IX.

    c. TMJ.

    d. ability to swallow.

10. The "H" test performed during the secondary assessment is meant to evaluate _____

    a. eyelid opening.

    b. peripheral vision.

    c. extraocular muscles.

    d. the corneal reflex.

11. When palpating the carotid arteries, you notice a left-sided thrill. Which procedure should you perform next to further investigate this finding?

    a. Auscultate for bruits.

    b. Percuss for dullness.

    c. Obtain a 12-lead ECG.

    d. Evaluate for egophony.

12. While reading your partner's PCR from the transport you just completed, you note that he documented that the sounds heard at the "PMI" were normal. This finding refers to what organ?

    a. Large intestine

    b. Heart

    c. Right lung

    d. Pancreas

13. You are assessing the distal pulse in your patient with a suspected spinal cord injury, and you find that it is strong and bounding. When you report this, you would characterize it as a pulse quality of

    _____

    a. 1+.   c. 3+.

    b. 2+.   d. 4+.

14. As you are conducting the physical examination on your patient, you note a large mass that pulsates. This finding is suggestive of a(n) _____

    a. malignancy.   c. sarcoma.

    b. aneurysm.   d. cyst.

15. A patient with ascites found during the secondary assessment will commonly have a history of

    _____

    a. brain injury.

    b. liver or renal disease.

    c. diabetes mellitus.

    d. tuberculosis.

16. The medical term for the "crunching" sound heard when manipulating a joint of an arthritis patient is

    _____.

    a. osteoarthritis.

    b. crepitus.

    c. bursitis.

    d. tendonitis.

17. Your patient has dysarthria. This is best described as a speech defect caused by _____

    a. vocal cord problems.

    b. damage to the cortex.

    c. motor deficits.

    d. psychotic disorder.

18. You are performing a secondary exam on a patient and have placed a familiar object—a key—into the patient's hand and asked him to identify it. This test is known as_____
    a. position sense.
    b. discrimination.
    c. vibration sense.
    d. spinothalamic testing.

19. To assess your patient's recent memory during the secondary assessment, ask him to
    a. add two numbers together.

b. describe his boyhood neighborhood.

c. describe his last meal.

d. give you his Social Security number.

20. When assessing the extremities during the secondary assessment, unilateral coldness suggests

_____
    a. an environmental problem.
    b. an arterial occlusion.
    c. a venous occlusion.
    d. shock.

See Answers to Review Questions at the back of this book.

References

1. Rock, M. "Underexposed: The Neglected Art of the Physical Exam." *JEMS* 2006;31(5): 40–43.
2. Ochoa, F. J., et al. "Competence of Health Professionals to Check the Carotid Pulse." *Resuscitation* 1998;37(3): 173–175.
3. Kantola, I., et al. "Bell or Diaphragm in the Measurement of Blood Pressure?" *J Hypertension* 2005;23(3): 499–503.
4. Bates, B., L. S. Bickley, and R. A. Hoekelman. *A Guide to Physical Examination and History Taking.* 9th ed. Philadelphia: Lippincott Williams & Wilkins, 2005.
5. Bledsoe, B. E. and F. Martini. *Anatomy and Physiology for Emergency Care.* 2nd ed. Upper Saddle River, NJ: Pearson/Prentice Hall, 2008.
6. Popov, T. "Review: Capillary Refill Time, Abnormal Skin Turgor, and Respiratory Pattern Are Useful Signs for Detecting Dehydration in Children." *Evidenced Based Nursing* 205;29(1): 2–19.
7. Seidel, H. M., et al. *Mosby's Guide to Physical Examination.* 6th ed. St. Louis: Mosby, 2006.
8. *Expert 10-Minute Physical Exams.* St. Louis: Mosby Lifeline, 1997.
9. Bradford, C. A. *Basic Ophthalmology for Medical Students and Primary Care Residents.* 8th ed. San Francisco: American Academy of Ophthalmology, 2004.
10. *Assessment Made Incredibly Easy.* 4th ed. Springhouse, PA: Springhouse Corporation, 2008.
11. Epstein, O., et al. *Clinical Examination.* 3rd ed. St. Louis: Mosby, 2003.
12. Sinisalo, J., et al. "Simplifying the Estimation of Jugular Venous Pressure." *Am J Cardiol* 2007;100(12): 1779–1781.
13. Pullen, R. L., Jr. "Assessing for Hepatojugular Reflex." *Nursing* 2006;36(2): 28.

Further Reading

Advanced Cardiac Life Support Manual. Dallas: American Heart Association, 2015.
American Heart Association. 2015 American Heart Association Guidelines for Cardiopulmonary Resuscitation and Emergency Cardiovascular Care Science. (Available at http://circ.ahajournals.org/content/vol122/18_suppl_3/. Accessed July 20, 2015.)
Bledsoe, B. E. and R. W. Benner. *Critical Care Paramedic.* Upper Saddle River, NJ: Pearson/Prentice Hall, 2006.
Bledsoe, B. E., B. J. Colbert, and J. E. Ankney. *Essentials of A&P for Emergency Care.* Upper Saddle River, NJ: Pearson/Prentice Hall, 2011.
Campbell, J. E. *International Trauma Life Support for Prehospital Care Providers.* 7th ed. Upper Saddle River, NJ: Pearson/Prentice Hall, 2012.
Foltin, G., et al. *Teaching Resource for Instructors in Prehospital Pediatrics for Paramedics.* New York: Center for Pediatric Medicine, 2002.
Limmer, D., M. F. O'Keefe, et al. *Emergency Care.* 12th ed. Upper Saddle River, NJ: Pearson/Prentice Hall, 2011.
Mistovich, J., et al. *Prehospital Emergency Care.* 9th ed. Upper Saddle River, NJ: Pearson/Prentice Hall, 2009.
Netter, F. H. *Netter's Atlas of Human Anatomy.* 6th ed. St. Louis: Mosby, 2014.
Prehospital Trauma Life Support, 7th ed. St. Louis: Mosby Lifeline, 2010.
Spaite, D. W., et al. "A Prospective Evaluation of Prehospital Patient Assessment by Direct In-Field Observation: Failure of ALS Personnel to Measure Vital Signs." *Prehosp Disaster Med.* 5 (1990): 325–333.
Tintinalli, J. E., et al. *Tintinalli's Emergency Medicine: A Comprehensive Guide.* 7th ed. New York: McGraw-Hill, 2010.
Yanoff, M., et al. *Ophthalmology.* 2nd ed. St. Louis: Elsevier Science, 2004.

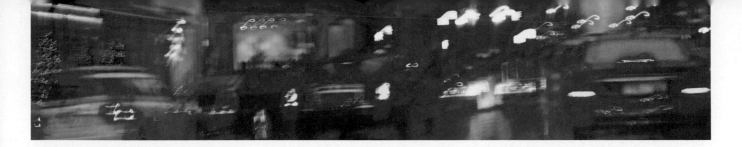

Chapter 6
Patient Monitoring Technology

Richard A. Cherry, MS, EMT-P

Bryan E. Bledsoe, DO, FACEP, FAAEM, EMT-P

Joseph R. Lauro, MD, EMT-P

STANDARD
Assessment

COMPETENCY
Integrate scene and patient assessment findings with knowledge of epidemiology and pathophysiology to form a field impression. This includes developing a list of differential diagnoses through clinical reasoning to modify the assessment and formulate a treatment plan.

 ## Learning Objectives

Terminal Performance Objective: After reading this chapter, you should be able to integrate patient monitoring technology into the patient assessment process.

Enabling Objectives: To accomplish the terminal performance objective, you should be able to:

1. Define key terms introduced in this chapter.

2. Discuss the purpose, applications, procedures, diagnostic information provided, and limitations for single-lead ECG monitoring.

3. Discuss the purpose, applications, procedures, diagnostic information provided, and limitations for 12-lead ECG monitoring.

4. Discuss the purpose, applications, procedures, diagnostic information provided, and limitations for pulse oximetry monitoring.

5. Discuss the purpose, applications, procedures, diagnostic information provided, and limitations for end-tidal capnography monitoring.

6. Discuss the purpose, applications, procedures, diagnostic information provided, and limitations for carbon monoxide monitoring.

7. Discuss the purpose, applications, procedures, diagnostic information provided, and limitations for methemoglobinemia monitoring.

8. Discuss the purpose, applications, procedures, diagnostic information provided, and limitations for total hemoglobin monitoring.

9. Discuss the purpose, applications, procedures, diagnostic information provided, and limitations for blood glucometry monitoring.

10. Discuss the purpose, applications, procedures, diagnostic information provided, and limitations for basic blood chemistry monitoring.

11. Discuss the purpose, applications, procedures, diagnostic information provided, and limitations for arterial blood gas monitoring.

12. Discuss the purpose, applications, procedures, diagnostic information provided, and limitations for bedside ultrasonography and FAST exam.

13. Given a scenario with diagnostic findings, discuss how this information can facilitate the determination of primary field impression and several differential diagnosis.

KEY TERMS

arterial blood gas, p. 214

artifact, p. 182

augmented leads, p. 185

B-natriuretic peptide, p. 211

bipolar leads, p. 176

blood tube, p. 208

carboxyhemoglobin, p. 198

creatine kinase, p. 210

deoxyhemoglobin, p. 191

depolarization, p. 175

Einthoven's triangle, p. 177

electrodes, p. 176

electrolyte, p. 211

glycogenolysis, p. 205

heme, p. 191

hemoconcentration, p. 210

hemolysis, p. 210

ischemia, p. 183

lactic dehydrogenase, p. 210

leads, p. 176

methemoglobin, p. 201

multidraw needle, p. 208

myocardium, p. 174

myoglobin, p. 211

oxyhemoglobin, p. 191

precordial (chest) leads, p. 186

pulse oximetry, p. 191

troponins, p. 211

ultrasound, p. 215

unipolar leads, p. 185

vacutainer, p. 208

Case Study

It had been years since Paul Cuzins was in the back of an ambulance. He had been a paramedic for most of his professional life, but that seemed like a lifetime ago. Now he lies on the stretcher en route to the hospital. His wife called because he had been experiencing some unusual weakness and upper abdominal discomfort. Paul had never imagined this day and especially had not thought he would ever be in the back of an ambulance.

As he watched the paramedics attach him to a very sophisticated-looking device, he felt as if he was in a Star Trek scenario. He reminisced about the old "Lifepak 4 and orange box telemetry unit" he used back in his day. Lead paramedic Rich Russell showed him their new device and told him everything they would monitor during the ride. He also explained how this new technology enables him to recognize and document dangerous trends in a patient's condition.

"OK, we're going to hook you up to our monitor, lead II, and see what your heart is doing." Paul was well versed on rhythm strip monitoring and waited with anticipation to learn of all the other capabilities of this new machine. "Looks like you're in normal sinus rhythm, but with your history of risk factors and your vague complaints, we're going to do a 12-lead as well." "Twelve-lead, are you serious?" remarked Paul. "Wow, things sure have changed since I retired."

"Yes, when 12-lead ECG capabilities first became available, not many EMS agencies used it but, in time, cardiologists and EMS medical directors convinced us that if we really wanted to help provide the earliest possible treatment for patients with acute coronary syndromes, we should use 12-lead ECGs." Paul's 12-lead showed some minor ST segment elevation in leads II, III, and aVF, suggesting ischemia in his inferior myocardial wall.

"We're going to administer some oxygen, start an IV line, and also put this noninvasive blood pressure cuff on your arm. It will automatically inflate every five minutes and measure your blood pressure for us. It's a real time saver because, as you know, it's difficult to hear blood pressures using stethoscopes in moving ambulances. So someone adapted an electronic BP device into our prehospital monitors." Paul was amazed at what he was hearing and seeing.

"Now, I'm sure you've seen one of these before," said Rich as he placed a spring probe on Paul's finger. "Sure, it's to measure my oxygen levels. I saw this on the Discovery Channel."

"Yes, pulse oximetry has been available since the mid-1980s, but this probe measures a lot more than that. These incredible bioengineers developed the technology to noninvasively and continuously monitor carboxyhemoglobin and methemoglobin, as well as pulse oximetry, using the same finger probe."

"That sound very impressive, but why would you want to?" asked Paul. Rich answered, "I asked the same question when it first came out. But being able to monitor carbon monoxide concentrations in a patient's blood eliminates the risk of misdiagnosing unsuspected carbon monoxide poisoning as flu or fatigue. Misdiagnosing either carbon monoxide or methemoglobinemia can have dire consequences.

"We're also going to monitor your carbon dioxide levels with this little device I'm putting on your nasal cannula," Rich said. "Capnography—why measure that?" asked Paul. "Well, we can watch your breathing and circulation effectiveness and be alerted to problems immediately. It's really a great tool."

"Is that all, or is there more?" asked this very impressed patient.

"Funny you should ask. It's also a manual defibrillator, an automatic external defibrillator, and an external cardiac pacemaker." "That's quite a machine. When I worked the streets I couldn't have even imagined such a device," said Paul. "Someday all these capabilities, and more, will be available in a handheld device the size of my PDA. What do you think about that?" asked paramedic Russell.

"It's just amazing the advances EMS has made over the years," said Paul. Rich replied, "Yes, we can save the emergency department staff a lot of time if we do these things in the ambulance. It's all about delivering the best patient care possible."

Customer Service Minute

Communication. Communication skills play a vital role in every customer interaction and often determine their evaluation of our service. How well do we communicate to our patients and their families? To our coworkers and other responding agencies? To other health care providers at nursing homes? To the emergency department staff? In all these instances, effective communication is the key to good relations.

Nonverbal communication may play an even more important role than the words we say. Communication studies demonstrate that often people will concentrate more on our nonverbal posture and the tone of our voices than on the actual words we speak. Watch your body language, your facial expressions, your gestures, and your tone. Make sure they match what you are trying to say.

The most important aspect of effective communication is eye contact. Your eyes are the mirror of your soul. It is what separates truly sincere people from the phonies. Look into the eyes of whomever you're talking with. It says "I am speaking to you and I care about you." There is no more effective way to communicate.

Introduction

The past 40 years have witnessed an explosion of new technology in EMS. This new technology has enabled you to do your job better by helping you to recognize dangerous trends occurring in your patient's condition, to better document those trends and the care you provided, and present that documentation and trending data to the emergency department staff. We have come an incredibly long way—and there is no reason to think this trend is waning. In fact, the opposite is true. There is every reason to be excited about the most recent advances in prehospital patient monitoring. A quick historical perspective serves to illustrate how far we have come technologically as an industry in the past 40 years.

You may remember the first manual defibrillators. They were monophasic, large, and heavy, and used paddles that had to be smeared with electrode jelly. And all they were capable of was monitoring your patient's rhythm and performing manual defibrillation. Compare them with today's units, with biphasic electrical technology and hands-off multifunction electrode pads that monitor as well as provide defibrillation, synchronized cardioversion, and external cardiac pacing. For years, only physicians could defibrillate. Now, any bystander with minimal training can safely and effectively perform automated defibrillation.

The first ECG monitors were primitive units that recorded only a single limb lead. Now you can acquire and transmit a 12-lead ECG directly to the hospital. In certain cases, this allows you to deliver your patient directly to the cardiac cath lab. This is a critical time and cardiac muscle-saving benefit for your acute coronary syndrome patients. From glucose dipsticks to easy, one-touch glucometers; from single function pulse oximetry finger probes to revolutionary multifunction probes that also accurately measure carbon monoxide and methemoglobin; from aneroid sphygmomanometers to automatic

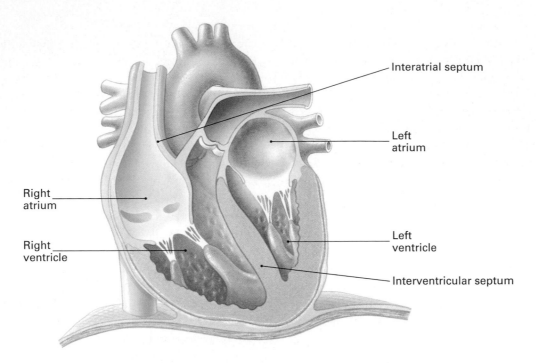

Interatrial septum

Left atrium

Right atrium

Right ventricle

Left ventricle

Interventricular septum

FIGURE 6-1 The chambers of the heart.

electronic blood pressure monitoring—we can only imagine what the future holds.

In this chapter, we discuss how to use this array of technology in everyday prehospital patient care. We take an in-depth look at the following:

- ECG monitoring
- 12-lead ECG acquisition
- Pulse oximetry
- Capnometry and capnography
- CO-oximetry
- Methemoglobin monitoring
- Total hemoglobin monitoring
- Glucometry
- Basic blood chemistries (cardiac biomarkers, electrolytes, arterial blood gases, and serum lactate)
- Ultrasound

For each device, we discuss the pertinent anatomy and physiology, explain the technology, discuss its limitations, and describe how and when to use it. As always, which technology you use in the field is always determined by your patient's situation and condition.

ECG Monitoring
Anatomy and Electrophysiology

The heart is a mechanical pump that runs on electricity. The mechanical component is composed of cardiac mus-

cle fibers that, when stimulated, contract in a uniform fashion to eject blood from its chambers. The heart is really two pumps (Figure 6-1). The right side, made up of the right atrium and right ventricle, receives oxygen-poor blood from the body's tissues and delivers it to the lungs. There, an extremely thin alveolar–capillary membrane facilitates the diffusion of oxygen into the capillary. Pulmonary veins transport this oxygen-rich blood to the left side of the heart, made up of the left atrium and left ventricle, which sends it out to the body to nourish the cells. A series of one-way valves keeps the blood moving forward and prevents backflow in this remarkably efficient pump (Figure 6-2).

The heart muscle itself is perfused by the coronary arteries (Figure 6-3) that lie on the surface of the **myocardium**. Like all other organs in the body, the heart must receive a constant supply of oxygen and nutrients and rid itself of carbon dioxide and waste products in order to function properly.

The electrical component consists of a unique system of specialized excitatory and conductive fibers. These fibers are designed to conduct electrical impulses quickly—400 times faster than the standard cell membrane—from one muscle fiber to the next (Figure 6-4). This speed allows cardiac muscle cells to function physiologically as a unit. That is, when one cell becomes excited, the action potential spreads rapidly across the entire group of cells, resulting in a coordinated muscle contraction.

The pacemaker for this system is the sinoatrial (SA) node located in the right atrium (Figure 6-5). The SA node has automaticity, a property that allows it to initiate an

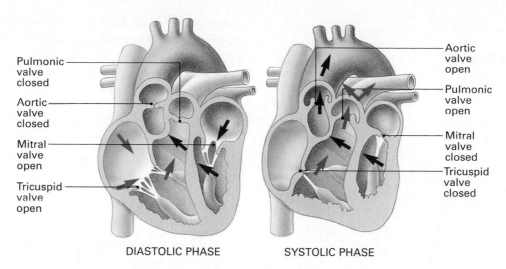

FIGURE 6-2 One-way valves prevent backflow during the cardiac cycles.

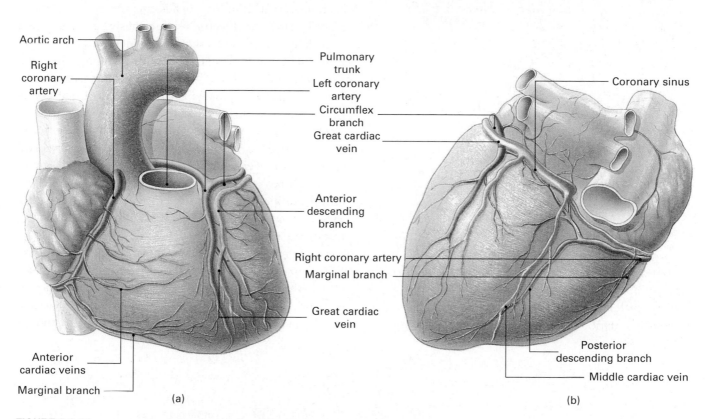

FIGURE 6-3 The coronary circulation: (a) anterior; (b) posterior.

electrical impulse. A process known as **depolarization**, in which electrolytes such as sodium and potassium cross cell membranes and cause a shift in cell polarity, generates this impulse. When a cardiac cell depolarizes, the inside of the cell becomes more positive and "charged." This impulse is conducted to all adjacent cells, which, in turn, become excited and depolarize. Intraatrial pathways connect the SA node to the atrioventricular (AV) node. These internodal pathways conduct the depolarization impulse to the

atrial muscle mass and through the atria to the AV junction. As the atrial muscle is depolarized, a wave of muscle contraction helps push blood into the ventricles. The AV junction actually slows the impulse, allowing the ventricles extra time to fill. Then, the impulse passes through the AV junction into the AV node and on to the AV fibers, which conduct the impulse from the atria to the ventricles.

In the ventricles, the AV fibers form the bundle of His. The bundle of His subsequently divides into the right and

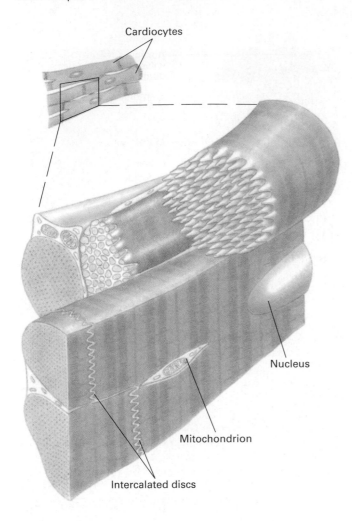

Cardiocytes

Nucleus

Mitochondrion

Intercalated discs

FIGURE 6-4 Microscopic appearance of cardiac muscle. The intercalated disks speed transmission of the electrical potential quickly from one cell to the next.

left bundle branches. The bundle branches deliver the impulse rapidly to the apex of the heart. From there, the Purkinje system spreads it across the myocardium in an inferior-to-superior direction. A wave of cardiac muscle

contractions follows these impulses and ejects blood from the right ventricle to the lungs and from the left ventricle to the body. This entire electromechanical process resembles a patterned series of falling dominoes.

Repolarization, or the return of polarity, occurs predominantly in the opposite direction. The electrocardiogram (ECG) records these electrical events on the rhythm strip.

The heart will continue to function day after day, year after year, unless there is a serious malfunction in either the mechanical or the electrical system.

Technology

The body acts as a giant conductor of electricity, and the heart is its largest generator of electrical energy. The ECG machine indirectly detects electrical voltage changes that are caused when the heart muscle depolarizes during each heartbeat. It accomplishes this through electrodes placed on the skin. **Electrodes** are adhesive pads designed to stick to your patient's skin; they contain conductive gel to facilitate the transmission of electrical impulses. The electrodes are connected by color-coded wires, also called **leads**, to the ECG machine. The electrical activity is recorded as tiny rises and falls in voltage. Because the electrical impulses on the skin surface have a very low voltage, the ECG machine amplifies these impulses and records them over time on ECG graph paper or a monitor.

The three types of ECG leads are bipolar, augmented, and precordial. **Bipolar leads**, the kind most frequently used, have one positive electrode and one negative electrode. Any electrical impulse moving toward the positive electrode will cause a positive (upward) deflection on the ECG paper or monitor. Any electrical impulse moving toward the negative electrode will cause a negative (downward) deflection. The absence of a positive or negative deflection means either that there is no electrical impulse

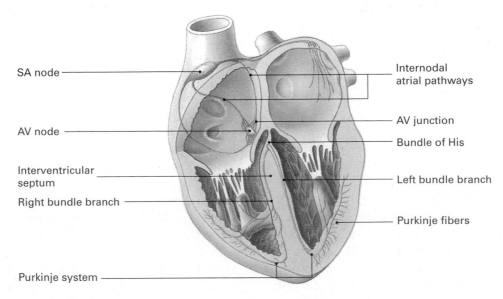

SA node
AV node
Interventricular septum
Right bundle branch
Purkinje system

Internodal atrial pathways
AV junction
Bundle of His
Left bundle branch
Purkinje fibers

FIGURE 6-5 The cardiac conductive system.

or that the impulse is moving perpendicular to the lead. The three bipolar leads are:

- *Lead I.* The negative electrode is placed on the right arm and the positive electrode is placed on the left arm. Thus, when the electrical current moves through the heart from the right arm toward the left arm, lead I will record a positive deflection.
- *Lead II.* The negative electrode is placed on the right arm and the positive electrode is placed on the left leg. Thus, when the electrical current moves through the heart from the right arm toward the left leg, lead II will record a positive deflection.
- *Lead III.* The negative electrode is placed on the left arm and the positive electrode is placed on the left leg. Thus, when the electrical current moves through the heart from the left arm toward the left leg, lead III will record a positive deflection.

A single monitoring lead can provide considerable information, including:

- Heart rate
- Regularity
- Time it takes to conduct the impulse through the various parts of the heart
- The identity of the pacemaker
- Major conduction abnormalities

The electrode placement sites for the three bipolar leads are based on **Einthoven's triangle**, named after the inventor of the ECG machine (Figure 6-6). The two arm and the left leg electrodes form the corners of the triangle.

Electrodes are typically attached to both legs. The right leg is normally used as a ground or a spare, as recordings obtained from either leg are virtually identical. (Usually, the leads are placed on the chest wall rather than the limbs.) Of these, lead II is used more frequently because most of the heart's electrical current flows toward its positive axis. This gives the best view of the ECG waves and best depicts the conduction system's activity. The direction from the nega-

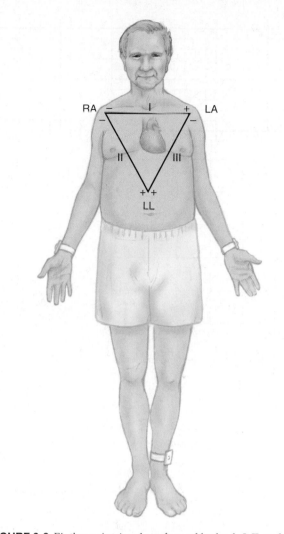

FIGURE 6-6 Einthoven's triangle as formed by leads I, II, and III.

tive to the positive electrode is the lead's axis. Each lead shows a different axis of the heart. Lead I, at the top of Einthoven's triangle, has an axis of 0°. Lead II forms the right side of the triangle and has an axis of 60°. Lead III forms the left side of the triangle and has an axis of 120°.

ECG graph paper is standardized to allow comparative analysis of ECG patterns. The paper moves across the stylus at a standard speed of 25 mm/sec (Figure 6-7). The

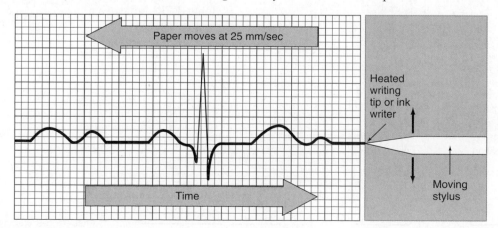

FIGURE 6-7 Recording of the ECG.

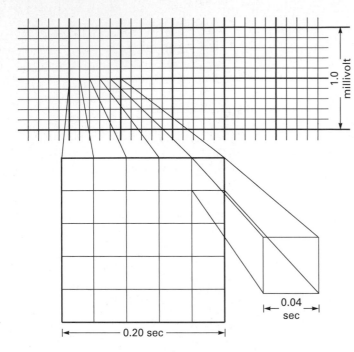

FIGURE 6-8 The ECG paper and markings.

amplitude of the ECG deflection is also standardized. When properly calibrated, the ECG stylus should deflect two large boxes when 1 millivolt (mV) is present. Most machines have calibration buttons, and a calibration curve should be placed at the beginning of the first ECG strip. Many machines do this automatically when they are first turned on. The ECG graph is divided into a grid of light and heavy lines. The light lines are 1 mm apart, and the heavy lines are 5 mm apart. The heavy lines thus enclose large squares, each containing 25 of the smaller squares formed by the lighter lines (Figure 6-8). The following relationships apply to the horizontal axis:

- 1 small box = 0.04 sec
- 1 large box = 0.20 sec (0.04 sec × 5 = 0.20 sec)

These increments measure the duration of the ECG complexes and time intervals. The vertical axis reflects the voltage amplitude in millivolts (mV). Two large boxes equal 1 mV.

In addition to the grid, ECG paper has time interval markings at the top. These marks are placed at 3-second intervals. Each 3-second interval contains 15 large boxes (0.2 sec × 15 boxes = 3.0 sec). The time markings measure heart rate.

The ECG tracing's components reflect electrical changes in the heart (Figure 6-9):

- *P wave.* The first component of the ECG, the P wave, corresponds to atrial depolarization. In lead II, it is a positive, rounded wave before the QRS complex (Figures 6-10 through 6-13).

- *PR interval (PRI).* The PR interval is the distance from the beginning of the P wave to the beginning of the QRS complex (Figure 6-14). It represents the time the impulse takes to travel from the atria to the ventricles. A normal PRI is 0.12 to 0.20 sec. A short PRI lasts less than 0.12 sec; a prolonged PRI lasts longer than 0.20 sec. A prolonged PRI indicates a delay in the AV node.

CONTENT REVIEW

➤ ECG Components
- P wave
- QRS complex
- T wave
- U wave

➤ ECG Time Intervals
- PR interval
- ST segment

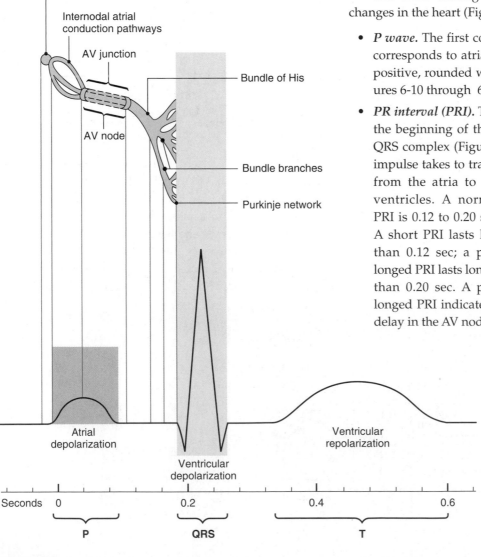

FIGURE 6-9 Relationship of the ECG to electrical activities in the heart.

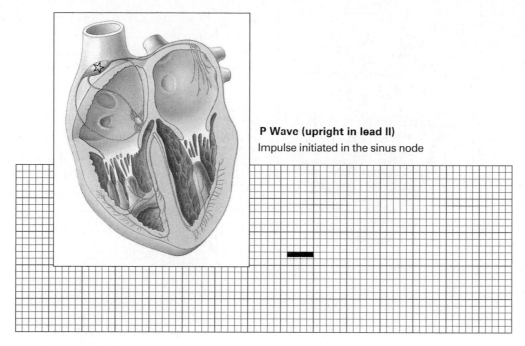

P Wave (upright in lead II)
Impulse initiated in the sinus node

FIGURE 6-10 Impulse initiation in the SA node.

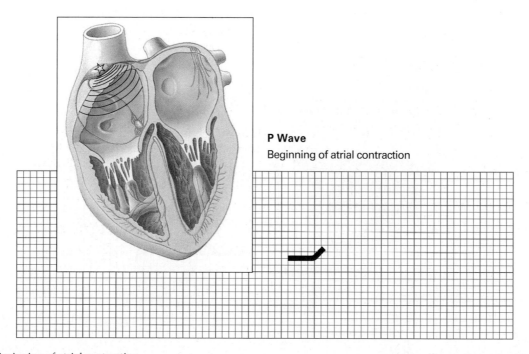

P Wave
Beginning of atrial contraction

FIGURE 6-11 Beginning of atrial contraction.

- *QRS complex.* The QRS complex reflects ventricular depolarization. The Q wave is the first negative deflection after the P wave, the R wave is the first positive deflection after the P wave, and the S wave is the first negative deflection after the R wave. Not all three waves are always present, and the shape of the QRS complex can vary among individuals (Figure 6-15).

- *ST segment.* The ST segment is the distance from the S wave to the beginning of the T wave. Usually it is an

isoelectric line; however, it may be elevated or depressed in certain disease states, such as ischemia.

- *T wave.* The T wave reflects repolarization of the ventricles. Normally positive in lead II, it is rounded and usually moves in the same direction as the QRS complex (Figure 6-16).

- *U wave.* Occasionally, a U wave appears. U waves follow T waves and are usually positive. U waves may be associated with electrolyte abnormalities, or they may be a normal finding.

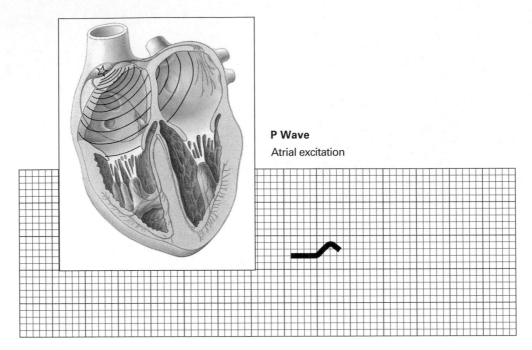

P Wave
Atrial excitation

FIGURE 6-12 Atrial excitation.

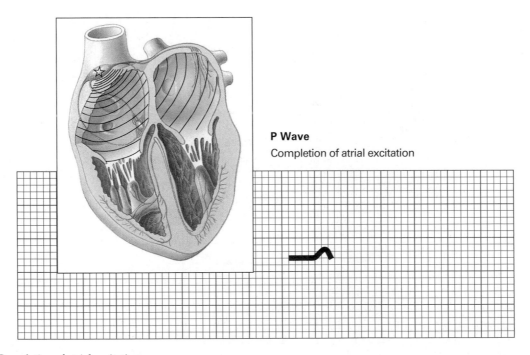

P Wave
Completion of atrial excitation

FIGURE 6-13 Completion of atrial excitation.

The cardiac monitor is essential in assessing and managing your patient's cardiac rhythm (Figure 6-17). The simplest prehospital machines monitor the electrical activity of the heart in three "leads" or positions. These "limb leads" adequately identify life-threatening cardiac rhythms. Twelve-lead ECGs, described later in this chapter, are becoming the standard of care for prehospital use. They are essential in gathering data to confirm a myocardial infarction and to lessen time to reperfusion therapy.

Most modern cardiac monitors also include the capability to perform manual and automated defibrillation, synchronized cardioversion in the presence of an unstable tachycardia, and transcutaneous pacing that provides an electrical impulse to stimulate cardiac contraction in cases of bradycardia and heart blocks. This is a temporary measure until a permanent pacemaker can be implanted. These machines use large multifunction electrode pads that allow you to perform all the aforementioned procedures. The newest multifunction machines also feature noninvasive monitoring capabilities for oxygen saturation, carbon dioxide, carbon monoxide, methemoglobin, and blood pressure.

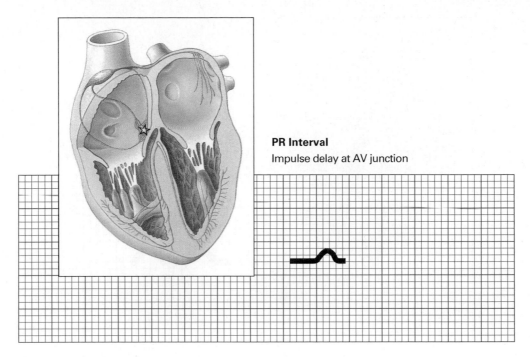

PR Interval

Impulse delay at AV junction

FIGURE 6-14 Impulse delay at the AV junction.

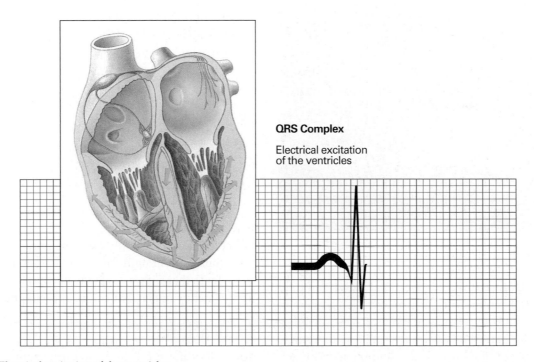

QRS Complex

Electrical excitation
of the ventricles

FIGURE 6-15 Electrical excitation of the ventricles.

Limitations

The cardiac monitor is a useful tool for measuring electrical activity. Electrodes placed on the skin measure voltage changes as they occur. Even using a single-lead rhythm strip, you can easily ascertain the heart rate and the regularity of the rhythm, measure the time it takes to conduct the impulse through the various parts of the heart, determine the pacemaker, and detect conduction problems and threats to perfusion. It has one major disadvantage, however: It cannot tell you whether the heart is pumping efficiently, effectively, or at all. The ECG reading you see does not necessarily correlate with the mechanical function of the heart. Electrical activity can exist with no mechanical contraction, or pulse. Always compare what you see on the monitor with your patient's pulse and blood pressure. These are important steps in developing your patient's clinical picture.

The most common lead used in prehospital care is lead II and is usually sufficient for identifying life-threatening

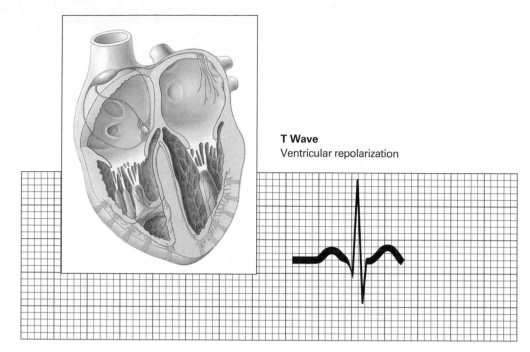

T Wave
Ventricular repolarization

FIGURE 6-16 Ventricular repolarization.

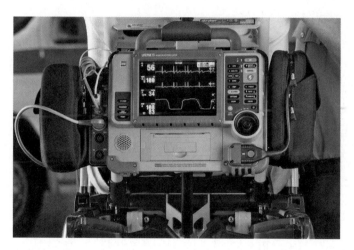

FIGURE 6-17 Cardiac monitor.

arrhythmias. Because it records electrical activity in only one direction (e.g., from the right arm to the left leg), however, sometimes it is impossible to make an accurate interpretation of your patient's ECG from a single lead. A single lead cannot confirm the presence or location of an infarct, axis deviation or chamber enlargement, right-to-left differences in conduction or impulse formation, or the quality or presence of pumping action.

If you suspect a myocardial infarction, a single lead cannot provide the necessary information to make a diagnosis. In both cases, additional leads are necessary to definitively identify the rhythm or the presence of cardiac ischemia or infarction. The 12-lead ECG has become the prehospital standard of care for screening patients for myocardial infarction. We discuss 12-lead ECGs in the next section.

Artifacts are deflections on the ECG produced by factors other than the heart's electrical activity. Artifacts can inhibit your ability to interpret the rhythm. It is important for ECGs to be free of artifacts. Common causes of artifacts include:

- Muscle tremors
- Shivering
- Patient movement
- Loose electrodes
- 60-hertz interference
- Machine malfunction

When an artifact is present, you must first try to eliminate it before recording the ECG. Loose electrodes should be replaced. Occasionally, patients may be quite diaphoretic, thus preventing the electrodes from adhering well to the skin. In these cases, you may need to wipe the skin and apply tincture of benzoin before applying the electrode.

Indications

You will perform cardiac monitoring routinely whenever you need to monitor the heart's rhythm. The most obvious cases involve patients complaining of chest pain, those with irregular pulses, those you suspect may be having a myocardial infarction, and anyone with a severe bradycardia or tachycardia. But the reality is that you will monitor the cardiac status of any patient receiving advanced life support measures, such as patients with difficulty breathing, syncope, altered mental status, major trauma, hypoperfusion, or other derangements of the ABCs. You will hear the following: "O_2 in the presence of hypoxia, IV, monitor" used together when describing routine management of patients with significant illness or injury.

Table 6-1 Bipolar Lead Placement Sites

Lead	Positive Electrode	Negative Electrode
I	Left arm	Right arm
II	Left leg	Right arm
III	Left leg	Loft arm

Procedure

Place the ECG monitor at the side of your patient and turn it on (Procedure 6-1a). Make certain the skin is clean and free of hair before you place the electrodes on the chest wall (Procedure 6-1b). Usually you should place the electrodes on the chest wall instead of the extremities (Procedure 6-1c). This helps to reduce artifacts from arm movement. (If you use the arms, place the lead as high as possible on the extremity to decrease movement.)

For lead II, the positive electrode is usually placed at the apex of the heart on the chest wall (or on the left leg) and the negative electrode below the right clavicle (or on the right arm). The third electrode, the ground, is placed somewhere on the left, upper chest wall (or on the left arm) (Table 6-1). Ask your patient to relax and lie still while you assess the rhythm (Procedure 6-1d). If necessary, obtain rhythm strip tracing (Procedure 6-1e). To change leads and view the heart from a different vector, simply push a button or turn a selector knob on the ECG machine. It's as easy as that.

One of your most important skills as a paramedic will be obtaining and interpreting ECG rhythm strips. Your patient's subsequent treatment will be based on rapid, accurate interpretation of these strips. At first, rhythm strips may seem difficult to read, for only through classroom instruction and repeated practice can you master their interpretation. Nor will every rhythm strip you encounter be a "textbook" example; you must be comfortable with all possible variants. With practice and a systematic approach, however, you will soon be skilled in their interpretation. Refer to the "Cardiology" chapter in Volume 3, Medical Emergencies, for ECG rhythm interpretation and for more information on this topic.

Twelve-Lead ECG Acquisition

Pathophysiology of Acute Coronary Syndromes

As stated earlier in this chapter, the heart is a mechanical pump that runs on electricity. The heart muscle is nourished by two major arteries—the right and left coronary arteries (Figure 6-3). They originate from the base of the aorta and are perfused during diastole, the resting phase of the heart. The left coronary artery (LCA) is the larger of the two and divides into the left anterior descending (LAD) and the left circumflex arteries. The LAD perfuses the anterior ventricular wall and the circumflex perfuses the posterior wall. The right coronary artery (RCA) supplies blood to the right ventricle, the inferior portion of the left ventricle, and the upper pacemaker sites (SA and AV nodes). Understanding the anatomy of the heart's perfusion will help you identify and anticipate the location of infarction.

The heart demands a constant supply of oxygen and nutrients. If the myocardium fails to receive oxygen as a result of coronary artery blockage, the muscle will become ischemic, suffer injury, and eventually die if the situation is not corrected. Because "time is muscle," it is critical to detect the signs and symptoms of a myocardial infarction as early as possible. The 12-lead ECG is the most important diagnostic tool we have to identify the ECG changes that occur when the myocardium becomes ischemic. The ECG changes must occur in two or more contiguous leads to be diagnostically accurate.

The three distinct zones of myocardial damage are ischemia, injury, and infarction (Figure 6-18).

- **Ischemia** occurs when the myocardium is deprived of oxygen for a period of time. Signs and symptoms include chest pain, anxiety, fatigue, and diaphoresis. ECG changes include ST depression, T wave inversion, and peaked T waves. ST depression must be at least one small box below the isoelectric line. This stage is reversible.

- *Injury* signifies damage from prolonged ischemia. Signs and symptoms may include increased chest pain, shortness of breath, increased anxiety, and pallor. ECG changes include ST elevation of 1 mm in two or more contiguous leads and/or T wave inversion. This stage is also reversible.

- *Infarction* means death of myocardial tissue. Signs and symptoms are similar to injury, but they are more significant. Your patient may also state a feeling of impending doom. ECG changes include a significant or pathological Q wave. A significant or pathological Q wave is at least 1 mm or 0.04 seconds wide or deeper than one-third the R wave in the same lead, which develops within 2 hours. It indicates the lack of depolarization through necrotic tissue. This stage is irreversible.

The goal of emergency services in managing the patient with chest pain is to stop the infarction process. The goal of prehospital providers is to acquire 12-lead ECGs on cardiac patients; treat them with aspirin, nitroglycerine, morphine, and oxygen; and deliver them to a facility at

Procedure 6-1 ECG Monitoring

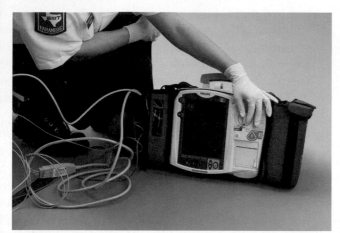

6-1a Turn on the machine.

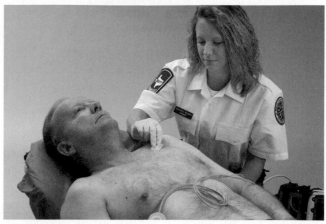

6-1b Prepare the skin.

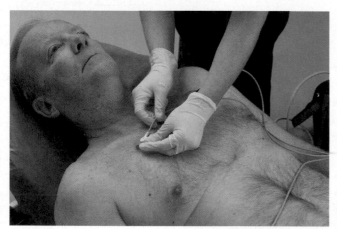

6-1c Apply the electrodes.

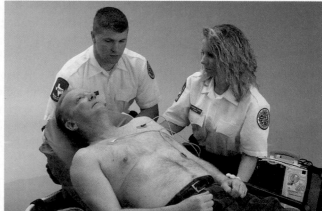

6-1d Ask the patient to relax and remain still.

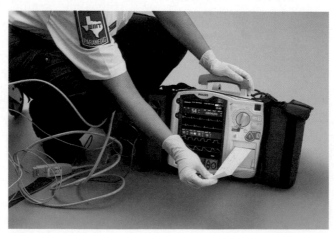

6-1e Obtain a tracing.

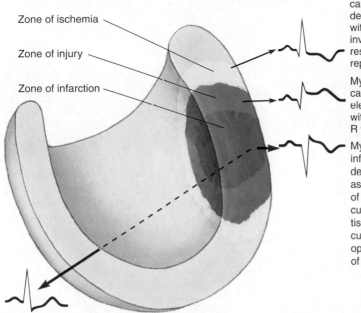

Zone of ischemia

Zone of injury

Zone of infarction

Myocardial ischemia causes ST segment depression with or without T wave inversion as a result of altered repolarization

Myocardial injury causes ST segment elevation with or without loss of R wave

Myocardial infarction causes deep Q waves as a result of absence of depolarization current from dead tissue and receding currents from opposite side of heart

FIGURE 6-18 The effects of myocardial ischemia, injury, and infarction.

which reperfusion therapy can occur as soon as possible (Figure 6-19). The therapy may be percutaneous coronary intervention in the cardiac cath lab or the administration of fibrinolytics.

Technology

There are a number of differences between a rhythm strip and a 12-lead ECG. A rhythm strip shows only one continuous look at the heart from a single direction. A 12-lead ECG shows the heart from 12 different directions and two different planes. A typical 12-lead ECG reading consists of short (2.5 seconds) segments containing only two or three complexes. Because of this, most machines also provide a

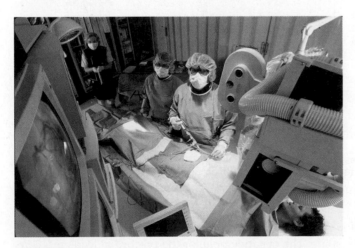

FIGURE 6-19 The goal of acquiring a 12-lead ECG is to deliver the patient to the cardiac cath lab for reperfusion therapy as soon as possible.

(© Getty Images, Inc.-Stone Allstock)

continuous rhythm strip at the bottom to adequately measure heart rate and rhythm.

The standard 12-lead ECG uses three bipolar leads (I, II, III); three unipolar, or augmented, leads (aVR, aVL, and aVF); and six chest, or precordial, leads (V1–V6) (Figure 6-20). The bipolar and unipolar leads are called *limb leads* because they are all obtained from the four electrodes you place on your patient's arms and legs.

The six limb leads view the heart from six directions in the frontal plane. They allow a different "look" at the heart by using two of the electrodes as a single electrode. To achieve this, two selected leads are combined in the ECG machine after each has been run through a resistor to reduce the current flow. This effectively provides a functional electrode halfway between the combined leads. The term *unipolar* refers to the resulting arrangement of one polarized (positive) electrode and the combined leads, which serve as a nonpolarized reference point (Figure 6-21). To increase the deflection's amplitude, the ground lead is disconnected—thus, the term **augmented lead**. The three **unipolar leads** are:

- *Lead aVR.* The positive electrode is placed on the right arm. The negative electrode is a combination of the left arm and left leg electrodes.

- *Lead aVL.* The positive electrode is placed on the left arm. The negative electrode is a combination of the right arm and left leg electrodes.

- *Lead aVF.* The positive electrode is placed on the left foot. The negative electrode is a combination of the right arm and the left arm electrodes.

All the limb leads are in the frontal plane. If you superimpose the direction of each of these leads on a single diagram, the six leads will constitute a complete 360° circle (Figure 6-22). By established convention, the direction toward the left arm is considered to be 0°. Some systems will use the full 360° circle to describe the axis of the lead in question. The radials increase clockwise in this system.

Other systems will divide the circle into positive and negative halves (semicircles). Using this system, moving clockwise, the radial coordinates are positive up to 180°. Moving counterclockwise from 0°, the radial coordinates are negative up to 180°. Each lead can be measured on this coordinate system. Table 6-2 lists the limb leads and the direction in which they point.

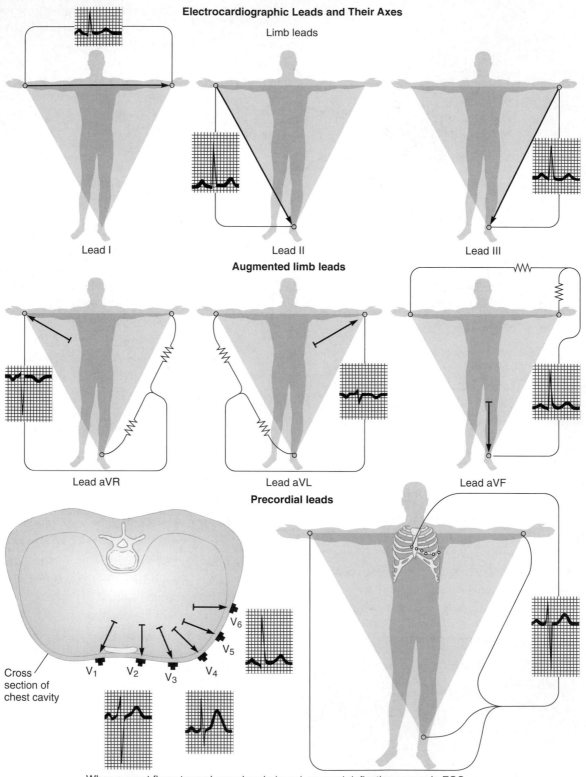

FIGURE 6-20 ECG leads and their axes.

The six chest, or **precordial, leads** are acquired by placing electrodes across your patient's chest. The precordial leads provide a look at the horizontal plane of the heart. The horizontal plane is the plane that results from a section taken from front to back, from the sternum to the spine. The negative pole for the precordial leads is a common ground arranged electronically within the ECG machine by connecting all limb leads together. The positive electrode is placed on the anterior surface of the chest in positions ranging from V1 to V6 (Figure 6-23). All 12 leads

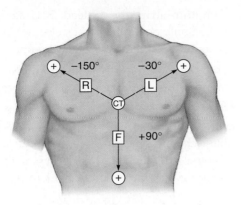

FIGURE 6-21 The pattern formed by the unipolar/augmented leads.

Table 6-2 12-Lead Angles

Lead	Full Circle	Semicircle
Lead I	0°	0°
Lead II	60°	+60°
Lead III	120°	+120°
aVR	210°	
aVL	330°	−30°
aVF	90°	+90°

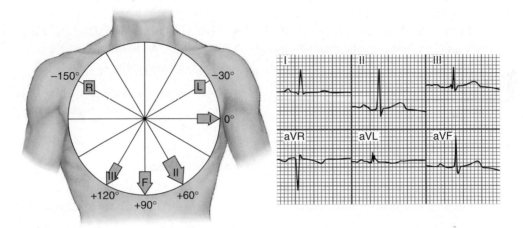

FIGURE 6-22 The hexaxial (six axes) reference system.

Lead V₁ The electrode is at the fourth intercostal space just to the right of the sternum.
Lead V₂ The electrode is at the fourth intercostal space just to the left of the sternum.
Lead V₃ The electrode is at the line midway between leads V₂ and V₄.
Lead V₄ The electrode is at the midclavicular line in the fifth interspace.
Lead V₅ The electrode is at the anterior axillary line at the same level as lead V₄.
Lead V₆ The electrode is at the midaxillary line at the same level as lead V₄.

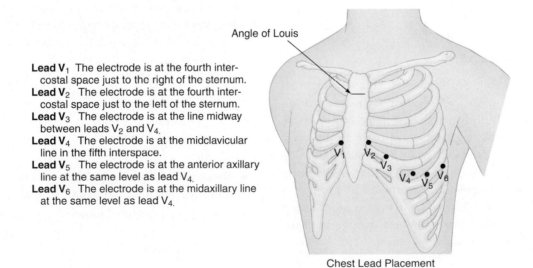

FIGURE 6-23 Proper placement of the precordial leads.

record exactly the same electrical events within the heart. Each lead, however, allows us to look at these events from a different perspective.

The classic 12-lead ECG is designed to detect the most common types of cardiac problems—usually those involving the left side of the heart and the left anterior descending coronary artery. However, problems that arise in the right

ventricle and the posterior wall of the left ventricle may not be readily visible on the standard 12 leads. Because of this, using a 15-lead or 18-lead ECG can increase the sensitivity of the test. These supplemental leads look specifically at the right ventricle and the posterior wall of the left ventricle.

By combining the different ECG leads, you can view different parts of the heart. For example, leads V1 through

Table 6-3 Overview of ECG Lead Groupings

Leads	Portion of the Heart Examined
I and aVL	Left side of the heart in a vertical plane
II, III, and aVF	Inferior (diaphragmatic) side of the heart
aVR	Right side of the heart in a vertical plane
V1 and V2	Right ventricle
V3 and V4	Interventricular septum and anterior wall of the left ventricle
V5 and V6	Anterior and lateral walls of the left ventricle

V4 view the anterior surface of the heart. Leads I and aVL view the lateral surface of the heart. The inferior surface of the heart can be visualized in leads II, III, and aVF. These leads can show ischemia, injury, and necrotic changes and can provide information about the corresponding heart surface (Table 6-3). For example, significant ST elevation in V1 and V4 may indicate anterior involvement, whereas elevation in leads II, III, and aVF may indicate inferior involvement.

The ST segment is usually an isoelectric line. Myocardial infarctions, which are caused by lack of blood flow to a part of the heart, produce changes in this line. The affected area is then electrically dead and cannot conduct electrical impulses.

As stated earlier, myocardial infarctions usually follow this sequence:

1. Ischemia (lack of oxygen)
2. Injury
3. Infarction (cell death)

Each of these stages results in distinct ST segment changes. Ischemia causes ST segment depression or an inverted T wave. The inversion is usually symmetrical. Injury elevates the ST segment, most often in the early phases of a myocardial infarction. As the tissue dies, a significant Q wave appears. As we noted earlier, small, insignificant Q waves may show up in normal ECG tracings. A significant Q wave is at least one small square wide, lasting 0.04 seconds, or is more than one-third the height of the QRS complex. Q waves may also indicate extensive transient ischemia.

Medical procedures (angioplasty) and drugs (fibrinolytics) can treat acute myocardial infarction (AMI). The earlier they are initiated, the better the patient's potential outcome. Earlier identification in the field of patients with AMI will allow for earlier interventions.

Limitations

A number of limitations should be considered when acquiring a 12-lead ECG. These include the following:

- Like a rhythm strip, the 12-lead ECG can provide information only about the heart's electrical activity. It tells us nothing about the mechanical pump.
- ECG changes may occur with postural changes that may cause changes in the position of the heart in the chest.
- An ECG represents a brief sample in time. Because unstable ischemic syndromes have rapidly changing supply-versus-demand characteristics, a single ECG may not accurately represent the entire picture.
- The standard 12-lead ECG also does not directly examine the right ventricle, and is relatively poor at examining the posterior basal and lateral walls of the left ventricle.
- Mistakes in interpretation are relatively common, and the failure to identify high-risk features has a negative effect on the quality of patient care.

In spite of these limitations, the 12-lead ECG stands at the center of risk stratification for the patient with suspected AMI.

Indications

Acquiring a 12-lead ECG is important in the early recognition and treatment of acute coronary syndromes (ACS), especially ST-segment elevation myocardial infarction (STEMI).[1] Studies have shown that when prehospital 12-lead ECG programs are in place, the time it takes to deliver reperfusion therapy to the patients after arrival at the hospital can be reduced by up to 1 hour.

The 12-lead ECG is used to classify MI patients into one of three groups:

- Those with ST segment elevation or new bundle branch block (suspicious for acute injury and a possible candidate for acute reperfusion therapy with thrombolytics or percutaneous coronary intervention [PCI]).
- Those with ST segment depression or T wave inversion (suspicious for ischemia).
- Those with a so-called nondiagnostic or normal ECG; however, a normal ECG does not rule out acute myocardial infarction.

In addition to patients exhibiting signs and symptoms of acute coronary events, indications for acquiring a 12-lead ECG include the following:

- Chest pain or anginal equivalents (e.g., dyspnea, syncope, near syncope, weakness, diabetic ketoacidosis [DKA], diaphoresis disproportionate to the environment, palpitations)
- Acute ischemic stroke (often associated with large anterior wall MIs and/or arrhythmias)

- Pre- and postcardioversion of stable patients
- Postcardioversion of unstable patients (including postarrest)
- Suspected electrolyte disturbances
- Overdose (unknown or suspected antidepressant)
- Blunt chest trauma (only after transport or more urgent care)
- Arrhythmia (to aid in the cause and diagnosis of the arrhythmia)
- Respiratory failure
- Ventricular failure (CHF)

Once you have acquired the 12-lead ECG, you should either communicate your interpretation or send the ECG itself to the receiving facility. The hospital should then prepare appropriately for the ACS patient. Acquiring and transmitting a 12-lead ECG in the field reduces the time to reperfusion therapy. This reduction in time saves cardiac muscle.

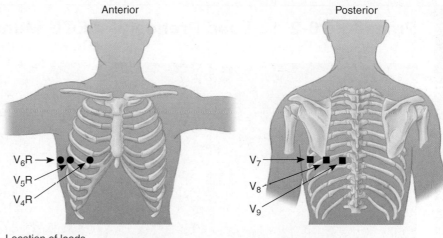

Anterior   **Posterior**

V_6R V_5R V_4R V_7 V_8 V_9

Location of leads

FIGURE 6-24 Supplemental lead placements for an 18-lead ECG.

Procedure

To become proficient in correct lead placement, it is important to follow some simple guidelines:

- Clean the area with an alcohol swab and allow it to dry (Procedure 6-2a).
- Shave any excess hair as needed.
- Dry the area or use benzoin spray as needed.
- Ensure proper placement. Improper lead placement can affect R wave progression through the chest leads.
- Make sure the conductive gel in the electrodes is pliable.

To acquire a standard 12-lead ECG, first have your patient lie supine and place the limb leads on his arms and legs, as described earlier (Procedure 6-2b). Then, place the chest leads as follows (Procedure 6-2c):

- Place lead V1 to the right of the sternum at the fourth intercostal space.
- Place lead V2 to the left of the sternum at the fourth intercostal space.
- Place lead V4 at the midclavicular line at the fifth intercostal space.
- Place lead V3 in a line midway between lead V2 and lead V4.
- Place lead V5 at the anterior axillary line at the same level as V4.
- Place lead V6 at the midaxillary line at the same level as V4.

To the standard 12 leads (I, II, III, aVR, aVL, aVF, and V1 through V6), the 18-lead ECG adds three right-sided chest leads (V4R, V5R, and V6R) and three posterior leads (V7, V8, and V9) (Figure 6-24). To look at the right side of the heart, simply mirror the left-sided lead placement:

- Place the V4R electrode in the fifth intercostal space at the right midclavicular line.
- Place the V5R level with V4R at the right anterior axillary line.
- Place the V6R level with V5R at the right midaxillary line.

To look at the posterior heart, extend the V7 to V9 electrodes in a horizontal line from V6 as follows:

- Place V7 lateral to V6 at the posterior axillary line.
- Place V8 at the level of V7 at the midscapular line.
- Place V9 at the level of V8 at the paravertebral line.

The 15-lead ECG is a subset of the 18-lead ECG, using V4R, V8, and V9 as additional leads to the standard 12-lead ECG.

Obtain your tracing and check the quality (Procedure 6-2d). Transmit the tracing to the receiving facility as per your local protocols (Procedure 6-2e). Refer to the "Cardiology" chapter in Volume 4, Medical Emergencies, for 12-lead ECG interpretation and for more information on this topic.

Pulse Oximetry

Anatomy and Physiology of Oxyhemoglobin

After oxygen diffuses across the alveolar–capillary membrane into a pulmonary capillary, about 97 percent of it binds to the hemoglobin molecule on the red blood cell.

Procedure 6-2 12-Lead Prehospital ECG Monitoring

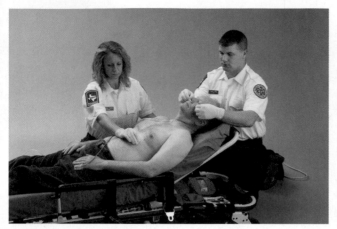

6-2a Prep the skin.

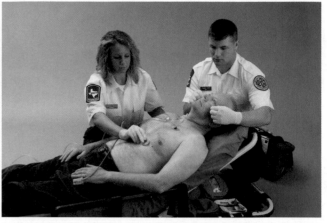

6-2b Place the four limb leads according to the manufacturer's recommendations.

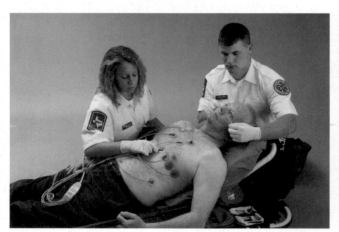

6-2c Ensure that all leads are attached.

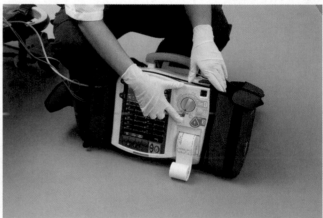

6-2d Check the quality of the tracing being received from each channel.

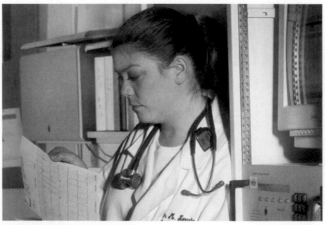

6-2e Transmit the tracing to the receiving hospital.

Hemoglobin, an iron-containing protein that transports oxygen, is essential for life. It is produced and contained within the red blood cells, which deliver oxygen to all body tissues. Hemoglobin is made up of four protein chains–normally, two alpha (α) and two beta (β) chains–each containing an iron-based structure called a **heme**. The heme structure is where oxygen binds to hemoglobin. Thus, each molecule of hemoglobin can bind four molecules of oxygen. When oxygen is bound to hemoglobin, the resultant molecule is called **oxyhemoglobin**. When oxygen is not bound, the molecule is called **deoxyhemoglobin**.

The effectiveness of oxygen transport depends on many factors. These include the number of red blood cells present, the PO_2, the hemoglobin's affinity for oxygen, the pH, the pCO_2, body temperature, and exercise. Let's look at each of these factors individually.

- The greater the number of red blood cells, the greater the potential oxygen-carrying capacity.

- As the pO_2 increases, so does the percentage of oxygen bound to hemoglobin. This is illustrated in the oxyhemoglobin dissociation curve (Figure 6-25). Normal pO_2 is approximately 95 mmHg. Based on this, the oxyhemoglobin dissociation curve indicates that normal oxygen saturation is about 97 percent.

- Other substances can compete with oxygen for hemoglobin's binding sites. The greater a substance's affinity for hemoglobin, the more readily it will bind with it. Carbon monoxide (CO) is an excellent example. CO has 200 times oxygen's affinity for hemoglobin and competes for the same binding sites. In carbon monoxide poisoning, when CO binds to one of the hemoglobin molecule's four binding sites, the hemoglobin molecule is altered so that the remaining three oxygen molecules are held more tightly. This inhibits oxygen release in the peripheral tissues, contributing to hypoxia, acidosis, and eventually shock.

- The lower the pH (i.e., the more acidic the blood), the more readily hemoglobin will release oxygen. This shifts the oxyhemoglobin dissociation curve to the right. In contrast, alkalosis makes hemoglobin bind to oxygen more tightly. This shifts the oxyhemoglobin dissociation curve to the left.

- The pCO_2 is directly related to the pH. In the lungs, as pCO_2 decreases with diffusion of CO_2 into the alveoli, the pH rises and the quantity of oxygen that binds with the hemoglobin increases. The opposite effect occurs when the blood reaches the tissues. There, waste CO_2 from the tissues diffuses into the blood and the pH falls, causing the hemoglobin to give up more oxygen to the tissues. This is called the *Bohr effect*.

- An elevation in body temperature causes a shift to the right of the oxyhemoglobin dissociation curve and a decrease in hemoglobin's affinity for oxygen. Conversely, a fall in body temperature causes hemoglobin to bind oxygen more tightly. During periods of hyperthermia and pyrexia (fever), hemoglobin's decreased affinity for oxygen means more offloading at the tissue level.

- Exercise has several effects on oxygen affinity. It causes the production and release of carbon dioxide and other acids, especially from the large muscles, and increases body temperature. Thus, both a decrease in pH and an increase in body temperature will cause hemoglobin to release oxygen more readily. This serves to enhance peripheral tissue oxygenation during strenuous exercise and work.

All these factors have an effect on oxygen saturation and in the overall transport of oxygen to the tissues.

Technology

Pulse oximetry is a noninvasive method of monitoring the oxygen saturation of your patient's hemoglobin. The pulse oximeter has a probe sensor and a monitoring unit with digital readouts (Figure 6-26). A sensor, or probe, is attached to a thin, translucent part of the patient's body where the light from the oximeter can shine through arterial blood flow. The most common placement is on a fingertip, but an earlobe or toe is also acceptable. One side of the probe has a pair of small light-emitting diodes (LEDs) that send out a red light with wavelength of 660 nm and an infrared light with a wavelength of 905, 910, or 940 nm. These lights travel through the tissue to the opposite side, where they are received by a photo sensor. The photo sensor absorbs the lights based on the color differences between oxyhemoglobin (bright red) and deoxyhemoglobin (dark red or blue). It then provides an immediate measurement of the percent of hemoglobin bound with oxygen. This reading is known as the SpO_2,

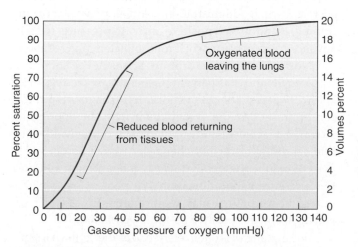

FIGURE 6-25 The oxygen–hemoglobin dissociation curve.

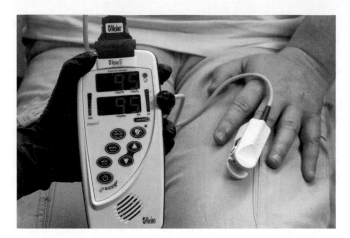

FIGURE 6-26 The pulse oximeter.

or the patient's oxygen saturation. Acceptable normal ranges for a patient breathing room air are from 95 to 100 percent, although values down to 90 percent are common. Patients with chronic obstructive pulmonary disease may exhibit oximetry readings as low as 85 percent on room air. Pulse oximeters display the SpO_2 and the pulse rate as detected by the sensors. Depending on the device, the display may be a number and/or a visual pulse waveform.

The monitored signal bounces in time with the heartbeat because the arterial blood vessels expand and contract with each heartbeat. By examining only the varying part of the absorption spectrum (essentially, subtracting minimum absorption from peak absorption), a monitor can ignore other tissues or nail polish (although black nail polish tends to distort readings), and discern only the absorption caused by arterial blood. Because of this, a pulse oximeter will not function unless it detects a pulse.

Limitations

The sensors can accurately measure the oxygen saturation only if blood flow through the tissue is adequate. A pulse oximeter requires a pulsating arterial blood flow to obtain an accurate reading. Anything that inhibits perfusion to the spot at which the probe is attached will alter your reading. Conditions that can produce an inaccurate reading include the following:

- Hypoperfusion caused by blood loss, dehydration, cold body temperature, or the use of vasopressors can provide inaccurate readings.
- A reduction in the number of red blood cells (anemia) will provide falsely high readings. The hemoglobin may be 100 percent saturated with oxygen but there are a decreased number of red blood cells.
- Incorrect sensor application, highly callused skin, and movement (such as shivering) can also provide inaccurate readings, especially during hypoperfusion.

- Hemoglobin can be bound to other gases, such as carbon monoxide, and still read high even though the patient is hypoxic. Pulse oximetry reads only the percentage of bound hemoglobin.
- The presence of methemoglobinemia characteristically causes pulse oximetry readings in the mid-80s. Cyanide poisoning can give a high reading because it reduces oxygen extraction from arterial blood (the reading is not false, as arterial blood oxygen is indeed high in early cyanide poisoning).

Oximetry is not a complete measure of respiratory sufficiency. A patient suffering from hypoventilation (poor gas exchange in the lungs) who is given 100 percent oxygen can have excellent blood oxygen levels while still suffering from respiratory acidosis owing to excessive carbon dioxide. Nor is it a complete measure of circulatory sufficiency. If there is insufficient blood flow or insufficient hemoglobin in the blood (anemia), tissues can suffer hypoxia despite high oxygen saturation in the blood that does arrive.

Learn to use the pulse oximeter as just another tool of patient assessment. Do not become so dependent on technology that you begin to trust it completely. For example, if the digital readout of the pulse rate or the pulsation wave does not match your patient's actual pulse, your reading may be inaccurate. Don't forget to use all your senses when assessing your patients.

Even with these limitations, pulse oximetry, when teamed with other patient assessment techniques, can be a useful tool in the prehospital setting.

Indications

A patient's need for oxygen is essential to life; no human can sustain life without oxygen. Measuring your patient's oxygen saturation is necessary if your patient's oxygen status is a concern or whenever you even remotely suspect hypoxia. With it you can determine your patient's baseline oxygenation status, guide his care, and quantify the effectiveness of therapies such as oxygen administration, ventilatory assistance, suctioning, continuous positive airway pressure (CPAP), advanced airway placement, bronchodilators, and sedation.

Normal oxygen saturation at sea level should be between 96 and 100 percent. Generally, if the reading is below 95 percent, suspect shock, hypoxia, or respiratory compromise. Provide your patient with the appropriate airway management and supplemental oxygen and watch him carefully for further changes. Any reading below 90 percent requires aggressive airway management and positive pressure ventilation with 100 percent oxygen. The unresponsive patient may require more invasive airway management and positive pressure ventilation.

Pulse oximetry is often referred to as the "fifth vital sign." It is designed to supplement your physical examination, not

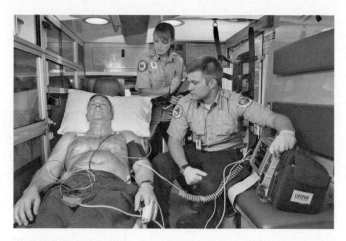

FIGURE 6-27 Many ECG machines come with built-in pulse oximetry.

to replace it. The information you receive must be considered within the context of your patient's overall condition.

Procedure

The procedure for monitoring your patient's pulse oximetry is as follows:

- Connect the probe to the monitor device.
- Attach the probe-sensor clip to your patient's finger, toe, or earlobe. In an infant, you can use the foot (Figure 6-27).
- Turn on the device and wait for the reading to appear. Match the pulse reading with your patient's actual pulse. If the heart rate is different, the SpO_2 will be inaccurate.
- If you get a poor signal or an "error" code, reposition the probe or try another location.
- Your patient's SpO_2 measurement should appear on the readout.
- Reassess and document every 5 minutes in the unstable patient and every 15 minutes for all others.
- Titrate oxygen administration to maintain a minimally acceptable SpO_2—usually 95 percent. Remember that excessive oxygen can manufacture toxic chemicals called *free radicals*, which can damage body tissues such as the brain and heart.

Capnography
Anatomy and Physiology of Carbon Dioxide Elimination

Carbon dioxide (CO_2) is a normal product of aerobic respiration. It is found in minute concentrations in atmospheric air, which is composed primarily of nitrogen (79 percent), oxygen (21 percent), and other gases in smaller concentrations. In the body, carbon dioxide is produced by metabolism at the cellular level in tissues. The blood transports

carbon dioxide mainly in the form of the bicarbonate ion (HCO_3^-). It carries approximately 70 percent as bicarbonate and approximately 20 percent combined with hemoglobin. Less than 7 percent is dissolved in the plasma.

Blood is delivered from the tissues to the right side of the heart by the venous system. From there, the pulmonary artery transports it to the lungs for gas exchange. CO_2 crosses the alveolar membrane, enters the tracheobronchial tree, and is exhaled through the oral/nasal passages. At this point, we can measure the concentration of carbon dioxide in the exhaled air. This is known as *end-tidal* CO_2 ($ETCO_2$).

$ETCO_2$ is a reflection of cellular metabolism, circulation, and ventilation.

- *Metabolism.* This refers to the amount of CO_2 produced by the cells. Conditions that increase CO_2 production include fever, burns, hyperthyroidism, and seizures. Increased levels can also be the result of bicarbonate therapy, return of spontaneous circulation, and the release of a tourniquet/reperfusion. Conditions that decrease CO_2 levels include hypothermia, sedation, and paralysis.
- *Circulation.* This refers to the amount of CO_2 that is transported to the lungs by the heart and pulmonary circulation. Conditions that decrease CO_2 transport to the lungs include decreased cardiac output, pulmonary embolism, hypotension, shock, and cardiac arrest.
- *Ventilation.* This refers to the amount of CO_2 that is exchanged in the alveoli and allowed to pass through the airways. Conditions that decrease CO_2 elimination include respiratory depression, respiratory muscle weakness, hypoventilation, bronchospasm, and airway obstruction. Hyperventilation increases CO_2 elimination.

$ETCO_2$ monitoring provides an immediate evaluation of metabolism, circulation, and ventilation. When these three components are working properly, the normal $ETCO_2$ is about 38 mmHg. This correlates well with PCO_2 levels in the blood (35–45 mmHg). $ETCO_2$ readings above 45 mmHg signify either increased CO_2 production, decreased CO_2 elimination, or a combination of both. This is known as *hypoventilation*. $ETCO_2$ readings below 35 mmHg signify either a decrease in CO_2 production, an increase in CO_2 elimination, or a combination of both. This is known as *hyperventilation*.

Carbon dioxide is a waste product and an acid that must be constantly eliminated so the body's pH range can remain stable between 7.35 and 7.45. An increase in CO_2 levels lowers the pH (acidosis), whereas a decrease in CO_2 levels raises the pH (alkalosis). Dramatic changes in pH can seriously alter normal bodily functions. In humans, a variation of only 0.4 of a pH unit in either direction from normal (6.9 or 7.8) can be fatal.

Because it provides an immediate evaluation of your patient's metabolic state, his circulatory status, and his ventilatory efficiency, monitoring your patient's $ETCO_2$ has become a vital tool in managing a critical patient effectively.

Technology

Capnometry provides a noninvasive measure of $ETCO_2$ levels, thus providing you with information about the status of systemic metabolism, circulation, and ventilation. The use of capnography has become commonplace in the operating room, in the emergency department, and in the prehospital setting.

When first introduced into prehospital care, $ETCO_2$ monitoring was used exclusively to verify proper endotracheal tube placement in the trachea. The presence of adequate CO_2 levels following intubation, through the presence of exhaled CO_2, confirms that the tube is in the trachea. $ETCO_2$ is detected by using either a colorimetric or an infrared device. $ETCO_2$ is measured just as the exhaled air leaves the oral/nasal cavity and has a high correlation with blood levels of CO_2. Here, we discuss two basic types of $ETCO_2$ monitoring systems: qualitative colorimetric devices and quantitative electronic devices. Both have their place in prehospital EMS systems.

Colorimetric Devices

The colorimetric device is a disposable $ETCO_2$ detector that was first designed simply to verify endotracheal tube (ETT) placement. It is basically a piece of litmus paper encased within a plastic chamber (Figure 6-28), which changes color based on the pH of the gas to which it is exposed. You simply place it in the airway circuit between the patient and the ventilation device. When the paper is exposed to CO_2, it will change color from purple to yellow, indicating a lower or more acidic pH.

As CO_2 is a product of aerobic respiration, we would expect that a properly placed ETT will cause a color change on the device. The color change is reversible and changes from breath to breath. This, of course, requires that the

patient is breathing, or being adequately ventilated (exhaling CO_2 in either case). A color scale on the device estimates the $ETCO_2$ level.

Electronic Devices

Electronic $ETCO_2$ detectors use an infrared technique to detect CO_2 in the exhaled breath. A heated element in the sensor generates infrared radiation. The CO_2 molecules absorb infrared light at a very specific wavelength and can thus be measured. Electronic $ETCO_2$ detectors may be either qualitative (i.e., they simply detect the presence of CO_2) or quantitative (i.e., they determine how much CO_2 is present). Quantitative devices are now routinely used in prehospital care. Most can provide a continuous digital waveform (capnogram) that reflects the entire respiratory cycle.

Electronic continuous waveform capnographs have the added benefit of displaying either a characteristic waveform or a numerical value, respectively, correlating to the expired CO_2 concentration. In addition to monitoring proper tube placement during transport, you can also assess the adequacy of respiration and ventilation. You can then use this number and/or waveform to guide the resuscitative efforts based on the anticipated clinical needs of your patient.

Initially, as noted earlier, $ETCO_2$ detection was originally used only to determine proper endotracheal tube placement. Typically, a qualitative colorimetric $ETCO_2$ device was applied to the airway circuit following intubation. If $ETCO_2$ levels were detected, then proper tube placement was verified. However, it is difficult to continuously monitor the airway with a qualitative colorimetric device. Now, continuous waveform capnography (Figure 6-29) is available and allows continuous monitoring of airway placement and ventilation for both intubated and nonintubated patients. By following trends in the capnogram, prehospital personnel can continuously monitor the patient's condition, detect trends, and document the response to medications.

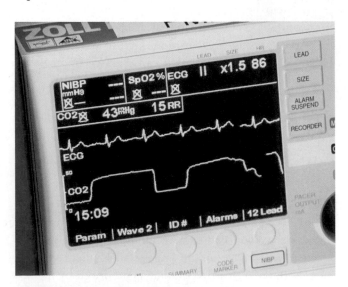

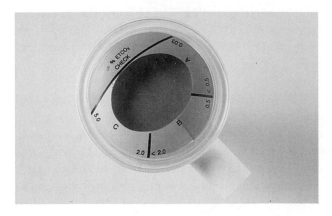

FIGURE 6-28 Colorimetric end-tidal CO_2 detector.

FIGURE 6-29 Continuous waveform capnography.

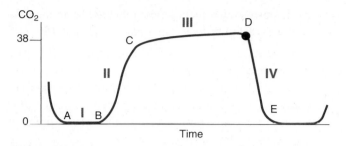

FIGURE 6-30 Normal continuous waveform capnogram.

The continuous waveform capnography device reflects CO_2 concentrations over time. It is typically divided into four phases (Figure 6-30):

- *Phase I* (AB in Figure 6-30) is the respiratory baseline. It is flat when no CO_2 is present and corresponds to the late phase of inspiration and the early part of expiration (in which dead-space gases without CO_2 are released).
- *Phase II* (BC in Figure 6-30) is the respiratory upstroke. This reflects the appearance of CO_2 in the alveoli.
- *Phase III* (CD in Figure 6-30) is the respiratory plateau. It reflects the airflow through uniformly ventilated alveoli with a nearly constant CO_2 level. The highest level of the plateau (point D in Figure 6-30) is called the $ETCO_2$ and is recorded as such by the capnometer.
- *Phase IV* (DE in Figure 6-30) is the inspiratory phase. It is a sudden downstroke and ultimately returns to the baseline during inspiration. The respiratory pause restarts the cycle (EA in Figure 6-30).

For patients who are not in cardiac arrest, studies of qualitative colorimetric $ETCO_2$ and quantitative capnography have demonstrated the ability to confirm proper ETT placement in the breathing patient.[2,3] This can be interpreted as a reliable measure that both the ETT is in the right place (the trachea, but does not preclude mainstem intubation) and the patient is ventilating. For patients in cardiac arrest, continuous waveform capnography is recommended in addition to clinical assessment as the most reliable method of confirming and monitoring correct placement of an endotracheal tube.[4]

Continuous waveform capnography shares the same sensitivities and specificities for confirming ETT placement as colorimetric CO_2 detection in the perfusing patient but has the added benefit of the following:

- Continuous monitoring of tube location during transport
- Monitoring effectiveness of resuscitation and adequacy of ventilation
- Altering the concentration of expired CO_2 in cases of suspected raised intracranial pressure (ICP)
- Predicting outcome in cardiac arrest patients and trauma victims

Limitations

The colorimetric devices, though inexpensive and easy to use, are fraught with limitations. These include the following:

- In low-flow states, such as diminished cardiac output or the ultimate low-flow state of cardiopulmonary arrest, one would expect diminished or absent color change. The sensitivity and specificity of the device fall in this population of patients.
- False positives (i.e., positive color change when the ETT is in the esophagus): If your patient arrested after enjoying a meal supplemented with carbonated beverages, an ETT in the esophagus may change color owing to the gases present in the stomach. This color change, however, is transient, as the patient is "ventilated" because there is not an active production of CO_2 coming into the stomach. Your device should not change with repeated ventilations, unlike a properly placed ETT in a ventilating, respiring patient.
- False negatives (i.e., no color change when the tube is in the right position): If your cardiac arrest patient has been apneic for a long enough period of time, then you would not expect color change. With appropriate CPR and, thus, production of CO_2, color change should then be encountered. Poor prognosis is universally encountered in the patient who is receiving appropriate CPR but is not causing a color change on the device.
- Colorimetric devices cannot detect hyper- or hypocarbia (increased or decreased CO_2 levels).
- If gastric contents or acidic drugs (e.g., endotracheal epinephrine) contact the paper in the device, subsequent readings may be unreliable.
- Although colorimetric CO_2 detection is vital in confirming tracheal ETT placement, its utility decreases over time. After the tube has been confirmed by repeated color change on the device, it should no longer be used to monitor placement. If you were to use the device for this purpose, it must be continually replaced.
- If the device should become wet with substances such as gastric contents, which have an acidic pH, you will see a false color change.
- There are no number, no waveform, and no alarm system, and it is difficult to read in the dark.

Quantitative devices accurately measure the $ETCO_2$ as either a number (capnometry) or a number and waveform (capnography). These devices require some degree of interpretation as compared with the qualitative devices, which are much easier to interpret. Capnography and the associated numerical values and waveforms give valuable information about adequacy of ventilation and pathological disease states. The qualitative colorimetric devices discussed previously do not yield as much information.

Prehospital $ETCO_2$ monitoring has many applications, including confirmation of ETT placement and assessing the quality of CPR and the adequacy of ventilation. However, providers should always use both clinical assessment and devices to confirm endotracheal tube location immediately after placement and throughout the resuscitation.[5] $ETCO_2$ monitoring has also been demonstrated to have prognostic value in victims of multiple trauma and head injury. Appropriate use of the device must be done with respect to its limitations and proper interpretation. It is only as good as the provider who is using it.

All confirmation devices should be considered adjuncts to other confirmation techniques. Application of this knowledge will result in a better clinician and subsequently better patient care.

Indications

Qualitative colorimetric $ETCO_2$ devices and continuous waveform capnography have many applications in the prehospital setting. The major prehospital indication for qualitative colorimetric $ETCO_2$ devices is to confirm ETT placement. An ETT placed in the trachea in a patient with intact circulation will change color from purple to yellow on repeated ventilations 100 percent of the time. This method of tube confirmation is superior to auscultating lung sounds, lack of epigastric sounds, and condensation in the tube in a patient with intact circulation. Your documentation after endotracheal intubation (ETI) should read, "Positive color change from purple to yellow with the CO_2 detector device on repeated ventilations." The statement regarding repeated ventilations corrects for the possible false positives discussed earlier. This method of confirmation should be used for every prehospital intubation, as unrecognized esophageal intubation is associated with disastrous consequences.

Although it has been demonstrated to be an effective, and perhaps definitive, objective measure of confirming endotracheal tube placement, continuous waveform capnography is useful in many other situations:

- Monitoring continuous waveform capnography during resuscitative efforts has been shown to have prognostic value regarding return of spontaneous circulation (ROSC). It has been demonstrated to be the earliest indicator of the ROSC in animal and human models. A rise in $ETCO_2$ can be detected even before a palpable pulse is noted. During effective CPR, $ETCO_2$ levels have been found to correlate well with cardiac output, coronary perfusion pressure, and even with the effectiveness of CPR compressions.

- Continuous waveform capnography can also be used to gauge the effectiveness of compressions. Effective CPR will cause a subsequent increase in cardiac output. This rise in cardiac output causes an increase in

tissue perfusion, which will be reflected as an increase in $ETCO_2$. $ETCO_2$ detection is also useful in CPR.

- In patients undergoing CPR, multiple studies have demonstrated that an $ETCO_2$ level of 10 mmHg or less measured 20 minutes after the initiation of ACLS accurately predicted death in adult patients with cardiac arrest. All patients who survived to hospital admission in these studies had higher average $ETCO_2$ levels, all greater than 10 mmHg. This can be used for termination of efforts in the field, as well as a prognostic indicator.

- Monitoring continuous waveform capnography is clinically applicable in victims of major trauma and head injury. Hypoventilation causing hypercarbia (increased CO_2 in circulating blood) is associated with cerebral vasodilation, increased intracranial pressure, and overall worse outcome. Overventilation is also associated with poor neurologic outcome in brain-injured patients. Consequently, the use of $ETCO_2$ can avoid both hypo- ($ETCO_2 > 50$ mmHg) and hyperventilation ($ETCO_2 < 30$ mmHg) in the brain-injured patient and victim of major trauma.[5,6,7]

- Continuous waveform capnography is useful in detecting accidental tracheal extubation, tube obstruction, or disconnection from a ventilation system during transport.

- Continuous waveform capnography is useful in monitoring the respirations of sedated patients. One study showed that the device detected acute respiratory depression before changes in respiratory rate and SpO_2 were observed.

- Patients with bronchospasm exhibit a particular waveform pattern known as a "shark fin," which indicates the severity of the bronchoconstriction. Continuous waveform capnography monitoring allows you to assess and quantify the efficacy of your bronchodilator therapy and identify trends during an asthma attack.

- $ETCO_2$ is an early indicator of hypoperfusion states. Low flow means less CO_2 is delivered to the lungs for gas exchange.

- $ETCO_2$ is a way to determine the degree of hypoventilation and possible respiratory failure.

Continuous waveform capnography is rapidly becoming a standard of care in EMS. Misplaced endotracheal tubes represent a significant area of liability in EMS, and the documentation provided by this technology can provide irrefutable evidence of proper endotracheal tube placement.

Procedure

The three basic applications for $ETCO_2$ monitoring in the prehospital setting are:

- Qualitative colorimetric $ETCO_2$ device for ETT placement verification

- Continuous waveform monitoring for ETT placement verification and subsequent patient monitoring
- Continuous waveform monitoring for a variety of nonintubated patients

The procedure for each device follows.

Qualitative Colorimetric $ETCO_2$ Device

Following placement of an endotracheal tube, simply place the device between the endotracheal tube and the ventilation device and ventilate your patient (Figure 6-31). A color scale on the device estimates the CO_2 level.

Continuous Waveform Monitoring (with ETT)

Following placement of an endotracheal tube, attach the inline sensor between the endotracheal tube and the ventilation device and ventilate your patient (Figure 6-32). Visualize the $ETCO_2$ number reading and the digital waveform that reflects the entire respiratory cycle.

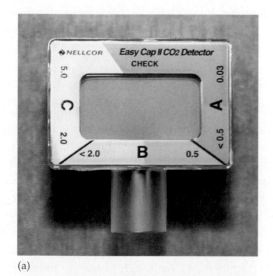

(a)

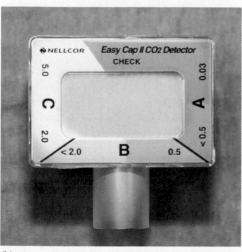

(b)

FIGURE 6-31 Color display on a colorimetric device (a) before and (b) after successful ventilation via endotracheal tube.

(Both photos: © Dr. Bryan E. Bledsoe)

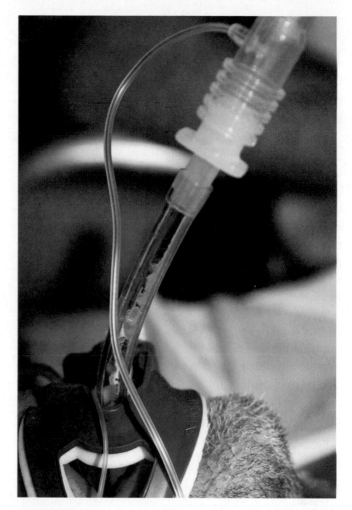

FIGURE 6-32 Confirming ET tube placement with an inline device.

(© Dr. Bryan E. Bledsoe)

Continuous Waveform Monitoring (Nonintubated Patients)

Nonintubated patients require a special nasal cannula with $ETCO_2$ sampling technology (Figure 6-33). It allows you to deliver oxygen and monitor $ETCO_2$ simultaneously.

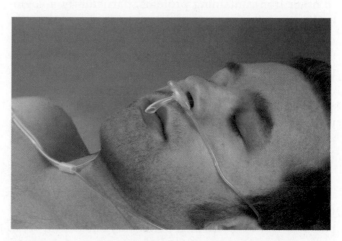

FIGURE 6-33 Capnography with a nasal cannula device.

Pulse CO-Oximetry

Pathophysiology of Carboxyhemoglobin

Carbon monoxide (CO) is the number-one cause of poisoning in industrialized countries. CO is an odorless, tasteless, colorless gas that is often the byproduct of incomplete combustion of carbon-containing compounds, such as wood and petroleum products. One carbon atom and one oxygen atom joined by a triple bond make up the carbon monoxide molecule. It is an extremely stable molecule.

As stated earlier in this chapter, each hemoglobin molecule contains four oxygen-binding sites. CO competes with oxygen for the oxygen-binding sites on hemoglobin. Because of its molecular structure, CO will bind to hemoglobin with an affinity 200 times greater than that of oxygen. The binding of CO to hemoglobin results in **carboxyhemoglobin** (COHb). As CO levels increase in the blood, oxygen molecules will actually be displaced from hemoglobin, releasing the remaining oxygen in the tissues prematurely. In addition, CO will prevent oxygen molecules from binding to hemoglobin. Carboxyhemoglobin cannot carry oxygen. As CO poisoning increases, and carboxyhemoglobin levels rise, the amount of hemoglobin that is saturated with oxygen, called oxyhemoglobin, is steadily diminished. This ultimately affects organ systems that are highly dependent on a constant supply of oxygen.

Once CO binds to hemoglobin and forms carboxyhemoglobin, it can be removed only when it is degraded and ultimately removed from the body. The normal half-life of carboxyhemoglobin, when the patient is breathing room air, is 4 to 6 hours. The half-life can be decreased to 80 minutes with the administration of 100 percent oxygen. With hyperbaric oxygen (HBO) therapy—administering oxygen under pressure—the half-life can be reduced to under 25 minutes.

In addition to binding to hemoglobin, CO also binds to other iron-containing proteins, particularly myoglobin. Myoglobin is an iron-containing protein found in muscles and serves as a storage site for oxygen. A reduction in functional myoglobin results in decreased oxygen levels in the heart. This could lead to cardiac ischemia, dysrhythmias, and other types of cardiac dysfunction. Chest pain, unstable tachycardias, and even ventricular fibrillation are all manifestations of CO poisoning. In fact, most deaths from CO poisoning are the result of ventricular fibrillation.

As a rule, CO causes nervous system depression, resulting in headache, dizziness, confusion, seizures, and, ultimately, coma. In approximately 10 to 30 percent of patients with CO poisoning, pulmonary edema will occur. This can result from the direct effect of CO on the alveolar membrane. It can also occur with left ventricular failure secondary to myocardial depression. Because CO is often associated with nausea and vomiting, consider the possibility of aspiration as a cause of acute pulmonary edema.

The signs and symptoms of carbon monoxide poisoning are vague and nonspecific, closely resembling those of other diseases. For this reason, CO poisoning is often misdiagnosed as a viral illness (e.g., influenza), acute coronary syndrome, or even migraine.

CO poisoning is typically classified as either acute or chronic. Acute CO poisoning results from short exposure to a relatively high level of CO. Chronic CO exposure results from long or recurrent exposures to relatively low levels of CO. The signs and symptoms of chronic CO poisoning are essentially the same as those of acute CO poisoning. However, their onset and severity may be delayed or extremely varied.

As a rule, the higher the level of COHb, the more severe the signs and symptoms will be (see Table 6-4). However, COHb levels do not always correlate with signs and symptoms, nor do they predict complications and outcomes. The cherry red skin color, though an unreliable sign, is usually associated with a significant CO exposure.

Technology

Pulse CO-oximetry is a monitoring technology that uses eight different wavelengths of light to measure levels of oxygen (SpO_2), carboxyhemoglobin (COHb), and methemoglobin (MetHgb) in the blood. Light waves are emitted from light-emitting diodes (LEDs), pass through a finger vascular bed, and are detected by photoreceptors on the other side. The amount of light received by these photoreceptors is fed into a processor, which then determines the percentage of carboxyhemoglobin present (SpCO) (Figure 6-34). Although pulse CO-oximetry is an indirect measure of carboxyhemoglobin levels, it corresponds well to actual carboxyhemoglobin levels in the blood. If you administer 100 percent oxygen to a patient with CO poisoning, you will see a steady decrease in SpCO readings.

Table 6-4 Signs and Symptoms of Carbon Monoxide Poisoning, by Severity

COHb	Severity	Signs and Symptoms
<15–20%	Mild	Headache, nausea, vomiting, dizziness, blurred vision
21–40%	Moderate	Confusion, syncope, chest pain, dyspnea, tachycardia, tachypnea, weakness
41–59%	Severe	Dysrhythmias, hypotension, cardiac ischemia, palpitations, respiratory arrest, pulmonary edema, seizures, coma, cardiac arrest
>60%	Fatal	Death

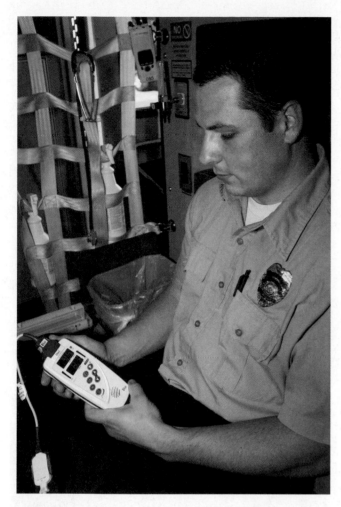

FIGURE 6-34 A CO-oximeter allows for the rapid detection of carbon monoxide poisoning through the noninvasive measurement of carboxyhemoglobin levels.

(© Dr. Bryan E. Bledsoe)

Limitations

The limitations of CO-oximetry are similar to those of pulse oximetry. The sensors can accurately measure the wavelengths only if blood flow through the tissue is adequate. To obtain an accurate reading, CO-oximetry requires a pulsating arterial blood flow. Anything that inhibits perfusion to the spot where the finger probe is attached will alter your reading. Conditions that can produce an inaccurate reading include the following:

- Hypoperfusion caused by blood loss, dehydration, cold body temperature, or the use of vasopressors
- A digital readout of the pulse rate or a pulsation wave that does not match your patient's actual pulse
- Incorrect sensor application, highly callused skin, and movement (such as shivering), especially during hypoperfusion

As stated earlier, make sure that the digital readout of the pulse rate or the pulsation wave matches your patient's actual pulse. If it doesn't, your reading may be inaccurate.

Indications

The detection and monitoring of SpCO levels have several applications and advantages for prehospital professionals. Until recently, it was impossible to diagnose CO poisoning in the prehospital setting. You had no option but to transport to the hospital any patient even remotely suspected of being poisoned. Obviously, many patients were transported who did not have CO poisoning. With CO-oximetry, you have the ability to triage exposed patients and send those with low SpCO levels home while routing those with elevated levels to the hospital for treatment.

During that same time, some patients with CO poisoning may not have been transported. It is clear from the medical literature that the earlier CO poisoning is diagnosed and treated, the better the ultimate outcome for your patient. Obtaining a fairly definitive diagnosis in the prehospital setting is critical.[8],[9],[10]

The ability to exclude CO poisoning as a diagnosis can help to prevent unnecessary transport and the associated expenses to the EMS system and your patients. The fire service often responds to calls involving CO detector alarm activations. Traditionally, firefighters have used monitors to assess the presence of CO in the air, but had no way to screen people for actual CO poisoning. With CO-oximetry, they are now able to accurately and safely determine whether the alarm detection poses a danger to building occupants.

As stated earlier, the clinical presentations of CO poisoning and cyanide poisoning are similar. If your patient was exposed to products of combustion and presented with chest pain and a tachydysrhythmia, CO-oximetry can help determine the exact diagnosis. If your patient has a relatively high SpCO, then CO is more likely the cause (although this does not necessarily rule out cyanide poisoning as well). If your patient has a relatively low SpCO but has significant signs and symptoms, cyanide may be more likely.

Now that a safe antidote (hydroxocobalamin) is available for cyanide poisoning, it is important to try to determine whether your patient may be suffering from cyanide poisoning. Because both toxins are often present, provide high-concentration oxygen.

Carbon monoxide poisoning is a major occupational hazard for firefighters. Premature cardiovascular death and neurologic diseases can be traced to both acute and chronic CO exposure. Because of this risk, the National Fire Protection Association (NFPA) has published a standard (NFPA 1584) that calls for medical monitoring of firefighters on the fire ground and in certain training situations. NFPA 1584 recommends the use of both pulse oximetry and CO detection. With the guidance of medical directors, fire departments are developing policies and procedures for CO monitoring and subsequent treatment if elevated CO levels are found.[11]

Historical trending of CO levels during prehospital care is another useful indication for CO-oximetry. Often you will detect an elevated SpCO in a patient, provide high-concentration oxygen therapy during assessment and transport, and deliver the patient to the ED with near-normal SpCO readings. This is because high-concentration oxygen therapy significantly increases the rate of carboxyhemoglobin elimination. Your ability to document the rate of SpCO decline will help the medical staff evaluate the degree of CO exposure and the response to treatment. It is important to point out that this goes beyond documentation issues. By administering high-concentration oxygen early, you also help prevent many of the serious effects (both short-term and long-term) of CO poisoning.

Procedure

The procedure for monitoring your patient's CO-oximetry is similar to obtaining his oxygen saturation, as described earlier in this chapter:

- Connect the probe to the monitor device.
- Attach the probe sensor clip to your patient's finger, toe, or earlobe. In an infant, you can use the foot (Procedure 6-3a).
- Turn on the device and wait for the SpO_2 reading to appear (Procedure 6-3b). Match the pulse reading with your patient's actual pulse. If the heart rate is different, the readings will be inaccurate.
- If you get a poor signal or an "error" code, reposition the probe or try another location.

Procedure 6-3 CO-Oximetry Monitoring

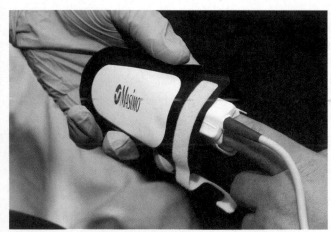

6-3a Place the probe on the patient's finger. Be sure the sensor is properly placed.

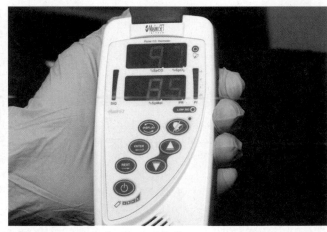

6-3b Measure the pulse rate and SpO_2.

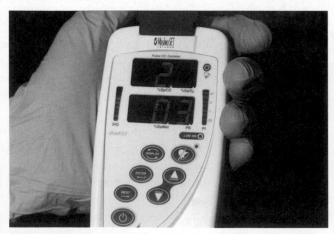

6-3c Press the SpCO button and measure the SpCO and the SpMet if applicable.

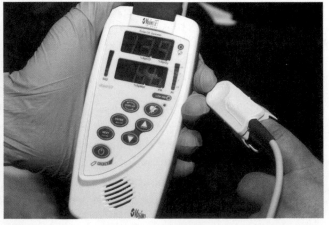

6-3d Some CO-oximeters have the capability to measure total hemoglobin (SpHb).

(All photos © Dr. Bryan E. Bledsoe)

- Your patient's SpCO measurement should appear on the readout (Procedure 6-3c).

- Reassess and document every 5 minutes for the unstable patient and every 15 minutes for all others.

Methemoglobinemia Monitoring

Pathophysiology of Methemoglobinemia

Earlier we discussed how hemoglobin, an iron-containing protein produced and contained within the red blood cells that transports oxygen, is essential for life. Heme is a metal (iron); therefore, it contains an electrical charge. When oxygen is not bound to the iron molecule, the iron molecule is in the ferrous (Fe^{2+}) charge state. When oxygen binds to the iron, a process called oxidation changes the charge to the ferric (Fe^{3+}) state. In the ferric state, iron cannot bind with oxygen until it is reduced back to the ferrous state.

Methemoglobin (MetHb) is hemoglobin that is oxidized. That is, the iron in the heme units of hemoglobin is in the Fe^{3+} (ferric state) instead of the Fe^{2+} (ferrous state). Hemoglobin must be in the reduced (Fe^{2+}) state to transport oxygen. Therefore, methemoglobin cannot transport oxygen. Hemoglobin contains four heme groups. The greater the number of these heme groups that are oxidized (converted from the Fe^{2+} to the Fe^{3+} state), the less oxygen will be transported by the hemoglobin molecule. Furthermore, the presence of a ferric (Fe^{3+}) heme group interferes with oxygen unloading by the other ferrous (Fe^{2+}) heme groups on the hemoglobin molecule. This decreases the oxygen-carrying capacity of hemoglobin and results in the oxyhemoglobin dissociation curve being shifted to the left.[12] Methemoglobin is produced continuously because of the oxidizing effects of oxygen. However, it is usually rapidly converted back to hemoglobin by the enzyme NADH-dependent methemoglobin reductase. This enzyme system is responsible for the removal of 90 percent to 95 percent of methemoglobin produced.

The remaining methemoglobin is removed by a similar enzyme system (NADPH-dependent methemoglobin reductase). Because of these, methemoglobin levels are normally less than 2 percent of total hemoglobin types. As methemoglobin levels rise, however, significant hypoxia can develop. This condition is known as *methemoglobinemia*.

There are two major causes of a rise in methemoglobin. One is an increase in methemoglobin production. Several drugs and toxins can induce methemoglobin production, including drugs used for local anesthesia (e.g., benzocaine and lidocaine), drugs used to treat cyanide poisoning (e.g., amyl nitrite and sodium nitrite), certain

---

Table 6-5 Agents Implicated in Acquired Methemoglobinemia

- Amyl nitrite
- Aniline derivatives
- Benzocaine
- Bismuth subnitrite
- Butyl nitrite
- Dapsone
- Lidocaine
- Menthol
- Naphthalene
- Nitrates
- Nitrites
- Nitroglycerin (NTG)
- Nitrophenol
- Phenacetin
- Phenols
- Phenytoin
- Propellants (for room deodorizers)
- Pyridium
- Quinones
- Silver nitrate
- Sodium nitroprusside
- Sulfonamides

---

antibiotics, nitroglycerin, and others (Table 6-5). These are typically oxidizing agents and will induce a change in the charge state of the iron, thus forming methemoglobin.[12]

The other cause is a decrease in the enzymes that convert methemoglobin to deoxyhemoglobin. Some people who are born with these deficiencies are identified at birth because of persistent cyanosis. In infants, methemoglobinemia can also result from systemic acidosis secondary to an infection, diarrhea, or dehydration. Rural infants, whose well water may be contaminated with nitrates, are especially susceptible. Usually, methemoglobinemia is caused by a combination of factors.

As methemoglobin levels increase, the amount of normal hemoglobin available for oxygen transport falls, and your patient will eventually exhibit the signs and symptoms of hypoxia. The areas most dependent on oxygen, such as the heart and the brain, will show the earliest and most severe symptoms.

The signs and symptoms of methemoglobinemia are quite similar to the signs and symptoms of CO poisoning (Table 6-6). Both decrease the oxygen-carrying capacity of

---

Table 6-6 Signs and Symptoms of Methemoglobinemia

SpMet	Signs and Symptoms
1–3%	Normal, asymptomatic
3–15%	Slight grayish-blue discoloration
15–20%	Cyanotic, but asymptomatic
25–50%	Headache, dyspnea, confusion, weakness, chest pain
50–70%	Altered mental status, delirium
70%	Fatal

the blood by increases in abnormal hemoglobin types. When methemoglobinemia and CO poisoning occur simultaneously, the signs and symptoms of hypoxemia increase markedly.

Most patients with methemoglobinemia do not require treatment. The administration of supplemental oxygen will help to fully saturate the oxygen binding sites on hemoglobin. Symptomatic patients may benefit from the administration of methylene blue, which reduces methemoglobin to deoxyhemoglobin.

Technology

You can measure methemoglobin levels with a multifunction pulse CO-oximetry finger probe (Figure 6-34). As described earlier, pulse CO-oximeters use multiple wavelengths of light to measure and distinguish the various types of hemoglobin present (deoxyhemoglobin, oxyhemoglobin, carboxyhemoglobin, and methemoglobin).

The pulse CO-oximeter processes the data and reports oxygen saturation (SpO$_2$), carboxyhemoglobin percentage (SpCO), and methemoglobin percentage (SpMet).[13],[14] With these findings, you can either rule out methemoglobinemia as a diagnosis or continue monitoring while you provide therapy. Some multifunction ECG monitors are equipped with this revolutionary CO-oximetry finger probe.

Limitations

The limitations of SpMet measuring are similar to those of pulse oximetry and CO-oximetry. The sensors can accurately measure the wavelengths only if blood flow through the tissue is adequate. Accurate readings require a pulsating arterial blood flow to obtain an accurate reading. Anything that inhibits perfusion to the spot where the finger probe is attached will alter your reading. Conditions that can produce inaccurate reading include the following:

- Hypoperfusion caused by blood loss, dehydration, cold body temperature, or the use of vasopressors
- Incorrect sensor application, highly callused skin, and movement (such as shivering), especially during hypoperfusion

As stated earlier, make sure that the digital readout of the pulse rate or the pulsation wave matches your patient's actual pulse. If it doesn't, your reading may be inaccurate.

Indications

First of all, methemoglobinemia is relatively uncommon. However, prehospital methemoglobin monitoring should be performed in the following situations:

1. Any case involving a persistent uncorrectable cyanosis. Because oxygen administration will improve your patient's oxygenation in most instances, you should include methemoglobinemia in your differential diagnosis when it doesn't.

2. Critical care transport of a patient receiving intravenous nitroglycerine or nitroprusside therapy. Nitrates can increase the production of methemoglobin.

3. The first two components of the cyanide antidote kit (amyl nitrite and sodium nitrite) induce the conversion of hemoglobin to methemoglobin (changes the heme groups from the ferrous [Fe^{2+}] to the ferric [Fe^{3+}] state). Cyanide then preferentially binds to methemoglobin instead of cytochrome, thus freeing up cytochrome for energy production. The third step in the cyanide antidote kit, sodium thiosulfate, converts cyanomethemoglobin to normal hemoglobin and thiocyanate. Thiocyanate is excreted. However, methemoglobin cannot transport oxygen. Thus, as methemoglobin levels rise, the oxygen-carrying capacity of the blood falls. This is especially important in patients who are small (e.g., children, women) or have preexisting disease. In addition, the concomitant poisoning with carbon monoxide will further decrease the oxygen-carrying capacity of the blood as carboxyhemoglobin (COHb) levels rise. Because of these factors, it is prudent to measure both SpMet and SpCO levels when administering the nitrite components of the cyanide kit. The cyanide antidote hydroxocobalamin does not induce methemoglobinemia.

4. Nitric oxide (NO) therapy is often used to treat newborns with hypoxic respiratory failure (HRF). NO is administered as a gas and causes pulmonary vasodilation through smooth muscle relaxation. This serves to increase the partial pressure of oxygen in arterial blood (PaO$_2$). Some centers are starting to use NO in adults with acute respiratory distress syndrome (ARDS). NO induces the oxidation of hemoglobin to methemoglobin. It is important to monitor methemoglobin levels during NO therapy—especially in neonates in whom levels of fetal hemoglobin (HgF) are elevated.

5. Any patient with elevated SpCO readings. Pulse CO-oximetry can report falsely elevated CO readings in the presence of significant methemoglobinemia. SpCO readings are not considered reliable when SpMet levels exceed 5 percent. Thus, you can use a low SpMet reading to confirm the accuracy of a significantly high SpCO measurement.

6. Elevated methemoglobin levels have been detected following the administration of benzocaine and lidocaine. In one study, signs and symptoms typically developed within 20 minutes. MetHb concentrations ranged from 19 percent to 75 percent. Deaths have been reported.[15]

7. The free-radical compound nitric oxide (NO) is produced when hemoglobin is converted to methemoglobin. Methemoglobin releases free heme and iron,

which activates the cells that line blood vessels (endothelial cells). These cells release NO, causing an inflammatory response. This inflammatory response, initiated by NO and other free radicals, is a cascade of events called *oxidative stress*. Oxidative stress has been linked to the development of numerous chronic conditions, including atherosclerosis, heart disease, Alzheimer's disease, Parkinson's disease, and other chronic conditions. Measurement of SpMet levels, especially over time, may help to identify those at increased risk of oxidative stress and the subsequent problems associated with this. In addition, methemoglobin oxidizes low-density lipoprotein (LDL or "bad cholesterol"), increasing the risk of arteriosclerosis.

Procedure

You will monitor your patient's pulse methemoglobin level with the same multifunction CO-oximetry finger probe. The procedure is identical to obtaining his SpO_2 and his SpCO, as described earlier in this chapter:

- Connect the probe to the monitor device.

- Attach the probe sensor clip to your patient's finger, toe, or earlobe. In an infant, you can use the foot (Procedure 6-3a).

- Turn on the device and wait for the SpO_2 reading to appear (Procedure 6-3b). Match the pulse reading with your patient's actual pulse. If the heart rate is different, the readings will be inaccurate.

- If you get a poor signal or an "error" code, reposition the probe or try another location.

- Your patient's SpMet measurement should appear on the readout (Procedure 6-3c).

- Reassess and document every 5 minutes for unstable patients and every 15 minutes for all others.

Total Hemoglobin Monitoring

Anatomy and Physiology of Hemoglobin

As stated earlier in this chapter, hemoglobin is a protein carried on red blood cells, which is responsible for transporting oxygen. It is essential for sustaining life. As hemoglobin levels decrease, so does the ability to oxygenate the body's tissues. Early recognition of impaired organ perfusion is important to avoid tissue hypoxia that ultimately could lead to organ failure. During circulatory shock, skin blood flow decreases to preserve vital organ perfusion. This results in the clinical signs of poor peripheral perfusion, such as cold, pale, clammy, and mottled skin.[16]

The ability to measure total hemoglobin (Hb) is an important assessment tool in the acute care setting. Although Hb is one of the most frequently ordered laboratory measurements, it is invasive and time consuming, and can provide only intermittent Hb measurements—a quick snapshot. Noninvasive and continuous Hb measurement using a finger probe offers many advantages in the assessment of both acute and chronic anemia in a variety of clinical settings. It provides a view of real-time Hb changes and assists the clinician in recognizing the onset and progression of anemia. It also provides an objective reassessment tool for the ongoing evaluation of therapy.

Technology

As discussed earlier in this chapter, new advances in pulse oximetry technology have led to the development of multiwavelength pulse CO-oximeters designed to measure multiple physiologic parameters. These include oxyhemoglobin, carboxyhemoglobin, and methemoglobin. Since 2008, we have the ability to measure continuous hemoglobin concentration (SpHb) using the same device. We can now continuously and noninvasively measure hemoglobin concentration in addition to the other common hemoglobin species, and therefore provide a significant expansion of existing physiologic monitoring technology. Rapid measurement of hemoglobin can be extremely useful in the prehospital setting. In combination with methemoglobin and carboxyhemoglobin measurements, it should allow for significant advances in patient care.[17]

The newest technology uses multiple (7+) wavelengths of light housed in a single, simple-to-apply sensor and sophisticated signal-processing technologies to accurately determine the dyshemoglobins SpCO and SpMet, as well as SpO_2, PI (perfusion index), Pleth Variability Index (PVI), and pulse rate.

The pulse CO-oximetry method discerns the distinctive light absorption characteristics of different hemoglobin species and applies proprietary algorithms to determine Hb levels. Pulse CO-oximetry SpHb measurement provides clinically acceptable accuracy compared with laboratory CO-oximeter tHb measurement in the 8 to 18 g/dL range.

Pulse oximetry is governed by a few basic principles. Oxyhemoglobin, deoxyhemoglobin, carboxyhemoglobin, and methemoglobin all differ in their absorption of visible and infrared light. The amount of arterial blood in tissue changes with your pulse (photoplethysmography). Therefore, the amount of light absorbed by the varying quantities of arterial blood changes as well. CO-oximetry uses a multiwavelength sensor to distinguish among oxygenated blood, deoxygenated blood, blood with carbon monoxide, blood with oxidized hemoglobin, and blood plasma.

Signal data are obtained by passing various visible and infrared lights through a capillary bed (for example, a

Table 6-7 Normal Hemoglobin Levels

Age	Normal Hb Level
Neonates ages 0–2 weeks	14.5–24.5 g/dL
Infants ages 2–8 weeks	12.5–20.5 g/dL
Infants ages 2–6 months	10.7–17.3 g/dL
Infants ages 6 months–1 year	9.9–14.5 g/dL
Children ages 1–6	9.5–14.1 g/dL
Adult men	14–17.4 g/dL
Adult women	12–16 g/dL

fingertip, a hand, or a foot) and measuring changes in light absorption during the blood pulsatile cycle. Dyshemoglobins and hemoglobin absorb different amounts of red (RD) and infrared (IR) light at various frequencies. The photodetector receives the light and converts it into an electronic signal. Once the device receives the signal, it calculates your patient's functional oxygen saturation (SpO$_2$), carboxyhemoglobin (SpCO), methemoglobin (SpMet), total hemoglobin concentration (SpHb), and pulse rate.

Normal values are age dependent (see Table 6-7). Abnormally high hemoglobin levels may be the result of dehydration, excess production of red blood cells, or severe chronic lung disease. Other factors include pregnancy, heavy smoking, and living at high altitudes. Abnormally low hemoglobin levels, which may lead to anemia, can be the result of many conditions. For prehospital providers, the most important issues are dehydration and hemorrhage.

In addition to total hemoglobin, two other methods for measuring your patient's perfusion are available with CO-oximetry: perfusion index (PI) and the Pleth Variability Index (PVI). PI is an objective method for measuring a patient's peripheral perfusion and is an early indicator of deterioration. PI can be used for any patient whose perfusion status must be monitored closely. Because there is a very strong relationship between PI and blood flow, as the PI increases, so does the perfusion to the site that is being measured.

PI works by comparing the ratio of the variable absorption (AC) to the nonvariable absorption (DC) of the infrared signal. The PI display ranges from 0.02 percent (very weak) to 20 percent (very strong). The normal for PI in the adult population is >1.4 percent. Abnormally low values mean that your patient has decreased perfusion to that area, an early sign of compensated shock.[18]

PVI is a measure of dynamic changes in PI that occur during the respiratory cycle. It is useful in monitoring the therapeutic effects of fluid administration versus adverse tissue edema during resuscitation. It can help the field provider determine how his patient is responding to fluid administration. PVI is a percentage from 1 to 100 percent, with 1 meaning no variability and 100 meaning maximum variability. As with the PI, the PVI is best used to detect trends in perfusion and ventilation. Both are good indicators of whether your patient is getting better or worse.

Indications

Total hemoglobin testing should be used to:

- Measure the presence of anemia in any patient with excessive bleeding, or dehydration
- Triage the severity of any patient with signs of hypoperfusion
- Detect internal bleeding before the signs of hypoperfusion present themselves
- Monitor the response to treatment of hyperperfusion
- Objectively document improvement or deterioration trends

Procedure

You will monitor your patient's pulse methemoglobin level with the same multifunctioning CO-oximetry finger probe. The procedure is identical to obtaining his SpO$_2$, his SpCO, and his SpMet, as described earlier in this chapter:

- Connect the probe to the monitor device.
- Attach the probe sensor clip to your patient's finger, toe, or earlobe. In an infant, you can use the foot (Procedure 6-3a).
- Turn on the device and wait for the SpO$_2$ reading to appear (Procedure 6-3b). Match the pulse reading with your patient's actual pulse. If the heart rate is different, the readings will be inaccurate.
- If you get a poor signal or an "error" code, reposition the probe or try another location.
- Your patient's SpHb measurement should appear on the readout (Procedure 6-3c).
- Reassess and document every 5 minutes for the unstable patient and every 15 minutes for all others.

Blood Glucometry
Anatomy and Physiology

The pancreas, located just behind the stomach and between the duodenum and spleen, is composed of both endocrine and exocrine tissues. The exocrine tissues, known as *acini*, secrete digestive enzymes essential to digestion of fats and proteins into a duct that empties into the small intestine. The endocrine tissues found within the pancreas are known as the *islets of Langerhans*. The three most important types of endocrine cells in the islets of Langerhans are termed alpha, beta, and delta (Figure 6-35). Each type produces and secretes a different hormone (Table 6-8).

Patient Monitoring Technology

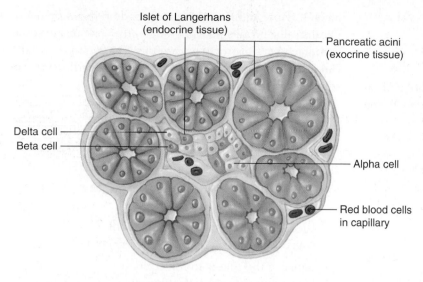

Islet of Langerhans
(endocrine tissue)

Pancreatic acini
(exocrine tissue)

Delta cell

Beta cell

Alpha cell

Red blood cells
in capillary

FIGURE 6-35 The internal anatomy of the pancreas.

Approximately 25 percent of islet tissue is made up of alpha cells, which produce the hormone glucagon. When the blood glucose level falls, alpha cells increase the secretion of glucagon. Glucagon stimulates the breakdown of glycogen, the storage form of glucose found mostly in the liver, into individual glucose molecules that are released into the blood. This process is known as **glycogenolysis**.

Glucagon also stimulates liver breakdown of body proteins and fats and chemically converts them into glucose. This second process, which produces glucose from nonsugar sources, is called *gluconeogenesis*. Both processes contribute to homeostasis by raising the blood glucose level.

Beta cells make up about 60 percent of islet tissue; they produce the hormone insulin. Insulin is the antagonist of glucagon. It lowers the blood glucose level by increasing the uptake of glucose by body cells. Insulin also promotes energy storage in the body by increasing the synthesis of glycogen, protein, and fat.

Insulin must be secreted constantly because the liver removes circulating insulin within 10 to 15 minutes from the time of secretion. This is necessary to maintain the proper balance of glucagon and insulin—a balance that results in a steady supply of glucose for immediate use as an energy source and for appropriate energy storage. Loss of functional beta cells leads to increased blood glucose levels, as seen in diabetes.

Table 6-8 Islets of Langerhans

Cell	Produce	Effect
Alpha	Glucagon	Increases blood glucose
Beta	Insulin	Decreases blood glucose
Delta	Somatostatin	Inhibits production of glucagon and insulin

Delta cells, which comprise about 10 percent of islet tissue, produce somatostatin. Somatostatin works within the islets to inhibit the secretion of glucagon and insulin.

Diabetes mellitus is a disease characterized by inadequate insulin production by the pancreas. Patients whose pancreas produces no insulin must take daily injections of insulin and monitor their caloric intake and their physical activity carefully. Maintaining normal blood glucose levels becomes a lifetime priority. Others, whose pancreases do not produce enough insulin, take daily doses of oral hypoglycemic agents to maintain normal blood glucose levels.

The normal blood glucose level is in the range of 80 to 140 mg/dL. Derangements in either direction can be life threatening. Hypoglycemia (<80 mg/dL) can result in severe brain damage from a lack of glucose. Hyperglycemia (>140 mg/dL), though not immediately life threatening, can, over time, result in life-threatening dehydration. With the glucometer, you can measure your patient's blood sugar level in a matter of a minute or so and begin to provide emergency therapy.

Technology

Inexpensive, user-friendly glucometers have had a remarkable impact on prehospital care. A number of different types of glucometers are available today. Although they all do relatively the same thing, their methods differ. Most glucometers used in prehospital care measure the glucose in whole blood.

The early glucometers used a test strip with a chemical that changes color when exposed to glucose in the blood. The darker the color change, the more glucose is present on the strip. The color variation is measured photometrically or colorimetrically to provide the glucose reading.

Newer glucometers use test strips containing a reagent, such as glucose oxidase and potassium ferricyanide. These reagents cause electrons to increase their electrical activity when exposed to glucose present on the strip. The more glucose, the more electrical activity generated. This electrical activity is measured to provide the glucose reading.

The newest glucometers are able to measure glucose extracted from the interstitial fluid in the skin. This means less painful testing. Many diabetic patients wear continuous monitoring systems that measure blood glucose at set time intervals.

In reality, most EMS agencies use the same glucometers that their patients purchase at their local drugstores. These devices, if properly maintained and calibrated, can provide consistently accurate blood glucose readings.

Limitations

The accuracy of glucometers is a common topic of clinical concern. A variety of factors can affect the accuracy of a test:

- Meter calibration. Glucometers must be calibrated on a regular basis with the coding strips provided by the manufacturers.
- Using an expired test strip.
- Improper cleaning of the test site. If you use an alcohol wipe to cleanse the skin in preparation, you must allow the alcohol to dry before testing. This prevents alcohol from being absorbed into the test strip, which can lead to a false reading.
- Waterless hand cleaners. Hands that have recently been cleaned with a waterless hand cleaner may also react with the test strip, so it is best to thoroughly clean the hands with soap and water, if possible.
- Environmental issues such as humidity, ambient temperature, and even a dirty meter.

Indications

The indications for using a glucometer include treating anyone you think may have an abnormal blood glucose level. It is a quick, simple test that should be performed on patients who display the following:

- Anyone with a history of diabetes who presents with the common signs and symptoms of hypoglycemia (e.g., altered mental status, diaphoresis, tachycardia, MedicAlert tag)
- Any unexplained altered mental status, syncope, or fall
- Seizures
- Head trauma
- Stroke
- Pregnant patients
- Chronic alcoholics
- Any overdose of lithium, acetaminophen, or antihistamines
- Hepatitis
- Patients taking beta-blockers, quinine, or prednisone
- Addison's disease
- Patients who took someone else's diabetes medications

This list is not all-inclusive. Glucometry is much too simple and fast not to use it whenever you want to know your patient's blood glucose levels.

Procedure

To perform this procedure, you will need a glucometer with test strips, a finger-stick device with sterile lancets, an alcohol wipe, and tissue or gauze pads (Procedure 6-4a). Because all glucometers work differently, you must read the manufacturer's instructions carefully. The slightest mistake can alter the measurement's accuracy. The following are some simple guidelines that pertain to all glucometers:

- Let your patient's arm hang down, to allow for better blood flow to the finger you will be using for the test.
- If the patient's fingers are cold, warm them briefly to provide better flow prior to testing.
- Always match the code number on the screen to the code number on your test strip vial.
- Cleanse the test site with an alcohol wipe (Procedure 6-4b). Make sure it dries completely before testing.
- Squeeze the finger to force blood into the tip. Use a lancet device to prick the fingertip (Procedure 6-4c).
- Place a drop of your patient's capillary blood from a finger stick onto a chemical reagent strip (Procedure 6-4d). Follow the manufacturer's instructions for placement of the test strip into the glucometer.
- Wait for the reading to appear on the screen (Procedure 6-4e).

Basic Blood Chemistries
Purpose

The laboratory analysis of blood can provide valuable information about your sick and/or injured patient. The concentrations of electrolytes, gases, hormones, or other chemicals in blood can often shed light on the underlying causes of vague complaints such as dizziness or generalized weakness. Additionally, blood evaluation can confirm suspected conditions. For example, elevated cardiac enzymes in a patient's blood can confirm a suspected myocardial infarction.

In the field, you often will be the first to assess and treat an ill or injured patient. Many of your interventions can alter the blood's composition and erase important information. If you obtain venous blood samples before performing those interventions, they will enable the physician to evaluate the patient's original status.

Venous blood is commonly obtained via venipuncture. As a paramedic who routinely initiates intravenous access, you can simultaneously obtain blood samples. Doing so saves considerable hospital time and avoids multiple needle sticks.

You should obtain venous blood in the following situations:

- During peripheral access
- Before drug administration
- When drug administration may be needed

Procedure 6-4 Blood Glucose Determination

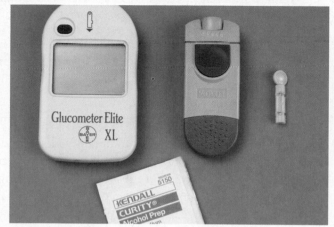

6-4a Glucometry equipment.

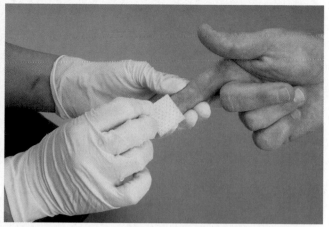

6-4b Cleanse the puncture site.

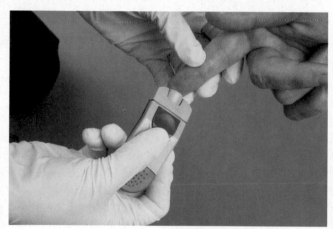

6-4c Perform the puncture with the lancet device.

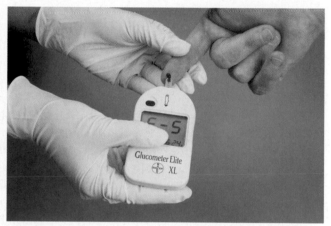

6-4d Apply the blood to the reagent strip in the glucometer.

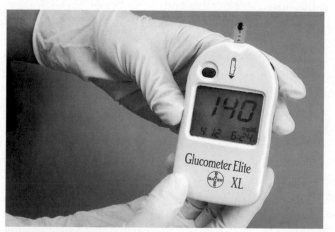

6-4e Read the blood glucose level on the meter.

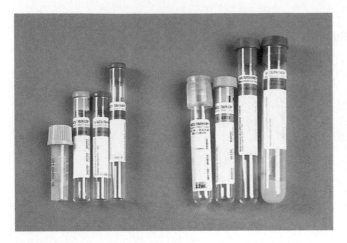

FIGURE 6-36 Color-coded tubes used for venous sampling.

Of course, never stop to draw blood if it will delay critical measures such as drug administration in cardiac arrest or transport in a multisystem trauma.

Technology

Blood tubes are made of glass and have color-coded, self-sealing rubber tops (Figure 6-36). Blood tube sizes for adults generally range from 5 to 7 mL; for pediatric patients, from 2 to 3 mL. They are vacuum packed, and some contain a chemical anticoagulant. The different-colored tops correspond to specific anticoagulants. A label on every blood tube identifies the type of additive and its expiration date. Do not use a blood tube after its expiration date, as both the anticoagulant and the vacuum lose their effectiveness.

Using blood tubes in their correct order is essential. If you do not follow the proper sequence, the various anticoagulants will cause cross-contamination, skewing the results and rendering the blood useless. Table 6-9 lists anticoagulants, the order in which you should use them, and the colors of the tubes' tops.

Depending on the technique you use to obtain venous blood, you will also need syringes, hypodermic needles, and commercially manufactured plastic sleeves called **vacutainers**.

Obtaining venous blood is a simple process; however, if the blood is to remain usable, you must pay strict attention to detail. You can obtain blood either from an angiocatheter or directly from the vein. The technique you use will depend on the situation. In either case, venous blood samples are best obtained from sturdy veins such as the cephalic, basilic, or median veins. Smaller veins, such as those on the back of the hand, are more likely to collapse during retrieval, making the procedure difficult to complete.

Table 6-9 Blood Tube Sequence

Anticoagulant	Color of Top
None	Red
Citrate	Blue
Heparin	Green
EDTA	Purple
Fluoride	Gray

The most convenient way to obtain venous blood is through an angiocatheter at the time of peripheral vascular access. In addition to blood tubes, you will need a tube holder (Figure 6-37) or vacutainer. A special adapter called a **multidraw needle** fits into the tube holder. The multidraw needle has a rubber-covered needle used to puncture the self-sealing top of the blood tube. The remaining portion of the multidraw needle protrudes from the tube holder and fits snugly into the hub of the angiocatheter.

Procedure

To obtain blood directly from the angiocatheter, use the following procedure:

- Assemble and prepare all equipment. Inspect the blood tubes for expiration or damage and insert the multidraw needle into the vacutainer. Never place blood tubes into the assembled vacutainer and multidraw needle until you are ready to draw blood. This will destroy the vacuum and render the blood tube useless.

- Establish IV access with the angiocatheter. Do not connect IV administration tubing.

- Attach the end of the multidraw needle adapter to the hub of the cannula.

- In correct order, insert the blood tubes so that the rubber-covered needle punctures the self-sealing rubber top (Table 6-9). Blood should be pulled into the blood tube.

- Fill all blood tubes completely, as the amount of anticoagulant is proportional to the tube's volume. Gently agitate the tubes to mix the anticoagulant evenly with the blood.

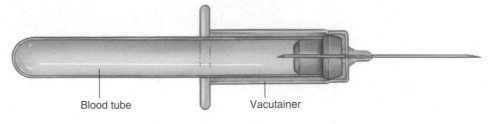

Blood tube   Vacutainer

FIGURE 6-37 Vacutainer with multisampling needle.

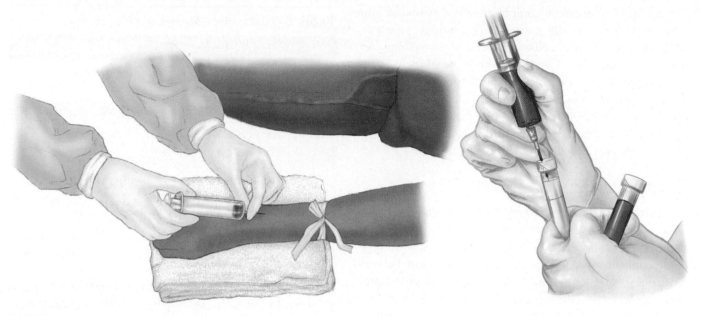

FIGURE 6-38 Obtaining a blood sample with a 20-mL syringe.

- Tamponade the vein and remove the vacutainer and multidraw needle. Attach the IV and ensure patency.
- Properly dispose of all sharps.
- Label all blood tubes with the following information:
  - Patient's first and last name
  - Patient's age and gender
  - Date and time drawn
  - Name of the person drawing the blood

If commercial equipment is not available, use a 20-mL syringe (Figure 6-38). Attach the syringe's needle adapter to the angiocatheter hub and gently pull back the plunger. Blood will fill the syringe. When the syringe is full, remove it from the angiocatheter and place the IV line into the angiocatheter. Carefully attach a hypodermic needle to the syringe to puncture the tops of the blood tubes. In the appropriate order, place the collected blood into the blood tubes and agitate gently. When finished, properly dispose of all sharps and label the blood tubes.

When IV access is difficult or unobtainable, you may draw blood directly from the vein with a hypodermic needle. This technique is useful for routine sampling that will not require further IV access. To draw blood directly from a vein, you will need the same equipment as for obtaining blood from an angiocatheter, but you will use a Luer sampling needle (Figure 6-39). A Luer

sampling needle is similar to a multidraw needle, but instead of an angiocatheter adapter it has a long, exposed needle. The Luer sampling needle screws into the vacutainer, and you insert the exposed needle directly into the vein. You will also need a constricting band and antiseptic wipes.

To obtain blood directly from a vein, use the following procedure:

- Assemble and prepare all equipment. Inspect the blood tubes for expiration or damage, and insert the multidraw needle into the vacutainer.
- Apply the constricting band and select an appropriate puncture site.
- Cleanse the site with alcohol or Betadine.
- Insert the end of the Luer sampling needle into the vein and remove the constricting band.
- In the correct order, insert each blood tube so that the rubber-covered needle punctures the self-sealing rubber top. Blood should be pulled into the tube.
- Gently agitate the tube to evenly mix the anticoagulant with the blood. Completely fill all blood tubes, as the anticoagulant is proportional to the volume of the tube.
- Place sterile gauze over the site and remove the sampling needle. Properly dispose of all sharps.
- Cover the puncture site with gauze and tape or an adhesive bandage.
- Label all blood tubes with the following information:
  - Patient's first and last name
  - Patient's age and gender
  - Date and time drawn
  - Person drawing the blood

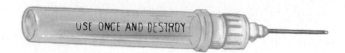

FIGURE 6-39 Single-use Luer sampling needle.

Again, if commercial equipment is not available, you may use a 20-mL syringe. When using a syringe, attach an 18-gauge hypodermic needle to the end of the syringe and insert it into the vein. Gently pull back the plunger to fill the syringe with blood. When the syringe is full, remove the syringe and dress the puncture site. In the appropriate order, inject the collected blood into the blood tubes and agitate gently. When you have finished, properly dispose of all sharps and label the blood tubes.

Complications

Complications from drawing blood include damage to the vein wall, inadvertent removal of the IV angiocatheter, and hemoconcentration and hemolysis of the blood sample. **Hemoconcentration** occurs when the constricting band is left in place too long, elevating the numbers of red and white blood cells in the sample.

Hemolysis is the destruction of red blood cells. When red blood cells are destroyed, they release hemoglobin and potassium, thus rendering the blood unusable. Causes of hemolysis include shaking the blood tubes vigorously after they are filled, using too small a needle for retrieval, or too forcefully aspirating blood into or out of a syringe.

Next, we discuss two basic blood chemistry laboratory tests that will be performed with your venous blood sample: cardiac biomarkers and electrolytes.

Cardiac Biomarkers

The measurement of enzymes and markers associated with cardiac disease is an important aspect of medical practice—especially emergency medicine and critical care transport. Numerous tests are used to help diagnose and classify cardiac disease.

When cells are damaged, enzymes within those cells are leaked into the circulatory system. Although these enzymes may not be tissue specific, various forms of the enzymes (called *isoenzymes*) can be tied to a specific tissue type. The most frequently encountered cardiac enzymes and markers are discussed next (see Table 6-10).

Creatine Kinase

Creatine kinase (CK or CPK; formerly called creatinine phosphokinase) is important in energy utilization. Almost all CK comes from muscle tissue, but it can be separated into three different isoenzymes:

- CK-I (BB): Produced primarily in the brain and in selected smooth muscle
- CK-II (MB): Produced primarily in the heart
- CK-III (MM): Produced primarily in skeletal muscle

An elevated CK may be caused by various factors, such as an IM medication injection or skeletal muscle

Table 6-10 Cardiac Enzymes and Biomarkers

Test	Normal Value
Creatine kinase (CK)	Men: 60–100 U/L Women: 40–150 U/L
CK–MB fraction	<12 U/L
Lactate dehydrogenase (LDH)	Adult: 40–90 U/L
Myoglobin	50–120 mcg/dL
Troponin I	<6 ng/mL,>1.5 ng/mL (MI)
Troponin T	>0.1–0.2 ng/mL (MI)
B-natriuretic peptide (BMP)	5–100 pg/dL

trauma. When the isoenzymes are isolated, however, the source of the elevation is known. CK is the first enzyme to elevate after acute myocardial infarction and is increased in 90 percent of infarctions (Figure 6-40).

The time sequence for CK after myocardial infarction is as follows:

- Begins to rise in 4 to 6 hours
- Peaks at 24 hours
- Returns to normal in 3 to 4 days

Lactic Dehydrogenase

Lactic dehydrogenase (LD or LDH) is found in heart muscle, skeletal muscle, liver, erythrocytes, kidney, and some types of tumors. It is increased in more than 90 percent of myocardial infarctions. However, it can be increased in diseases of any of the previous organs or hemolysis. There are five LDH isoenzymes:

- LDH1: Heart, erythrocytes, renal cortex
- LDH2: Reticuloendothelial system

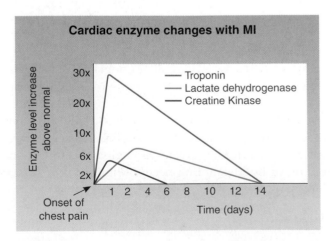

FIGURE 6-40 Cardiac enzyme changes associated with myocardial infarction.

- LDH3: Lung tissue
- LDH4: Placenta, kidney, pancreas
- LDH5: Skeletal muscle, liver

Reversal of the LDH1/LDH2 ratio is characteristic of an acute myocardial infarction, with 80 percent to 85 percent sensitivity.

The time sequence of LD after myocardial infarction is as follows:

- Begins to rise in 24 hours
- Peaks in 3 days
- Returns to normal in 8 to 9 days

Myoglobin

Myoglobin is found in striated muscle and contains iron. It stores oxygen and gives muscle its red color. Damage to skeletal or cardiac muscle releases myoglobin into the circulation. Myoglobin rapid assay kits are available that allow testing in the prehospital critical care and emergency department settings.

The following is the time sequence for myoglobin after myocardial infarction:

- Rises quickly (2 hours) after MI
- Peaks at 6 to 8 hours
- Returns to normal in 20 to 36 hours
- False positives seen with skeletal muscle injury and renal failure

Troponin

The **troponins** are the contractile proteins of the myofibril. The cardiac isoforms are very specific for cardiac injury and are not present in serum from healthy people. Troponin I is the form frequently assessed. There is a new form (Troponin L) that may be detected earlier. Troponin rapid assay kits are available that allow testing in the prehospital, critical care, and emergency department settings.

The time sequence for troponin after myocardial infarction is as follows:

- Rises 4 to 6 hours after injury
- Peaks in 12 to 16 hours
- Stays elevated for up to 10 days

B-Natriuretic Peptide

B-natriuretic peptide (BNP) is a peptide found in the ventricles of the heart. Levels increase when ventricular filling pressures are high. It can be used to detect congestive heart failure.

Electrolytes

Electrolytes are chemical substances that take on a charge when dissolved in water. The four most com-

Table 6-11 Conversion of Milligrams to Milliequivalents

Measurement of Weight	Measurement of Chemical Activity
23 mg sodium (Na⁺)	1 mEq
39 mg potassium (K⁺)	1 mEq
36 mg chloride (Cl⁻)	1 mEq
30 mg bicarbonate (HCO₃⁻)	1 mEq

monly measured electrolytes are sodium, potassium, chloride, and bicarbonate. Less commonly measured electrolytes are calcium, magnesium, and phosphate. Sodium, chloride, and bicarbonate are the principal electrolytes in the extracellular fluid. Potassium, magnesium, and phosphate are the principal electrolytes in the intracellular fluid.

Electrolytes are measured in milliequivalents per liter (mEq/L) instead of milligrams because milligram units measure only the weight of the chemical element or compound, not its chemical activity. The standard of equivalents is based on the number of grams of an element or compound that liberate or combine with 1 gram of hydrogen. A milliequivalent is 1/1000 of an equivalent. Table 6-11 details this relationship.

Electrolytes that take on a positive charge are called *cations* and include sodium, potassium, magnesium, and calcium. Electrolytes that take on a negative charge are called *anions* and include chloride, bicarbonate, and phosphate. There must be a constant balance between the positively and negatively charged ions. This is referred to as *chemical electrical neutrality*. Thus, when the concentration of one of the electrolytes changes, other electrolytes shift to maintain chemical electrical neutrality.

For example, when metabolic acids are introduced into the body, bicarbonate ions are used as buffers. When the bicarbonate ions are eliminated, a negative ion deficit is left. To maintain chemical electrical neutrality, chloride ions (Cl⁻) are shifted out of the cells.

Although most electrolytes can be measured easily, some cannot be. When cations and anions in the serum are measured, there appears to be a deficit in the number of anions, which is referred to as the *anion gap*. This gap is made up of unmeasured anions such as organic acids, sulfates, and phosphates. To calculate the anion gap, add the measured cations and subtract the measured anions. The difference in the anion gap is usually about 12 to 14 mEq.

The anion gap is important in that it is increased in certain metabolic acidosis states. Thus, an increase in the anion gap helps identify the type of metabolic acidosis present.

The most frequently occurring cations include the following.

Sodium

Sodium (Na^+) is the most prevalent cation in the extracellular fluid. It plays a major role in regulating the distribution of water because water is attracted to and moves with sodium. In fact, it is often said that "water follows sodium." Sodium is also important in the transmission of nervous impulses. An abnormal increase in the relative amount of sodium in the body is called *hypernatremia*, whereas an abnormal decrease is referred to as *hyponatremia*.

Potassium

Potassium (K^+) is the most prevalent cation in the intracellular fluid. It is also important in the transmission of electrical impulses. An abnormally high potassium level is called *hyperkalemia*, and an abnormally low potassium level is referred to as *hypokalemia*.

Calcium

Calcium (Ca^{2+}) has many physiologic functions. It plays a major role in muscle contraction as well as nervous impulse transmission. An abnormally increased calcium level is called *hypercalcemia*, whereas an abnormally decreased calcium level is called *hypocalcemia*.

About half the calcium in the serum is loosely associated with proteins. The other half (which is the metabolically active portion) is called *ionized calcium*. The usual methods for measuring calcium measure the total calcium level (bound + free). *Ionized calcium* is measured when other factors complicate the interpretation of the normal serum calcium test. For example, if the levels of binding proteins are increased or decreased (for example, in the presence of abnormal amounts of albumin or immunoglobulins), the amount of serum calcium will appear to be increased or decreased, because it is the free calcium that is regulated hormonally by the body. In these circumstances, ionized calcium is a more reliable measure of calcium levels.

Magnesium

Magnesium (Mg^{2+}) is necessary for several biochemical processes that occur in the body and is closely associated with phosphate in many processes. An abnormally increased magnesium level is called *hypermagnesemia*; an abnormally decreased magnesium level is called *hypomagnesemia*.

The most frequently occurring anions include the following.

Chloride

Chloride (Cl^-) is an important anion. Its negative charge balances the positive charge associated with the cations. It also plays a major role in fluid balance and renal function. Chloride has a close association with sodium.

Bicarbonate

Bicarbonate (HCO_3^-) is the principal buffer of the body. This means that it neutralizes the highly acidic hydrogen ion (H^+) and other organic acids.

Phosphate

Phosphate (HPO_4^{3-}) is important in body energy stores. It is closely associated with magnesium in renal function. It also acts as a buffer, primarily in the intracellular space, in much the same manner as bicarbonate.

Many other compounds carry negative charges. Among these are some of the proteins, certain organic acids, and other compounds.

Serum Lactate

Aerobic metabolism, which supplies 90 percent of the body's energy needs, requires oxygen. If oxygen is not readily available to body cells, anaerobic metabolism occurs, with lactic acid as a byproduct. A serum lactate level measures the amount of lactic acid in the blood and is a fairly sensitive and reliable indicator of tissue hypoperfusion and hypoxia.

Any disorder that causes an imbalance between lactate production and clearance can lead to lactic acidosis, a serious and sometimes life-threatening condition. Lactic acid production can increase with any condition that results in anaerobic metabolism, such as hemorrhagic shock or pulmonary embolism. Normally, the liver clears most lactic acid from the blood, but hepatic dysfunction decreases lactic acid clearance.

The laboratory evaluation of electrolytes is known commonly as a CHEM-7. The status of the electrolytes can provide a great deal of information about the patient's condition.

Point-of-Care Testing

Point-of-care (POC) testing takes obtaining basic blood chemistries in the field to another level. Instead of bringing samples of your patient's blood to the hospital for analysis, you can, via a finger stick and a portable analytical device, obtain instant results from a variety of tests. EMS providers have been using POC testing for decades. Blood glucose, pulse oximetry, capnometry, and cardiac rhythm strips are just some of the bedside testing that aids paramedics in making a field diagnosis and determining emergency care. With the newest generation of analyzers, you can obtain results of some of the previously mentioned blood tests in just a few minutes. Because of that, you can provide emergency treatment in a more timely and precise manner. In addition, it allows you to objectively monitor your patient's improvement or deterioration en route to the hospital.

Expanded POC testing helps you to make better patient assessments and provide more specific treatments after obtaining a history and performing a physical examination. In many cases, such as caring for patients with altered mental status, these tests may be the only information available besides the physical examination. Obtaining early blood chemistry results also helps to determine the most appropriate destination for your patient and, upon arrival to the emergency department, can result in better triage and earlier treatment. Simply put, in a properly coordinated system, prehospital POC testing translates into better patient care.

Technology

There are two devices that offer comprehensive blood analysis, the i-STAT® and the epoc® Blood Analysis System (Figure 6-41). Although technologically different, they both offer bedside testing in electrolytes, hemoglobin and hematocrit, troponin, and serum lactate. They work similarly to blood glucose testing in that a few drops of blood are placed onto or into a cartridge that is inserted into the analyzer. The results are displayed within minutes. Prehospital POC testing simplifies the process of obtaining blood samples. Less blood is drawn and fewer tubes will be filled. This saves valuable on-scene time and lessens the risk of provider contamination through blood contact.

Prehospital POC testing also streamlines the reporting and documentation process because the data can be downloaded directly to a patient report and, ultimately, to the patient's medical chart. Being able to transmit test results in a printed or electronic format reduces the possibility of communication errors.

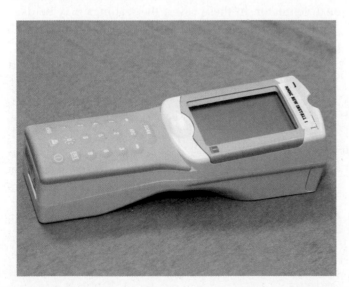

FIGURE 6-41 Point-of care testing is possible with portable iSTAT Blood Analysis System device.

(© Dr. Bryan E. Bledsoe)

Limitations

Any POC blood testing mechanism will have the same limitations as stated in the section on blood glucose testing. The major limitation in using POC technology isn't the technology itself, but rather how the prehospital POC testing system is configured.

Government standards for laboratory testing are regulated by the Clinical Laboratory Improvement Amendments (CLIA), established in 1988 to ensure public safety and accuracy in blood testing. It is imperative that prehospital systems become familiar with CLIA regulations before designing their POC testing system. For example, according to CLIA, the prehospital POC testing system must use the same methodology as the hospital system. In other words, the tests must be performed in the same manner. If different methods are used, the devices are most likely calibrated differently. This renders trending results from one system to another impossible.

It is also essential that the prehospital system coordinate with the receiving hospitals to determine whether the devices can download data to the hospital system. Ideally, prehospital providers would be able to download automatically into the patient's electronic medical record via wireless technology because POC bedside testing can make a significant difference in patient care.

Indications

- *Potassium.* To ensure adequate cardiac function, it is necessary to maintain the level of potassium between 3.5 and 5 mEq/L. Hypokalemia and hyperkalemia can cause life-threatening emergencies, even in a healthy person. If your patient has end-stage renal disease or maintains his potassium levels with supplements, he is at a higher risk for a potassium-related emergency.

- *Sodium.* To ensure adequate hydration, it is necessary to maintain the level of sodium between 135 and 145 mEq/L. Administering or withholding IV fluids, for example, is no longer left to guessing. Paramedics can recognize a minor issue before it becomes a major issue, as both hyponatremia and hypernatremia can cause significant neurologic emergencies.

- *Hemoglobin and hematocrit.* To ensure adequate oxygen-carrying capabilities of the blood, it is necessary to maintain the level of hemoglobin between 14 and 18 g/dL and the hematocrit between 35 and 45 percent. These values will not affect care in the field, but early recognition will facilitate better critical care in the hospital.

- *Troponin.* The troponin test measures the levels of certain proteins, troponin T and troponin I, in the blood.

These proteins are released when the heart muscle has been damaged, such as in a heart attack. The more damage there is to the heart, the greater the amount of troponin T and I there will be in the blood. If your patient has chest pain, but no ST elevation, a rise in troponin (anything over 10 mcg/L) would indicate a trip to the cardiac cath lab.

- *Lactate.* Any condition that results in anaerobic metabolism (hypovolemia, sepsis) leads to increased lactic acid levels. Anything greater than 4 mmol/L indicates a significant illness or injury. Lactate is a measure of tissue perfusion and can tell you how well the cells are being oxygenated regardless of the blood pressure. Early recognition and reporting leads to more timely care in the hospital, especially in septic shock.

Arterial Blood Gases

An **arterial blood gas (ABG)** analysis provides information regarding your patient's ventilation and perfusion status, as well as data concerning the overall acid–base balance status. This test analyzes the SaO_2, PaO_2, pCO_2, pH, and bicarbonate levels in the arteries (see Table 6-12 for normal ABG values). In an ABG blood draw, which is typically not a prehospital skill, arterial blood is drawn from a direct arterial puncture, most often from the radial artery or an existing arterial catheter (art line). The blood is then sent to the lab, or a portable ABG unit can be used at the bedside.

Arterial blood gas analysis is particularly important in the critical care setting, and any paramedic performing critical care transports must have a good understanding of this. The arterial blood gas generally consists of the following variables:

- *Oxygen saturation (SaO2).* The oxygen saturation provides information concerning the percentage of hemoglobin that is saturated with oxygen. This should be identical to readings obtained through the use of pulse oximeters. This reading is important because most oxygen is transported bound to hemoglobin.

- *PaO_2.* The partial pressure of oxygen in the blood reflects the amount of oxygen dissolved in the serum. Most oxygen (approximately 98 percent) is transported by hemoglobin. However, there is a direct, yet complex, relationship between PO_2 and hemoglobin saturation.

- *$PaCO_2$.* The partial pressure of carbon dioxide reflects the amount of carbon dioxide present in the arterial system. Carbon dioxide is transported in the serum, although some is combined with water to form carbonic acid (H_2CO_3).

- *pH.* The pH simply reflects the hydrogen ion concentration of the arterial blood. The greater the concentration, the lower the pH. It is important to remember that pH is a logarithmic relationship. A change in units reflects a 10-fold change in hydrogen ion concentration (Figure 6-42).

- *Bicarbonate (HCO3−).* The bicarbonate ion is one of the principal metabolic buffers. Abnormalities in the amount of bicarbonate present tell a great deal about any acid–base derangements. An excess of bicarbonate ion is called a *base excess*, whereas a decreased amount of bicarbonate is called a *base deficit*.

- *Hemoglobin (Hgb).* Most arterial blood gas units will provide a spot hemoglobin reading because anemia can affect oxygen transport. This should correspond to any measurements obtained during the complete blood count.

Often, critically ill patients will have undergone multiple arterial blood gas readings, especially if the patient is on a ventilator. In these cases, the readings may be displayed sequentially or graphically by the hospital information system.

Table 6-12 Normal ABG Values

• SaO_2	94–99%
• PaO_2	80–100 mmHg
• $PaCO_2$	35–45 mmHg
• pH	7.35–7.45
• HCO_3^-	22–26 mEq/L
• Hgb	12–18 g/DL

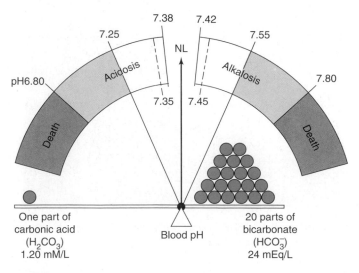

FIGURE 6-42 Arterial blood gas changes.

Ultrasound

Introduction

Ultrasound has become an important diagnostic tool in the emergency department. This technology now allows emergency physicians to make clinical diagnoses at the bedside, resulting in faster and more accurate care of patients who present with conditions requiring timely intervention.[19] The natural extension of this technology to the prehospital arena is made possible by portable ultrasound machines that are small, lightweight, and durable.[20] Ultrasound has come a long way since the grainy, hazy images of the past. These new battery-operated machines deliver high-resolution images that allow paramedics to easily identify anatomical landmarks and pathological abnormalities. A study by Heegaard in 2010 demonstrated a 100 percent agreement between paramedic ultrasound assessments and physician diagnosis.[21]

Emergency ultrasound has many prehospital clinical applications that would reduce morbidity and improve outcomes of patients with life-threatening conditions. It can improve paramedic diagnostic accuracy and provide crucial information to guide management and help triage patients to the most appropriate destination. EMS trauma protocols to date indicate that ultrasound is normally used on the way to the hospital in a moving ambulance. For cardiac arrest, when transport is not the priority, paramedics can take the ultrasound unit to the patient for immediate detection of cardiac wall movement to help rule out the presence of pulseless electrical activity (PEA). You can easily scan the heart and inferior vena cava without interrupting CPR or ventilations. The real value of paramedic ultrasound may be similar to obtaining a 12-lead ECG. It does not drastically change field care but does expedite the patient to the most appropriate location and the most effective treatment.

Technology

Ultrasound, also called *ultrasonography*, is a medical imaging technique that uses high-frequency sound waves (and the resultant echoes) to visualize structures within the body. The sound frequency is typically higher than that heard by humans. A transducer is applied to the skin (using a conductive gel) and emits high-frequency waves that bounce off internal structures. The same transducer captures the echoes. The information from the sound waves and echoes is processed by a computer to provide real-time imaging of the internal structures. These images can be viewed in various formats, including conventional two-dimensional (2-D), three-dimensional (3-D), and even four-dimensional (4-D) formats.

Ultrasound provides a rapid assessment of internal body structures and is sensitive in detecting blood and fluid in body cavities. Fluid produces a black image, and scattered waves indicate air or gas. The monitor's transducer projects an ultrasound beam on the monitor screen, exhibiting a slice of the body anatomy in the shape of a flattened cone. In addition, ultrasound is often used for measuring blood flow and direction using a Doppler technique.

Limitations

Ultrasound technology itself is nearly limitless. With it, a paramedic can easily see the location, size, and orientation of organs. He can identify the presence of an abnormal amount of air or fluid in a particular area. He is able to detect degrees of tissue alteration and he can watch, in real time, how the walls of the heart move. The limitations of ultrasound lie with the EMS system and the paramedics using the machine. The initial training, continuing education, medical oversight, scope of practice, and protocols will determine the degree of success or failure of using ultrasound.

Several studies have demonstrated that paramedics can easily acquire the necessary skill in ultrasound use with training sessions varying from one hour and 15 minutes to two days, depending on the type of ultrasound application being learned.[22–24] Obviously, a wider focus of use requires more training time. As reported in a different study by Heegaard et al., paramedics underwent six hours of structured ultrasound training and were able to adequately obtain and interpret prehospital FAST (exam for internal bleeding, explained under "Hemoperitoneum" and "Procedure" below) and abdominal aortic (AA) ultrasound images with 100 percent interpretation agreement with physician overreader.[21] Other published reports also support the successful training of paramedics in ultrasound use in the prehospital setting.[25] As with any skill, continued practice is necessary to maintain competence and confidence.

Oversight and continuous quality improvement activities by the system medical director is essential to ensure that the public is receiving high-quality performance. The EMS system must consistently evaluate whether the protocols fit the needs of the community. The use of telesonography, transmitting ultrasound images from scene to ED for expert review of images and interpretation is an effective option in EMS systems that lack advanced-level providers, or in rural EMS systems. Cellular and satellite networks allow for the transmission of real-time ultrasound images from the field to the ED without affecting the quality of the images.[26]

These off-line issues will determine the success of the program. Poor training, inadequate oversight, and an overreaching scope of practice and protocols will eventually undermine any efforts to use this game-changing technology.

Indications

There is an ever-growing number of trauma and medical applications for prehospital ultrasound. The following list of indications is by no means all-inclusive, but does represent a variety of common, everyday uses for this increasingly popular technology.

- *Hemoperitoneum.* The first and most common emergency ultrasound application is the focused abdominal sonography for trauma (FAST) exam, which is used to assess internal bleeding. An experienced examiner can detect as little as 200 to 250 mL of peritoneal fluid using the FAST exam (Figure 6-43). In one multicenter study of 202 trauma patients, prehospital focused abdominal sonography for trauma (PFAST) performed at the trauma scene had much higher sensitivity, specificity, and accuracy of detecting free blood in the abdomen when compared to regular physical examination (93%, 99%, and 99%, respectively, compared with 93%, 52%, and 57%).[22]

- *Abdominal aortic aneurysm.* Ultrasound can be used to quickly evaluate the intraabdominal aorta for aneurysm and measure the diameter and character of any aneurysms detected.

- *Cardiac emergency.* Ultrasound can detect the presence or absence of cardiac wall motion, normal to severely impaired ventricular function, right ventricular dilatation, and pericardial tamponade. In patients undergoing CPR, ultrasound use demonstrated cardiac wall motion in 13 out of 37 patients (35%) whose initial ECG diagnosis was asystole, which correlated with increased survival to hospital admission.[27]

- *Suspected pneumothorax.* Prehospital ultrasound use in trauma patients with suspected pneumothorax may be useful in preventing harm from unnecessary field intervention such as needle thoracostomy. When

thoracic ultrasound was used to detect lung sliding sign (pleural sliding indicating respirations in the absence of a pneumothorax) in the emergency department in patients after prehospital needle thoracostomy, 15 out of 57 (26%) trauma patients "appeared not to have had a pneumothorax originally nor to have had one induced by the needle thoracostomy."[28] In these cases, ultrasound may prevent an unnecessary invasive procedure and subsequent harm to patients.

- *Heart failure.* Prehospital ultrasound can improve the accuracy of diagnosing pulmonary edema as the cause of acute dyspnea. In a study of 218 patients presenting with acute dyspnea (heart failure or COPD/asthma related), ultrasound findings were determined to be the strongest predictors for the diagnosis of heart failure in the prehospital setting.[29]

- *Shock.* Prehospital ultrasound can be useful in differentiating between cardiogenic and noncardiac etiologies of shock. Adding ultrasound to prehospital shock management can help rule out the presence of life-threatening conditions such as clinically significant pericardial effusion or abdominal aortic aneurysms.[27,30,31]

- *Confirming endotracheal tube placement.* Continuous waveform capnography remains the gold standard method for ETT correct placement confirmation. It also offers prehospital providers another method for ETT confirmation and for differentiating between main tracheal intubation and right mainstem intubation. However, there is an evolving body of research demonstrating that endotracheal tube placement can be effectively confirmed with ultrasound.

Other possible uses include identifying early pregnancies and ectopic pregnancies, monitoring fetal conditions, delivery position, placenta location, cardiac capture during pacing, acute ischemic stroke, and confirming fractures.

Procedure

The most common emergency ultrasound examination is the focused assessment in trauma (FAST). This exam takes less than a minute and includes the following:

- *Right Upper Quadrant.* The probe is placed on the right side of the abdomen (with the probe indicator toward the head). (Review Figure 6-43.) The following structures should be identified: diaphragm, inferior pole of the right kidney, and hepatorenal interface (Morrison's pouch).

- *Left Upper Quadrant.* The probe is placed in the left side of the abdomen (with the probe indicator toward the head). The following structures should be identified: diaphragm, inferior pole of left kidney, inferior tip of spleen, and splenorenal interface.

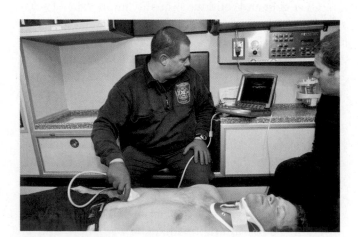

FIGURE 6-43 Ultrasound can be used in the prehospital setting to assess internal bleeding and evaluate abdominal aortic aneurysms.

(© Edward T. Dickinson, MD)

- *Suprapubic.* The probe is placed just above the pubic bone (with the probe indicator to the patient's right) and the following structures identified: outline of urinary bladder and uterus (if patient is female).

- *Cardiac.* The probe is placed in the parasternal or subxiphoid area (with the probe indicator to the patient's right) and the following structures identified: cardiac wall motion, pericardial space, and hepatocardiac interface.

A variant of the FAST exam is the extended focused assessment with sonography for trauma (eFAST). With the eFAST, the examiner also examines the thoracic cavity. A subxiphoid approach can be used to evaluate the pericardial space to evaluate for cardiac motion and the presence of fluid within the pericardial space. A second view through the second or third intercostal space in a midclavicular line in a sagittal orientation allows for rapid assessment of possible pneumothorax.

Summary

As you begin your career as a paramedic, you should become familiar with each piece of equipment available to you in the service(s) for which you work. It is imperative that you know how each piece of equipment works and what can cause false or skewed readings. You should also know how to troubleshoot the equipment in the heat of the moment.

As with all things mechanical, your tests, machines, and monitors can and will fail you at times. Whatever you do, *do not* allow the equipment and monitors to replace sound physical assessment and common sense. If your monitor is showing you something abnormal with the patient, but your physical assessment and all other signs disagree, *treat your patient and not your monitor*.

New and evolving technologies are revolutionizing the practice of prehospital care. Paramedics are no longer making uninformed decisions for patient care based on limited assessment abilities and experience. The tools and technologies available at their fingertips give them the ability to get definitive answers to a variety of questions while ruling out specifics of the differential diagnosis. This helps make critical decisions for patients while significantly improving patient outcomes. There is no doubt that technology will continue to improve and increase the paramedic's abilities to diagnose patient conditions and thereby treat them more effectively and rapidly than ever before.

You Make the Call

You respond to a reported "unknown medical problem". Upon arriving at the scene, you find an adolescent male unresponsive on the ground outside a high school gymnasium. School staff members report that they found the 16-year-old young man unconscious about 10 minutes ago and called 911. He has a patent airway, adequate breathing, a rapid pulse, and pale, cool, and diaphoretic skin. His medical history is unknown, and there are no obvious signs of trauma. As you prepare to package the patient for transport, you begin to consider all possible causes for his altered mental status.

1. What technological monitoring devices would you use for this patient?

See Suggested Responses at the back of this book.

Review Questions

1. According to Einthoven's triangle, lead II is characterized by _____
   a. right leg negative, left arm positive.
   b. left leg positive, right arm negative.
   c. right leg positive, left arm negative.
   d. left leg negative, right arm positive.

2. Which of the following can be obtained from a single-lead ECG reading?
   a. The presence of an infarct
   b. Cardiac output
   c. Chamber enlargement
   d. Heart rate

3. On the vertical axis of a standard ECG graph paper, a deflection of two large boxes signifies

   _____

   a. 1 mV of amplitude.

   b. 10 mV of amplitude.

   c. 0.08 seconds duration.

   d. 0.4 seconds duration.

4. On the horizontal axis of a standard ECG graph paper, a deflection of one large box signifies

   _____

   a. 1 mV of amplitude.

   b. 10 mV of amplitude.

   c. 0.2 seconds duration.

   d. 0.04 seconds duration.

5. Which of the following may produce artifact on the ECG?

   a. Muscle tremors   c. 60-Hz interference

   b. Loose electrodes   d. All of the above

6. Which of the following information is *not* obtained by cardiac monitoring?

   a. Strength of myocardial contraction

   b. Actual heart rate

   c. Depolarization time of the ventricles

   d. Identification of dysrhythmias

7. ST segment elevation in a 3- or 4-lead (single-lead) ECG signifies _____

   a. injury.   c. infarction.

   b. ischemia.   d. none of the above.

8. To properly understand the numeric display of the pulse oximeter, you should recall that most of the oxygen that enters the bloodstream is carried

   _____

   a. in plasma.

   b. in a bonded form with hemoglobin.

   c. as a bicarbonate molecule.

   d. by the nucleus in the red blood cell.

9. An acceptable normal SpO_2 range for a patient breathing room air is _____

   a. under 95 percent.   c. 85 to 95 percent.

   b. 95 to 100 percent.   d. 80 to 85 percent.

10. Under which of the following conditions should you suspect that a displayed pulse oximeter reading may be incorrect?

    a. Severe anemia   c. CO poisoning

    b. Hypovolemia   d. All of the above

11. In which of the following cases will the oxygen saturation and partial pressure be high, yet the patient may possibly die of hypoxia?

    a. Carbon monoxide poisoning

    b. Hypothermia

    c. Hypertension

    d. All of the above

12. To understand capnography correctly, you should know that the majority of carbon dioxide is carried in the body _____

    a. dissolved in the plasma.

    b. bound with hemoglobin.

    c. as bicarbonate.

    d. combined with carbon monoxide.

13. Which of the following would *not* typically increase a patient's $PaCO_2$?

    a. Hyperventilation

    b. Hypoventilation

    c. Airway obstruction

    d. Muscle exertion

14. While evaluating a set of blood gases during a transport between medical facilities, you note that the pH is 7.32, the $PaCO_2$ is 54 mmHg, and the PaO_2 is 92 mmHg. Given these findings, what should you suspect?

    a. Respiratory alkalosis

    b. Respiratory acidosis

    c. Metabolic alkalosis

    d. Metabolic acidosis

15. An acceptable PaO_2 for a healthy adult breathing room air is _____ mmHg.

    a. 60   c. 35–45

    b. 80–100   d. >100

16. The normal $PaCO_2$ for a healthy adult breathing room air is _____ mmHg.

    a. 60–80   c. 35–45

    b. 80–100   d. 7.35–7.45

17. To properly interpret the patient's methemoglobin level, you should recall that _____

    a. methemoglobin can bind with oxygen under certain circumstances.

    b. the antidote for methemoglobinemia is amyl nitrite and sodium thiosulfate.

    c. local anesthetics can cause methemoglobinemia.

    d. methemoglobin is metabolized by cholinesterase.

18. If you are reviewing a CHEM-7 analysis, you are evaluating what aspect of the patient?

    a. Electrolyte levels

    b. Cardiac biomarkers

    c. Complete blood cell counts

    d. Arterial blood gases

19. Increased blood levels of myoglobin, troponin, and creatine kinase indicate that what may be occurring?

    a. Peripheral hypoxia

    b. Cardiac injury

    c. Profound peripheral anaerobic metabolism

    d. Hypoglycemia

20. Hemoconcentration can occur when _____

    a. leaving a tourniquet on the arm too long.

    b. failing to use the proper blood tube for the test.

    c. failing to fill blood tubes in the proper order.

    d. destruction of the red blood cells occurs.

See Answers to Review Questions at the back of this book.

References

1. Garvey, J. L., et al. "Pre-hospital 12-Lead Electrocardiography Programs." *J Am Coll Cardiol* 47 (2006): 485–491.

2. Grmec, S. "Comparison of Three Different Methods to Confirm Tracheal Tube Placement in Emergency Intubation." *Intensive Care Med* 28 (2002): 701–704.

3. Takeda, T., K. Tanigawa, H. Tanaka, et al. "The Assessment of Three Methods to Verify Tracheal Tube Placement in the Emergency Setting." *Resuscitation* 56 (2003): 153–157.

4. 2010 American Heart Association Guidelines for Cardiopulmonary Resuscitation and Emergency Cardiovascular Care. (Available at http://circ.ahajournals.org/cgi/content/full/122/18_suppl_3/S729; accessed April 10, 2011.)

5. Silvestri, S., G. A. Ralls, B. Krauss et al. "The Effectiveness of Out-of-Hospital Use of Continuous End-Tidal Carbon Dioxide Monitoring on the Rate of Unrecognized Misplaced Intubation within a Regional Emergency Medical Services System." *Ann Emerg Med* 45 (2005): 497–503.

6. Brain Trauma Foundation. Management and Prognosis of Severe Traumatic Brain Injury Guidelines. (Available at http://www2.braintrauma.org/guidelines/downloads/btf_ guidelines_management.pdf; accessed April 29, 2006.)

7. Grmec, S. and S. Mally. "Prehospital Determination of Tracheal Tube Placement in Severe Head Injury." *Emerg Med J* 21(4) (2004): 518–520.

8. Sunar, S., et al. "Non-Invasive Pulse CO-Oximetry Screening in the Emergency Department Identifies Occult Carbon Monoxide Toxicity." *J Emerg Med* 34(4) (2008): 441–450.

9. Coulange, M., et al. "Reliability of New Pulse CO-Oximeter in Victims of Carbon Monoxide Poisoning." *Undersea Hyperb Med* 35(2) (2008): 107–111.

10. Piatkowski, A., et al. "A New Tool for the Early Diagnosis of Carbon Monoxide Intoxication." *Inhalation Toxicol* 21(13) (2009): 1144–1147.

11. Augustine, J. J. "More Than Just a Standard: NFPA 1584 Defines the Rehab Process." *JEMS* 33(5) (2008): 106–117.

12. Bledsoe, B. E. and M. McEvoy. "What Is Methemoglobin?" *JEMS* 34(3) (2009): 9–13.

13. Barker, S. J., et al. "Measurement of Carboxyhemoglobin and Methemoglobin by Pulse Oximetry: A Human Volunteer Study." *Anesthesiology* 105(5) (2006): 892–897.

14. Soeding, P., et al. "Pulse-Oximetric Measurement of Prilocaine-Induced Methemoglobinemia in Regional Anesthesia." *Anesthes Analges* 111(4) (2010): 1065–1068.

15. Abu-Laban, R. B., J. Zed, R. A. Purssell, and K. G. Evans. "Severe Methemoglobinemia from Topical Anesthetic Spray: Case Report, Discussion and Qualitative Systematic Review." *Can J Emerg Med* 3(1) (2003): 51–56.

16. Bond, R. F. A. "Review of the Skin and Muscle Hemodynamics during Hemorrhagic Hypotension and Shock." *Adv Shock Res* 8 (1982): 53–70.

17. Macknet, M. R., et al. "Non-Invasive Measurement of Continuous Hemoglobin Concentration via Pulse CO-Oximetry." *Anesthesiology* 107 (2007): A1545.

18. Lima, A. P., P. Beelen, and J. Bakker. "Use of Peripheral Perfusion Index Derived from the Pulse Oximetry Signal as a Noninvasive Indicator of Perfusion." *Crit Care Med* 30(6) (2002): 1210–1213.

19. D. Plummer, D. Brunette, R. Asinger, and E. Ruiz, "Emergency department echocardiography improves outcome in penetrating cardiac injury," Annals of Emergency Medicine, vol. 21, no. 6, pp. 709–712, 1992.

20. B. P. Nelson and K. Chason, "Use of ultrasound by emergency medical services: a review," International Journal of Emergency Medicine, vol. 1, no. 4, pp. 253–259, 2008.

21. Heegaard, William, et al: Prehospital Ultrasound by Paramedics: Results of Field Trial. Academic Emergency Medicine, Volume 17, Number 6, June 2010 , pp. 624–630.

22. F. Walcher, M. Weinlich, G. Conrad et al., "Prehospital ultrasound imaging improves management of abdominal trauma," British Journal of Surgery, vol. 93, no. 2, pp. 238–242, 2006.

23. C. Roline, W. Heegaard, J. Moore et al., "Feasibility of bedside thoracic ultrasound in the helicopter emergency medical services setting," Air Medical Journal, vol. 32, no. 3, pp. 153–157, 2013.

24. E. J. Chin, C. H. Chan, R. Mortazavi et al., "A pilot study examining the viability of a Prehospital Assessment with UltraSound for Emergencies (PAUSE) protocol," The Journal of Emergency Medicine, vol. 44, no. 1, pp. 142–149, 2013.

25. M. Brooke, J. Walton, and D. Scutt, "Paramedic application of ultrasound in the management of patients in the prehospital setting: a review of the literature," Emergency Medicine Journal, vol. 27, no. 9, pp. 702–707, 2010.

26. C. Ogedegbe, H. Morchel, V. Hazelwood, W. F. Chaplin, and J. Feldman, "Development and evaluation of a novel, real time mobile telesonography system in management of patients with abdominal trauma: study protocol," BMC Emergency Medicine, vol. 12, article 19, 2012.

27. R. Breitkreutz, S. Price, H. V. Steiger et al., "Focused echocardiographic evaluation in life support and peri-resuscitation of emergency patients: a prospective trial," Resuscitation, vol. 81, no. 11, pp. 1527–1533, 2010.

28. M. Blaivas, "Inadequate needle thoracostomy rate in the prehospital setting for presumed pneumothorax: an ultrasound study," Journal of Ultrasound in Medicine, vol. 29, no. 9, pp. 1285–1289, 2010.

29. G. Prosen, P. Klemen, M. Strnad, and S. Grmec, "Combination of lung ultrasound (a comet-tail sign) and N-terminal pro-brain natriuretic peptide in differentiating acute heart failure from chronic obstructive pulmonary disease and asthma as cause of acute dyspnea in prehospital emergency setting," Critical Care, vol. 15, no. 2, article R114, 2011.

30. D. I. Ward, "Prehospital point-of-care ultrasound use by the military," Emergency Medicine Australasia, vol. 19, no. 3, article 282, 2007.

31. P. M. Brun, H. Chenaitia, J. Gonzva, J. Bessereau, X. Bobbia, and M. Peyrol, "The value of prehospital echocardiography in shock management," The American Journal of Emergency Medicine, vol. 31, no. 2, pp. 442.e5–442.e7, 2013.

Further Reading

Beasley, B. *Understanding 12 Lead EKGs: A Practical Approach*. Upper Saddle River, NJ: Pearson/ Prentice Hall, 2010.

Bledsoe, B. E. and R. W. Benner. *Critical Care Paramedic*. Upper Saddle River, NJ: Pearson/Prentice Hall, 2006.

Bledsoe, B. E. and M. McEvoy. "Where There's CO, There's Not Always Fire." *JEMS* (March 2009): 5–8.

Clinical Research Updates. (Available at http://www.oridion.com/eng/learning-center/clinical-research-updates.asp.)

Page, R. *12-Lead ECG*. Upper Saddle River, NJ: Pearson/Prentice Hall, 2005.

Phalen, T. *The 12-Lead ECG in Acute Coronary Syndromes*. St. Louis: Mosby Lifeline, 2011.

Tintinalli, J. E., ed. *Emergency Medicine, A Comprehensive Study Guide*, 7th ed. New York: McGraw-Hill, 2010.

Umbreit, J. "Methemoglobin—It's Not Just Blue: A Concise Review." *Am J Hematol* 82 (2007): 134–144.

Walraven, G. *Basic Arrhythmias*, 7th ed. Upper Saddle River, NJ: Pearson/Prentice Hall, 2010.

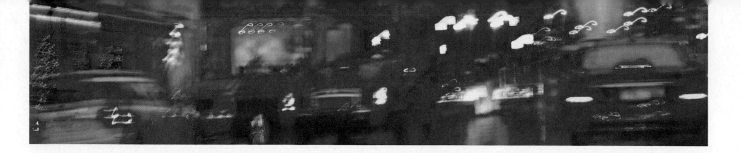

Chapter 7
Patient Assessment in the Field

Richard A. Cherry, MS, EMT-P

STANDARD
Assessment

COMPETENCY
Integrate scene and patient assessment findings with knowledge of epidemiology and pathophysiology to form a field impression. This includes developing a list of differential diagnoses through clinical reasoning to modify the assessment and formulate a treatment plan.

 Learning Objectives

Terminal Performance Objective: After reading this chapter, you should be able to integrate scene size-up, primary assessment, patient history, secondary assessment, and monitoring technology to plan and perform patient assessment in the field setting.

Enabling Objectives: To accomplish the terminal performance objective, you should be able to:

1. Define key terms introduced in this chapter.

2. Identify the importance of being able to perform a comprehensive, problem-oriented assessment of varied patient presentations to establish priorities of patient care.

3. Briefly review the major phases of patient assessment (scene size-up, primary assessment, secondary assessment, and reassessment).

4. Discuss how to adapt the major phases of patient assessment for a patient suffering from a major traumatic event.

5. Discuss how to adapt the major phases of patient assessment for a patient suffering from a minor traumatic incident.

6. Discuss how to adapt the major phases of patient assessment for an unresponsive or critical patient suffering from a medical emergency.

7. Discuss how to adapt the major phases of patient assessment for a responsive or noncritical patient suffering from a medical emergency.

8. List and define the five steps of the critical decision-making process.

9. Given a scenario from various traumatic events and medical emergencies, identify how to use a process of clinical reasoning to guide and interpret the assessment findings in the field.

KEY TERMS

Case Study

En route to the scene, paramedic Carl Marchetti and EMT Mike Gambino think about how many times they have responded to on-campus emergencies that seldom were. This time, though, they feel it could be something serious. The call came in as a severe allergic reaction at a noontime conference in a well-known lecture hall at State University.

On arrival, they find an 18-year-old female student in obvious distress. She is attended by a conference administrator and a campus police officer. She sits bent over a bowl containing a copious amount of her saliva. She is in obvious respiratory distress and is having difficulty swallowing. As Mike prepares to obtain her vital signs, Carl gets the story from bystanders. The girl has allergies to nuts, and she inadvertently ate a sandwich containing peanut butter. She has a history of severe asthma attacks, for which she uses an albuterol metered-dose inhaler, and takes diphenhydramine as needed. Although she has never had an anaphylactic reaction, she states that this reaction "feels different, more severe."

Her vital signs are respirations 26 and labored, pulse 100 and strong, blood pressure 138/78 mmHg, oximetry 91 percent on room air, skin warm and pink. She has diffuse expiratory wheezes, accessory muscle use, and retractions. Carl instructs his partner to administer a combination of albuterol and ipratropium via nebulizer to their patient while he starts an IV.

Following the treatment, her vital signs return to normal and her breathing effort eases. She feels much better, except for the scratchy throat. They get ready to transport, but the patient says she doesn't want to go to the hospital. She just wants to go back to her dorm room and relax. She may take a Benadryl if she needs to, but she'll be all right.

Carl, knowing what he does about allergic reactions, is aware that he can't allow his patient to refuse transport. He explains to his patient, "I know you're feeling better now, but reactions like these can sometimes get a lot worse hours later. You need to be seen by a physician and monitored until they feel it's safe for

you to return to your dorm. I've seen cases where people have died just a few hours after their reaction appeared to have totally subsided. I don't want that to happen to you. Why don't you let us take you up to the emergency department, where we all can be sure you're going to be all right?"

The girl agrees to be transported to the ED, which is 20 minutes away. En route, Carl continues to monitor her mental status, her respiratory rate and effort, her oximetry, her pulse rate, and her blood pressure every 5 minutes. Her airway remains patent, her vital signs stabilize, her oximetry on room air is 97 percent, and she says she feels fine.

About 10 minutes into the ride, Carl begins to notice the patient's pulse oximetry dropping. It reads 91 percent, so he places his patient back on supplemental oxygen until it rises above 95 percent. The patient then starts complaining of her chest tightening up again. Carl listens to her lungs and notes that the wheezing has returned. He administers another nebulizer treatment as they approach the ED entrance.

Carl and Mike transfer their patient to the ED staff. After completing the patient care report and cleaning and restocking their ambulance, they make their way back to the station. Later on, they receive a call from Dr. Fullagar, who congratulates them on convincing the patient to be transported. She went into respiratory arrest at the hospital; she recovered but was admitted for testing.

These types of calls are called your "moment of truth." This is when you are confronted with a situation that requires the sum total of your training and experience. At times like these, the sacrifices and dedication to learning your craft pay off. Had Carl and Mike allowed their patient to sign off and refuse transport, they may very well have responded to her dorm room later for an "unconscious person" and found their former patient in full cardiac arrest. Instead, their knowledge of allergic reactions and their sincere persistence in convincing her to go to the ED literally saved her life.

Introduction

Patient assessment means conducting a problem-oriented evaluation of your patient and establishing priorities of care based on existing and potential threats to human life. In the previous six chapters, you studied all the techniques of assessing the scene, conducting a primary assessment, taking a comprehensive patient history and physical exam, and using modern technology to monitor your patient's condition. Now, you will use your foundation of knowledge, skills, and tools to assess the acutely ill or injured patient. With time and clinical experience, you will learn which components of the comprehensive exam apply to each particular patient. It's time to put it all together.

Your patient's condition will determine which components you use and how you use them. For example, for trauma patients with a significant mechanism of injury, you will perform a primary assessment followed by a rapid secondary assessment (a head-to-toe exam aimed at traumatic signs and symptoms) and, if time allows, a more detailed secondary assessment en route to the hospital. For patients with minor, isolated trauma, a primary assessment followed by a problem-oriented exam is warranted. For the responsive medical patient, you will conduct a primary assessment followed by a focused history and physical exam. Finally, for the unresponsive medical patient, you will perform a primary assessment followed by a rapid secondary assessment (a head-to-toe exam aimed at medical signs and symptoms). In all cases, you will reassess your patient en route to the hospital to detect changes in patient condition.

Your proficiency in performing a systematic patient assessment will determine your ability to deliver the highest quality of prehospital **advanced life support** (ALS) to sick and injured people. Paramedic patient assessment is a straightforward skill, similar to the assessment you might have performed as an EMT. It differs, however, in depth and in the kind of care you will provide as a result.

Your assessment must be thorough, because many ALS procedures are potentially dangerous. Safely and appropriately performing advanced procedures such as administration of drugs, defibrillation, synchronized cardioversion, needle decompression of the chest, or endotracheal intubation will depend on your assessment and correct field diagnosis. If your assessment does not reveal your patient's true problem, the consequences can be devastating.

As always, common sense dictates how you proceed in the field. When you assess the responsive medical patient, the history reveals the most important diagnostic information and takes priority over the physical exam. For the trauma patient and the unresponsive medical patient, the reverse is true. However, trauma may cause a medical emergency, and, conversely, a medical emergency may cause trauma. Only by performing a thorough patient assessment can you discover the true cause of your patient's problems. This chapter provides problem-oriented patient assessment examples based on the information and techniques presented in the previous six chapters. You will need to refer to those chapters for the details of taking a history and conducting a physical exam.

Let's review the basic components of a patient assessment in the field.

Scene Size-Up

Scene size-up is the essential first stage of every emergency call (Figure 7-1). Sizing up an emergency scene is a series of timely decisions you will make to ensure that you and your crew remain safe and to begin to secure the necessary resources to manage the scene and care for your patient. You will base these informed, critical decisions on judgment and instinct—the sum total of your education and experience. They will be some of the most important decisions you will ever make as a paramedic.

Never skip this crucial component of an emergency run just because the scene appears to be safe. The components of a scene size-up include ensuring a safe environment, taking the necessary precautions for personal protection, determining what resources are needed, locating all patients, and assessing the mechanism of injury or nature of a medical illness.[1] Although you must consider all the elements of scene size-up important, circumstances

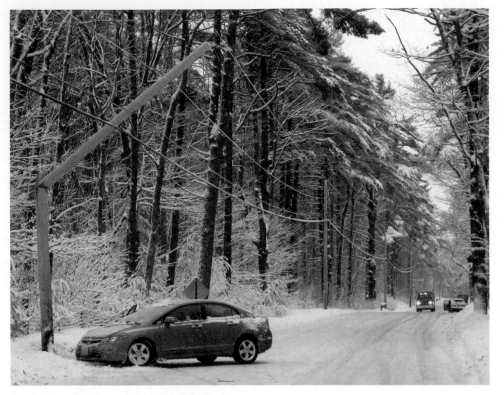

FIGURE 7-1 Perform a scene size-up on every emergency call.

(© Daniel Limmer)

will determine the priority you give to each one. Most likely, you will perform your scene size-up as the situation dictates and make critical decisions about the scene as it reveals itself to you. Refer to the "Scene Size-Up" chapter for more details.

Primary Assessment

First, determine whether your patient "looks dead or doesn't look dead." If your patient looks dead, quickly assess his responsiveness and breathing. Now, your primary assessment changes from ABC to CAB. If your patient is unresponsive and is apneic or has agonal respirations, quickly feel for a pulse and, if it is absent, begin chest compressions immediately. Continue the standard CPR sequence of 30 compressions and 2 quick breaths. If your patient shows any signs of life, such as moaning, groaning, moving, or if he shows a significant breathing effort, conduct the standard primary assessment (ABC).

In the standard primary assessment (Figure 7-2), your goal is to iden-

CONTENT REVIEW

➤ Steps of Primary Assessment
1. Form general impression
2. Stabilize cervical spine as needed
3. Assess baseline mental status
4. Assess airway
5. Assess breathing
6. Assess circulation
7. Assign priority

tify and correct immediately life-threatening patient conditions of the airway, breathing, or circulation (ABCs). If you find these conditions during this part of your assessment, treat them at once. For example, open a closed airway, provide ventilation, or control hemorrhage before moving on. Immediately following the primary assessment, decide priority regarding immediate transport or further on-scene assessment and care.[1]

The primary assessment consists of the following steps:

- Forming a general impression
- Stabilizing the cervical spine as needed
- Assessing a baseline mental status
- Assessing and managing the airway
- Assessing and managing breathing
- Assessing and managing circulation
- Determining priorities of care and transport

The primary assessment should take less than 1 minute, unless you must intervene with lifesaving measures. Perform the primary assessment as part of your reassessment throughout the patient contact, especially after any major intervention or whenever your patient's condition changes.

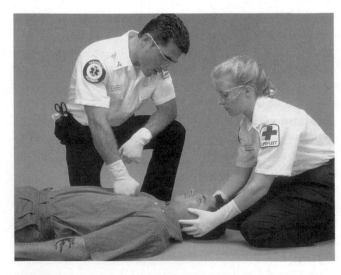

FIGURE 7-2 Manually stabilize the head and neck on first patient contact.

Once you have conducted a primary assessment, determine your patient's priority. If his primary assessment suggests a serious illness or injury, conduct a rapid head-to-toe assessment to identify other life threats and transport him immediately to the nearest appropriate facility that can deliver definitive care. Do not delay transport for detailed assessments and procedures that you can provide en route to the hospital. Refer to the "Primary Assessment" chapter for more details.

Secondary Assessment

The secondary assessment is the next stage of patient assessment. It begins with a full set of vital signs, followed by a **focused history and physical exam**—a problem-oriented process based on your primary assessment and your patient's chief complaint. It also includes any monitoring technology you apply, such as ECG monitoring, oximetry, blood glucose testing, and capnography.

How you proceed with the secondary assessment is based on which of four general categories your patient's initial presentation falls under:

- Major trauma patient with a significant injury or altered mental status
- Minor trauma patient with an isolated injury
- Responsive medical patient
- Unresponsive medical patient

Each type of patient requires a vastly different approach. For example, the major trauma patient with a significant mechanism of injury should receive a rapid secondary assessment, consisting of a rapid head-to-toe exam, and rapid transport. The patient with isolated, minor trauma, such as a cut finger or sprained ankle, should receive a physical exam focused on his particular problem or area. The responsive medical patient requires a history and physical exam that focuses on his chief complaint and vital signs. The unresponsive medical patient requires a rapid secondary assessment, consisting of a rapid head-to-toe exam and rapid transport.

Let's look at each of these patient categories separately. Refer to the preceding Patient Assessment chapters for more detailed information on eliciting a history and performing a secondary assessment and reassessment.

The Major Trauma Patient

The **major trauma patient** is one who has sustained a significant mechanism of injury or has an altered mental status from the incident. For serious trauma patients, you will conduct a primary assessment followed by a rapid secondary assessment, package your patient, provide rapid transport to the emergency department, and perform a reassessment as well as any treatments en route, in that order.

After acquiring a full set of vital signs (respiratory rate and quality; pulse rate and quality; blood pressure; skin color, temperature, and moisture), continue your secondary assessment by reconsidering the mechanism of injury (Figure 7-3). Although trauma poses a serious threat to life, its appearance often masks your patient's true condition. Extremity injuries, for example, are frequently obvious and grotesque, yet they rarely cause death. Conversely,

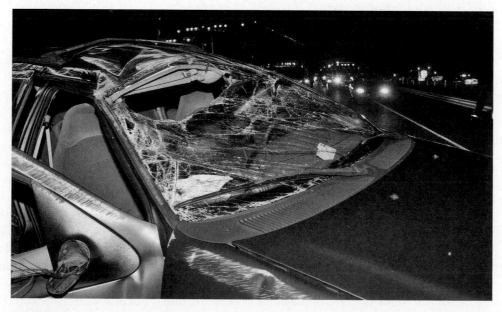

FIGURE 7-3 Evaluate the trauma scene to determine the mechanism of injury.
(© Daniel Limmer)

life-threatening problems such as internal bleeding and rising intracranial pressure often occur with only subtle signs and symptoms.

Your assessment of trauma patients must look beyond obvious injuries to the mechanism of injury for evidence that suggests life-threatening situations. Certain mechanisms predictably cause serious internal injury:

- A fall from 20 feet for an adult and 10 feet for a child
- Automobile crash with intrusion >12 inches into occupant site or >18 inches into any site
- Partial or complete ejection from automobile
- Death in same passenger compartment
- Vehicle telemetry data consistent with high risk of injury
- Automobile versus pedestrian
- Bicyclist thrown, run over, or with significant (>20 mph) impact
- Motorcycle crash >20 mph

For a more detailed illustration of trauma triage, refer to the Centers for Disease Control 2011 Guidelines for Field Triage in the chapter "Primary Assessment."

The presence of these mechanisms suggests a high index of suspicion for serious injury. Quickly transport patients to a trauma center when either the mechanism of injury or your patient's clinical presentation indicates a likelihood of internal injury.

Other significant mechanisms of injury can result from seat belts, air bags, and child safety seats. Do not rule out serious injury just because your patient wore a seat belt. Seat belts can actually cause injuries, even when worn properly. Always ask your patient whether he wore a seat belt and look for bruises across the chest or around the waist. If they are present, expect hidden internal injuries.

In general, air bags have been effective devices in preventing serious injury by protecting passengers from hitting the windshield, steering wheel, and dashboard. Originally, they deployed only when the front of the car hit another object. Many autos now have installed side air bags that deploy when the car is struck from the side. They are not without complications, however. For example, they are designed to cushion the chests of large adults. If the passenger is a child or a short adult, the air bag will hit him in the face, possibly causing injury. Furthermore, air bags are designed to deflate automatically within seconds after inflation, which may allow passengers to be propelled into the steering wheel or dashboard. For this reason, they may not be effective without the seat belt.

Always lift the deployed air bag and inspect the steering wheel for deformity. If you discover a bent steering wheel, suspect serious internal injury (Figure 7-4). There is also danger of the bag not deploying in the crash. It may

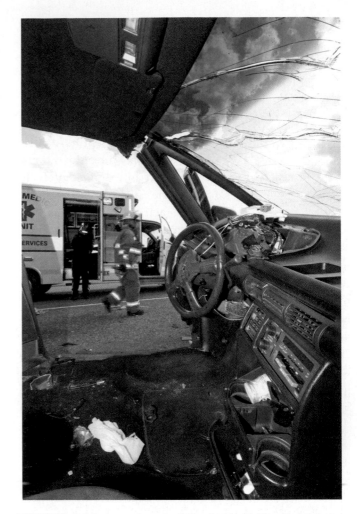

FIGURE 7-4 A bent steering wheel signals potentially serious injuries.
(© Kevin Link/Science Source)

deploy during the rescue operation, putting rescuers in danger of serious injury.

A child safety seat, when used appropriately, also can save a life. But if the safety seat is not securely fastened to the car seat, it can come loose and be thrown when the collision occurs, causing severe head, neck, and body cavity trauma to its occupant. If the harness straps are not tight on the child, the child may come out of the seat during the crash. If the safety seat is used in the car's front seat, the child can suffer a serious injury when the air bag deploys.

If your primary assessment rules out any immediate life threat, examine the suspected area of trauma. Physical signs of trauma, such as abrasions or contusions, confirm your index of suspicion. If you do not identify any physical evidence, reexamine the mechanism of injury and reevaluate your patient's vital signs. You will miss many serious injuries if your index of suspicion is too low. Usually you will distinguish between patients who need on-the-scene stabilization and those who need rapid transport after your primary assessment and rapid secondary assessment.

Whether to transport your patient immediately or to attempt more extensive on-the-scene assessment and care is among your most difficult decisions, but the care you provide will be more effective if you decide quickly. As a rule, patients who experience the mechanisms of injury listed earlier or who display serious clinical findings should be transported quickly, with intravenous access and other procedures attempted en route. Remember, you often arrive at the patient's side only minutes after the crash. He may not yet have lost enough blood internally to demonstrate signs of shock or progressive head injury. If in doubt, transport to an appropriate medical facility without delay. It is always best to err on the side of precaution.

Rapid Secondary Assessment

The **rapid secondary assessment** is designed to identify all other life-threatening conditions. Every trauma patient with a significant mechanism of injury, altered mental status, or multiple body-system trauma should receive a rapid secondary assessment. If your patient is responsive, ask him about symptoms as you proceed with your exam. Do not, however, focus totally on the areas your patient identifies as his chief problem. A patient with multiple injuries usually complains about his most painful injury. Sometimes, this may not be his most serious problem.

Assess your patient systematically and avoid the tunnel vision invited by dispatch information, first responders' reports, and your patient's chief complaint. Assume that any trauma patient has a spinal injury if he has injuries above the shoulders, has a significant mechanism of injury, or complains of weakness, numbness, or spinal pain. Maintain spinal immobilization throughout your rapid trauma exam.

As you proceed through the exam and discover additional information about your patient, reconsider your decision to transport. Things can change unexpectedly, especially with children. For example, your child patient who appeared stable may deteriorate suddenly, requiring you to expedite transport to the closest appropriate facility. The hallmark of an experienced paramedic is the ability to improvise, adapt to new situations, and overcome obstacles that hinder good patient care.

The rapid secondary assessment is not a detailed physical exam but a fast, systematic assessment for other life-threatening injuries. Because you perform it before packaging your patient for transport, you must conduct it quickly. First, reassess your patient's mental status using the AVPU mnemonic and compare your findings with the baseline mental status from your initial assessment. Pay special attention to the head, neck, chest, abdomen, and pelvis. Injuries in these areas can occur with limited signs and symptoms, yet they may rapidly lead to patient deterioration and death.

When inspecting an area for injury, keep in mind that the discoloration of contusions will develop over time and may not be apparent at first. Remember, your major concern may not be the injury you see, but rather the internal injuries beneath the superficial wounds. Palpate to identify other signs, such as tenderness, deformity, crepitus, symmetry, subcutaneous emphysema, or paradoxical movement. Compare muscle tone and tissue compliance from each side of the body or from one limb to another.

Some common signs of injury for which you are looking during most of this assessment include deformities, contusions, abrasions, penetrations, burns, tenderness, lacerations, and swelling.

HEAD Assess the head for injuries and crepitus (Procedure 7-1a). The scalp is extremely vascular and lacks the protective vasospasm mechanism that helps control bleeding. Thus, even the most minor lacerations tend to bleed profusely. Inspect the scalp for lacerations that are hidden under hair matted with clotted blood. Look for blood flowing into the hair and examine your gloved fingers periodically for blood or other body fluids (Procedure 7-1b). If you detect uncontrolled bleeding from the scalp, apply a direct pressure dressing immediately. A simple scalp laceration can cause a life-threatening hemorrhage.

Palpate the skull for open wounds, depressions, protrusions, lack of symmetry, and any unusual warmth. Use cupped hands and do not probe with your fingers. If you feel a depression, stop palpating it, because this risks pushing a broken piece of bone into the brain. If you find an impaled object, stabilize it in place with bulky dressings. If your patient presents with an altered mental status and any abnormality in the structure of the skull, consider this a serious emergency and expedite transport while you continue your assessment and treatment.

NECK Inspect and palpate the neck for injuries and crepitus (Procedure 7-1c). Immediately cover any lacerations that may involve the major blood vessels, such as the carotid arteries and jugular veins, with an occlusive dressing. This is a high-pressure area and your patient can suffer significant blood loss quickly. Because inspiration generates negative pressures in the chest, the jugular veins may draw in air. This can result in a massive air embolus that prevents the heart from pumping blood.

Examine the jugular veins for abnormal distention. In a patient lying supine without circulatory compromise, these veins should distend slightly. If they do not, your patient may be hypovolemic. In the **semi-Fowler's position** (sitting up at 45 degrees), the veins should not distend. Distention beyond 45 degrees is significant because something is inhibiting blood return to the chest. In the trauma patient, this may be the result of cardiac tamponade or tension pneumothorax.

Inspect and palpate the trachea just superior to the sternal notch. It should lie midline and remain fixed during the breathing cycle. Tugging to one side during inspiration suggests a pneumothorax on that side. Displacement

Procedure 7-1 Rapid Secondary Assessment—The Head and Neck

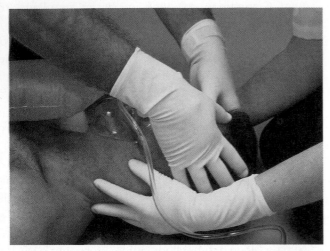

7-1a The first step in the rapid secondary assessment is to palpate the head.

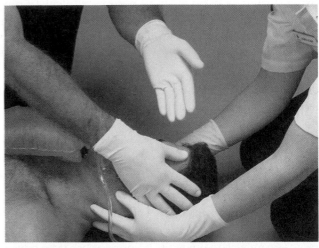

7-1b Periodically examine your gloves for blood.

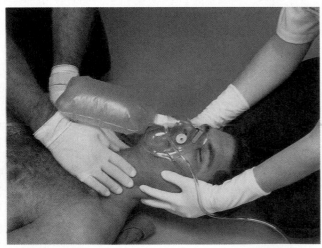

7-1c Inspect and palpate the anterior neck. Pay particular attention to tracheal deviation and subcutaneous emphysema.

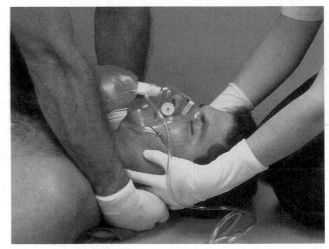

7-1d Inspect and palpate the posterior neck. Note any tenderness, irregularity, or edema.

to one side may indicate a tension pneumothorax on the opposite side as the entire mediastinum is pushed away from the injury.

Finally, inspect and palpate the neck for **subcutaneous emphysema**, the crackling sensation caused by air just underneath the skin. This condition is the result of air leaking from the respiratory tree into the tissues of the neck. It strongly indicates a serious neck or chest injury.

Palpate the posterior neck for evidence of spinal trauma (Procedure 7-1d). Gently feel the spinous processes and note any deformities, swelling, and tenderness. If you feel a muscle spasm, consider it a reflex sign following injury somewhere along the spinal column. When a corroborating mechanism of injury is present, suspect a significant spinal injury requiring spinal motion restriction. At this point, you can apply a cervical spinal immobiliza-

tion collar (CSIC). Have someone maintain head and neck stabilization even after applying the collar until your patient is fully fastened to a long board, vacuum mattress, vacuum stretcher, or other appropriate device as directed by local protocols.[2,3]

CHEST Look for signs of acute respiratory distress. If your patient has an upper airway obstruction, he may need to create tremendous negative pressures within his chest just to draw in air. To do so, he will use accessory muscles in his neck and chest to help lift the chest wall. These negative pressures may cause suprasternal, supraclavicular, and intercostal retractions. A patient with a lower airway obstruction may have difficulty moving air out. To do so, he may use his abdominal muscles to force the diaphragm upward and inward. He also may purse

Procedure 7-2 Rapid Secondary Assessment—The Chest

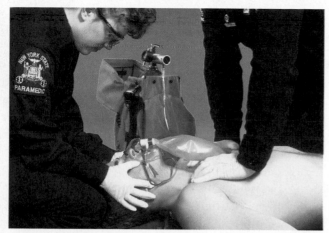

7-2a Palpate the clavicles.

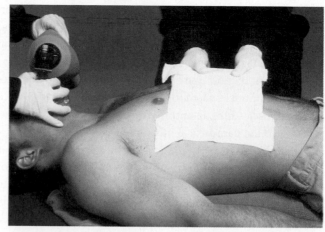

7-2b Stabilize a flail chest.

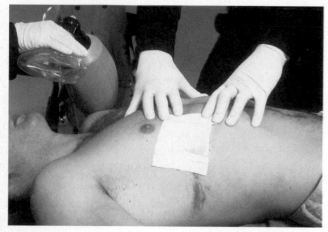

7-2c Seal any sucking chest wound with tape on three sides.

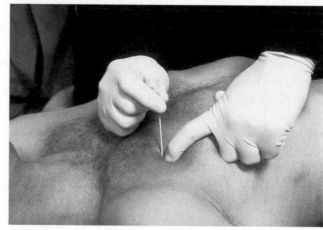

7-2d Perform needle decompression to relieve tension pneumothorax if authorized.

his lips during exhalation in an attempt to maintain a back pressure to keep the airways open. Infants and small children grunt to maintain this back pressure. Accessory muscle use always indicates a patient in respiratory distress owing to a difficulty in moving air. Assist these patients with positive-pressure ventilation and supplemental oxygen as needed.

Quickly inspect and then palpate the chest. Begin palpating at the clavicles and work down and around the rib cage, checking for stability. Palpate the clavicles over their entire length, bilaterally (Procedure 7-2a). These bones, which fracture more frequently than any other bone in the human body, are located directly over the subclavian artery and vein and the superiormost aspect of the lung. Their fracture and displacement may lacerate the vessels or puncture lung tissue, leading to hemothorax, pneumothorax, hypovolemia, or all three.

Be especially careful when palpating the ribs. Beneath each rib lies an artery, a vein, and a nerve that overaggressive palpation can easily damage. Classical soft-tissue injury signs may not be present because the ecchymotic coloration of bruising likely will not have had time to develop. Look for erythema caused by impact to the ribs.

The first three ribs are well supported by muscles, ligaments, and tendons. Because of the energy required to fracture them, you should suspect major damage to the underlying organs, especially vascular structures, when they are broken. If you notice the crackling of subcutaneous emphysema during chest palpation, suspect pneumothorax or a tracheobronchial tear. This condition results when air collects in the soft tissues. Subcutaneous air will normally flow from the upper chest to the neck and head. In some cases, it will drastically change your patient's facial features before your eyes.

Observe for equal, symmetrical, effortless chest rise. The chest should rise with inhalation and fall with exhalation. An abnormality in the chest wall may inhibit this process. For example, a patient with a rib fracture hesitates to expand his chest because it hurts. The fracture of two or more adjacent ribs in two or more places causes an unstable flail (floating) segment, which may be evidenced by paradoxical chest wall movement. Paradoxical movement may not appear early in a flail segment because the muscles surrounding the fractured ribs may contract spasmodically, securing the ribs in place. As the muscles fatigue and relax, the flail segment becomes obvious in the paradoxical movement.

A flail chest greatly reduces air movement. The underlying lung contusion and subsequent decreased tidal volume limit the air available for gas exchange. To ensure enough air movement for adequate gas exchange, assist ventilation with a bag-valve mask and supplemental oxygen. If the flail segment is loose, stabilize it to the chest wall with a large pad and tape (Procedure 7-2b).

Inspect your patient's chest and back for open wounds. The lungs expand because they adhere to the inner chest wall. This adherence is made possible by the presence of two thin membranes: the visceral pleura, which covers the lungs, and the parietal pleura, which covers the inner chest wall. A film of liquid between these two layers creates a negative-pressure bond that forces the lungs to expand with the chest wall. Any opening in this system can disrupt adherence and cause the lung to collapse.

Because air follows the path of least resistance, it may enter the chest cavity through the hole instead of through the respiratory tract. Thus, you should seal any open wounds with an occlusive dressing, such as Vaseline gauze, at the end of exhalation. Tape the dressing on three sides only to create a "one-way valve" effect, allowing air to escape but not be drawn in (Procedure 7-2c). Remember to check carefully under the armpits and back for knife and small-caliber gunshot wounds. You can easily miss these because the elastic skin closes quickly over the wound and limits external bleeding.

Auscultate both lungs quickly at each midaxillary line for equal and adequate air movement. Unequal air movement may indicate the presence of a collapsed lung from a pneumothorax or hemothorax. Absent sounds on one side and diminished sounds on the other may suggest a life-threatening condition known as *tension pneumothorax*. This condition also presents with severe respiratory distress, accessory muscle use, retractions, tachycardia, hypotension, narrowing pulse pressure, and distended neck veins. Tracheal deviation may be a late sign of tension pneumothorax. If authorized, perform needle decompression immediately. Insert a large-bore IV catheter into the pleural space at the second intercostal space over the top of the third rib, midclavicular line, allowing the trapped air to escape and release the tension (Procedure 7-2d).

Only through practice and repetition will you gain the confidence to recognize the difference between adequate and diminished lung sounds. Again, for patients with inadequate lung sounds or hypoxia (pulse oximetry below 95 percent), administer 100 percent oxygen and assist ventilation with a bag-valve mask and intubate as needed.

ABDOMEN Inspect and palpate the abdomen for injuries and crepitus. Note any areas of bruising and guarding. Exaggerated abdominal wall motion to assist respiration may result from spinal injury, airway obstruction, or respiratory muscle failure. Solid organs, such as the kidneys, liver, and spleen, can bleed enough into the abdominal cavity to cause profound shock.

Two characteristic areas for bruising are over the umbilicus (**Cullen's sign**) and over the flanks (**Grey Turner's sign**). Both signs indicate intraabdominal hemorrhage but usually will not occur until hours after the injury. Perform deep palpation over each quadrant and note any tenderness, rigidity, and guarding. Be careful, because deep palpation sometimes can aggravate the problem.

Avoid spending time needlessly trying to make a specific diagnosis. You need only to recognize the possibility that an intraabdominal hemorrhage exists and that your patient requires immediate transport to an appropriate medical facility for surgery.

Hollow organs such as the stomach and intestines, when injured, spill their toxic contents into the abdomen, irritating the peritoneum, the inner abdominal lining. Testing for rebound tenderness will help you determine whether your patient's peritoneum is irritated. Gently palpate an area and let your hand up quickly. If your patient experiences pain with this release, it is likely the result of peritoneal irritation. If you suspect intraabdominal hemorrhage, provide oxygen and expedite transport. En route to the hospital, provide IV fluid resuscitation as needed.

PELVIS Examine the pelvis for injuries and crepitus. The importance of a stable pelvic ring cannot be overemphasized. A patient with a pelvic fracture or dislocation risks lacerating the iliac arteries and veins, major blood vessels running through that area. He can easily lose a significant amount of blood into the pelvic cavity.

Evaluate the pelvic ring at the iliac crests and symphysis pubis. With the palms of your hands, direct pressure medially and posteriorly (Procedures 7-3a and 7-3b). Then press posteriorly on the symphysis pubis, being careful not to entrap the penis or cause injury to the urinary bladder. Any pain, instability, or crepitus suggests a pelvic fracture.

Always immobilize the pelvis before transport to prevent movement and a possible circulatory catastrophe. Many devices are available to immobilize an unstable

Procedure 7-3 Rapid Secondary Assessment—The Pelvis and Extremities

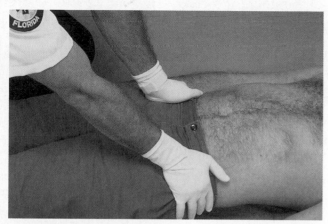

7-3a Assess the integrity of the pelvis by gently pressing medially on the pelvic ring.

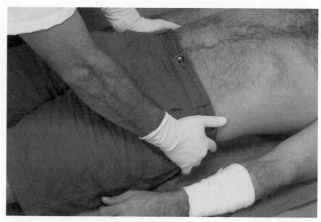

7-3b Compress the pelvis posteriorly.

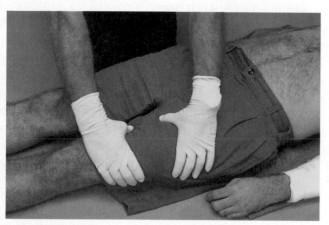

7-3c Palpate the legs.

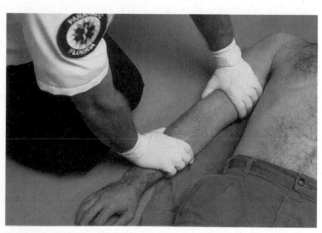

7-3d Palpate the arms.

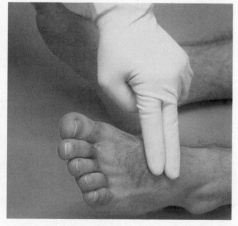

7-3e Palpate the dorsalis pedis pulse to evaluate distal circulation in the leg.

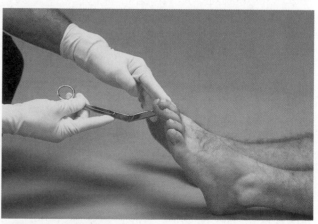

7-3f Assess distal sensation and motor function.

pelvic fracture. These include the pneumatic anti-shock garment, air and vacuum splint devices, and even blankets and pillows. Use whichever technique does the job.

EXTREMITIES Inspect and palpate all four extremities for injuries and crepitus (Procedures 7-3c and 7-3d). Splint fractures en route to the hospital if your patient is unstable. Do not spend time splinting fractures on the scene.

Before placing your patient on a backboard and immobilizing his spine, evaluate distal neurovascular function by checking for pulses, sensation, and the ability to move (Procedures 7-3e and 7-3f). If you cannot locate a pulse, determine the adequacy of perfusion by assessing the temperature, color, and condition of the skin of the extremity. Assume vascular compromise if pulse is absent, the extremity is cool, or the skin is ashen or cyanotic.

The inability to feel and move both legs indicates complete spinal cord disruption. Diminished sensation, paresthesias, or diminished motor ability may indicate a partial disruption. Weakness or disability on only one side of the body suggests brain injury due to a stroke or head injury. Evaluate these functions again after spinal immobilization to make certain they have not changed. Report and record all extremity function tests. Check for MedicAlert tags, which will identify a medical condition that may complicate the injury (Figure 7-5).

POSTERIOR BODY Log-roll the patient onto his side to inspect the posterior body. If you suspect a spinal injury, carefully maintain manual stabilization of the head and spine during this procedure. Then inspect and palpate the posterior trunk for injuries and crepitus (Figure 7-6). Particularly note any tenderness in the spinal area. Palpate the buttocks to rule out hemorrhage, contusion, or other injury. Though predominantly soft tissue, this area is a large mass and can conceal considerable internal blood loss. Next, log-roll the patient into a supine position on a long spine board while maintaining manual stabilization of the head and neck. He is now ready to be secured to the spine board, as directed by local protocols, and transported.

HISTORY The history consists of four elements: the chief complaint, the history of present

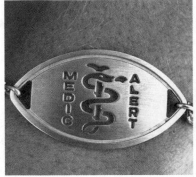
(a) Front

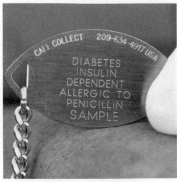
(b) Back

FIGURE 7-5 MedicAlert tags can give important information about the patient's condition and medical history.

illness, the past history, and the current health status. (Refer to the chapter "History Taking" for a detailed description of taking a history.) For major trauma cases when time is critical, use an abbreviated format that forms the acronym SAMPLE: Symptoms, Allergies, Medications, Pertinent past medical history, Last oral intake, and Events leading up to the incident. This handy mnemonic is especially useful for eliciting a quick history from your trauma patient. If your patient cannot provide this information, attempt to elicit it from family, friends, and bystanders.

The case described in "In the Field" here is an example of an assessment of a serious automobile crash victim. It includes the scene size-up, the primary assessment, and rapid secondary assessment.

> **CONTENT REVIEW**
> ➤ SAMPLE History
>   • **S**ymptoms
>   • **A**llergies
>   • **M**edications
>   • **P**ertinent past medical history
>   • **L**ast oral intake
>   • **E**vents leading up to the incident

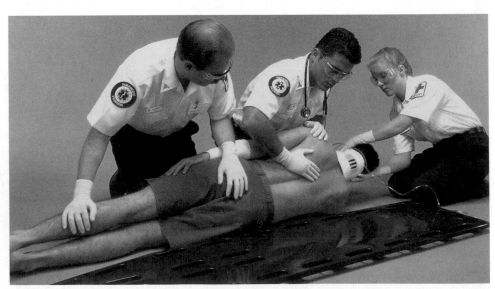

FIGURE 7-6 Inspect and palpate the posterior body.

In the Field

Major Trauma Case

You are dispatched to a motor vehicle crash, one car into a telephone pole.

Scene Size-Up. En route you assess that because it is midday, traffic flow in the area of this incident will not be significant. Weather conditions will not complicate rescue operations. Fire department rescue and law enforcement are also responding.

You imagine the mechanism of injury of one car into a pole at moderate speed with resulting head, neck, and chest injuries. You recall the conditions that suggest rapid transport to a trauma center, such as intrusion into the occupant site, ejection, and death in the same passenger compartment.

On arrival, your suspicions are confirmed. There is one car that crashed head-on into a wooden pole with significant front end vehicle damage and intrusion into the driver's space. Law enforcement personnel have arrived and are placing traffic cones strategically. You park safely off the road and exit your vehicle.

You don the appropriate gear for working in an automobile crash hazard zone (turnout, helmet, safety glasses, work gloves). Because no hazards are evident, such as leaking fluids, and the car is stable on the ground, you are free to approach the car. You note one person in the car, who appears alert but in moderate distress. Although his air bag deployed and he is wearing a seat belt, significant mechanisms of injury can still exist. You look for seat belt strap bruises across the neck and chest or around the waist and find none. You do, however, discover a bent steering wheel and suspect serious internal injury.

You decide that it is safe to have your partner enter the backseat and manually stabilize your patient's head and neck as you introduce yourself and provide reassurance. You begin your primary assessment.

Primary Assessment. You note your patient's alertness and his ability to speak in full sentences. You ask him his name, where he is, what day it is, and what happened. He is alert and oriented times four. You ask him about complaints, and he says he is having some difficulty breathing. There are no abnormal breathing noises, so his airway is patent.

His breathing is rapid, shallow, and somewhat labored. Because of this, you open his shirt and examine his neck and chest. He is using neck muscles during inhalation and has minor supraclavicular and substernal retractions. His neck veins are minimally distended. His trachea is midline, and no subcutaneous emphysema is noted. He has a reddish bruise to the right side of his chest, and when you palpate that area, it feels spongy and he complains of tenderness. You worry about fractured ribs, flail chest, lung contusion, pneumothorax, and worse.

You auscultate both sides of his chest and note diminished sounds over the left lung. Anticipating hypoxemia, you quickly apply oxygen as you continue your primary assessment and arrange for a rapid extrication from the vehicle and rapid transport to the trauma center. He has strong radial pulses, and his skin is warm and pink. There is no external bleeding, and his capillary refill time is 2 seconds. For now, he is hemodynamically stable—but you are concerned about his breathing.

Usually you will distinguish between patients who need on-the-scene stabilization and those who need rapid transport after your primary assessment and rapid secondary assessment. Whether to transport your patient immediately or to attempt more extensive on-the-scene assessment and care is among your most difficult decisions, but the care you provide will be more effective if you decide quickly.

As a rule, patients who experience significant mechanisms of injury or who display serious clinical findings should be transported quickly with IV access and other procedures attempted en route. If in doubt, transport to an appropriate medical facility without delay. It is always best to err on the side of precaution. In this case, you extricate him from the vehicle, fully secure him to the backboard, as directed by local protocols, and conduct your rapid secondary assessment before loading him into the ambulance. Just prior to securing him to the backboard, you inspect and palpate his back for wounds and deformities. You find none.

Secondary Assessment. The secondary assessment is aimed at identifying injuries that may not have been obvious during the primary assessment.

Head. You assess the head for injuries and crepitus. You palpate the cranium from front to back for symmetry and smoothness. You notice no tenderness, deformities, or areas of unusual warmth. You inspect and palpate the scalp for open wounds, depressions, protrusions, lack of symmetry, and any unusual warmth. You find none. You inspect and palpate the facial bones for stability and symmetry and do not find crepitus or loose fragments.

Neck. You inspect and palpate the neck for injuries and find increasing neck muscle use, deeper retractions, and more prominent jugular venous distention. From these findings, you suspect increasing problems in the chest, possibly a growing pneumothorax. The trachea remains midline.

You palpate the posterior neck for evidence of spinal trauma by gently feeling the spinous processes for deformities, swelling, and tenderness. You find no abnormalities, and your patient does not complain of tenderness in the area.

Chest. You quickly inspect and palpate the chest again. You find that the spongy area has more movement and you suspect a flail segment. At this point, you prepare to administer positive pressure ventilation with a bag-valve mask to prevent the impending hypoxemia from hypoventilation. On auscultation, you also note that the lung sounds on the right side are barely detectable, indicating a large pneumothorax. You will watch this carefully for the development of a tension pneumothorax.

Abdomen. You inspect and palpate the abdomen for injuries and crepitus. You find some bruising over the umbilicus. This is known as Cullen's sign and suggests intraabdominal hemorrhage. He also exhibits guarding of his abdomen and some rebound tenderness. At this point, avoid spending time needlessly trying to make a specific diagnosis. You need only to

(continued)

recognize the possibility that an intraabdominal hemorrhage exists and that your patient requires immediate transport to an appropriate medical facility for surgery.

Pelvis. You examine the pelvis for injuries and crepitus. The importance of a stable pelvic ring cannot be overemphasized. A patient with a pelvic fracture or dislocation risks lacerating the iliac arteries and veins, major blood vessels running through that area. His pelvic region is stable.

Extremities. You inspect and palpate all four extremities for injuries and crepitus. Before placing your patient on a backboard and immobilizing his spine, you evaluate distal neurovascular function by checking for pulses, sensation, and the

ability to move. Your patient has good neurovascular function in all four extremities.

Vital Signs. You take a baseline set of vital signs just before loading. His heart rate is 110 and strong, blood pressure 100/60 mmHg, respirations 34 and shallow, skin cool and pale. At this point you believe that your patient has a flail chest, a pneumothorax, and an intraabdominal bleed, and is in compensated shock. You will watch him closely en route to the hospital.

Monitoring Technology. You assess his pulse oximetry, monitor his ECG rhythm, and use capnography to detect immediate changes in his cardiorespiratory status.

History. Your patient has no pertinent findings.[4]

The Minor Trauma Patient

Some trauma patients sustain an isolated injury, such as a cut finger or sprained ankle. These patients have no significant mechanism of injury and show no signs of systemic involvement, such as poor peripheral perfusion, altered mental status, tachycardia, or breathing problems. They do not require an extensive history or comprehensive physical exam.

To treat the trauma patient with an isolated injury, first ensure his hemodynamic status via the primary assessment. Then conduct your secondary assessment on the specific isolated injury. Evaluate the injured area and take a full set of vital signs. Then, if time allows, this is an excellent opportunity to use some of the advanced assessment techniques you have learned in the chapter "Secondary Assessment."

After your exam of the isolated injury, take a SAMPLE history. Remember that some trauma patients may complain of an isolated problem but actually have more signifi-

cant injuries. Avoid tunnel vision and develop a low threshold for suspecting other injuries based on the mechanism of injury and your patient's story. The minor trauma cases described in "In the Field" in this section are three examples of assessing patients with isolated injuries and no life-threatening systemic involvement.

In the Field

Minor Trauma Case: Patient 1
Your patient is a young football player who twisted his knee and lies on the ground, complaining loudly of knee pain. After a quick primary assessment and injury assessment, you conclude that your patient is in stable condition with no signs or symptoms of systemic involvement and good distal neurovascular function.

Before splinting your patient's leg, you decide to elicit more information through a detailed exam of the knee. You inspect the normal concavities for evidence of excessive fluid in the joint by "milking the knee joint" on one side and looking for a fluid wave on the opposite side. Next, you palpate the medial and lateral collateral ligaments for tenderness. Then, if doing so does not cause your patient undue pain, you examine the stability of the collateral ligaments with the "side-to-side" test and the cruciate ligaments with the "drawer test." Finally, you assess the knee's passive range of motion (flexion and extension) and note any limitations.[5]

In the Field

Minor Trauma Case: Patient 2
Your patient sustains a laceration to the palm of his hand from a bread knife. After you have controlled the bleeding and ensured no systemic involvement or major loss of blood, you decide to examine the hand further before bandaging it. You inspect and palpate the hand for injury and note that distal neurovascular function is intact. Knowing that the flexor tendons all run through the palm of the hand, you examine each tendon's function through a full range-of-motion exam. You ask your patient to make a fist, then open his hand and extend all of his fingers. You note any abnormalities, pain, or limitations in the range of motion.[2]

In the Field

Minor Trauma Case: Patient 3
Your patient is a teenager who was punched in the eye during a minor altercation with a classmate. After determining that he had no loss of consciousness and that he is alert and oriented with stable vital signs, equal and reactive pupils, and no signs or symptoms of serious head injury, you may conduct a more detailed exam of the injured eye.

First, you inspect the external structures for discoloration, deformity, or swelling, and find all three. You palpate the orbit of the eye for tenderness and deformity. You look for evidence of hyphema (blood in the anterior chamber), indicating severe blunt trauma. You then examine your patient's visual acuity with a visual acuity card. With a penlight, you check for direct and consensual response to light and for the near–far reflex and accommodation. Finally, you assess the integrity of the extraocular muscles with the H test.[3]

The Responsive Medical Patient

Assessing the responsive patient with a medical emergency is entirely different from assessing the trauma patient, for two reasons. First, the history takes precedence over the physical exam. This is because, in the majority of cases, you will formulate your field diagnosis from your patient's story. The physical exam serves mostly to support your diagnostic impression. Second, your physical exam is aimed at identifying signs of medical complications, such as inflammation, infection, and edema, rather than signs of injury.

The secondary assessment evaluates pertinent areas suggested by the history. Remember that you will begin treatment as you conduct your assessment. For example, while interviewing your patient who complains of chest pain, simultaneously take vital signs, administer oxygen if the patient is hypoxic, provide cardiac monitoring, and start an IV if appropriate (Figure 7-7). The following secondary assessment pertains to the responsive medical patient. For a more detailed description of the information and techniques outlined here, refer to the chapters "Therapeutic Communications," "History Taking," and "Secondary Assessment."

History

Conscious, alert patients can usually tell you a great deal about their illness. Remember the old medical adage, "Listen to your patient; he will tell you what is wrong." Ask questions and then listen intently to your patient's answers. Because children may not be able to describe their illness and medical history clearly, look to their parents for this information. Elderly patients may pose several obstacles to the clear communication of medical information. They are more likely to be confused, have poor short-term and long-term memory, and have hearing, speech, or sight difficulties. Obtaining an accurate history from such patients requires patience, empathy, and outstanding communication skills.

The history consists of five elements: the chief complaint, the present problem, the past medical history, the family/social history, and the review of systems.

CONTENT REVIEW

➤ History for the Responsive Medical Patient
- Chief complaint
- Present problem
- Past medical history
- Family/social history
- Review of systems

CHIEF COMPLAINT   The **chief complaint** is the pain, discomfort, or dysfunction that caused your patient to request help. Ask your patient, "What seems to be the problem?"

When documenting the chief complaint, use your patient's own words—for example, "My chest hurts," "I can't breathe," or "I think I broke my arm."

PRESENT PROBLEM   Discover the circumstances surrounding the chief complaint, following the acronym OPQRST–ASPN:

- *Onset.* What was your patient doing when the problem/pain began? Did emotional or environmental factors contribute to the problem?
- *Provocation/Palliation.* What makes the problem/pain worse or better?
- *Quality.* Can your patient describe the problem/pain?
- *Region/Radiation.* Where is the problem/pain, and does it radiate anywhere?
- *Severity.* How bad is the problem/pain? Can your patient rate it on a scale of 1 to 10?
- *Time.* When did the problem/pain begin? How long does the pain last?
- *Associated Symptoms.* Is your patient having any other problems?
- *Pertinent Negatives.* Are any likely associated symptoms absent?

PAST MEDICAL HISTORY   The past medical history may provide significant insights into your patient's chief complaint and your field diagnosis. It includes your patient's general state of health, childhood and adult diseases, medications, allergies, psychiatric illnesses, accidents and injuries, and surgeries and hospitalizations. If your history taking reveals significant medical problems, investigate in more detail. Note when your patient first recognized the problem and how it affected him. How frequently did it happen, and what medical care did he seek? Was the treatment effective or did the problem recur?

FAMILY/SOCIAL HISTORY   A family history of serious disease may be a "red flag" in the case of, say, the chest

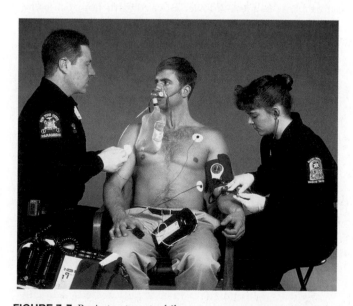

FIGURE 7-7 Begin treatment while you assess your responsive medical patient.

pain patient whose brother died of a heart attack at an early age. Social history includes the use of drugs (e.g., alcohol, tobacco, illicit drugs) and lifestyle (e.g., sedentary lifestyle, high stress, loneliness).

REVIEW OF SYSTEMS The review of systems is a system-by-system list of questions that are more specific than those asked during the basic history. Again, the patient's chief complaint, condition, and clinical status determine how much, if any, of the review of body systems you will use. For example, if your patient complains of chest pain, you may want to review the respiratory, cardiac, gastrointestinal, and hematologic systems. If your patient complains of a headache, you may want to review the HEENT (head, eyes, ears, nose, and throat), neurologic, peripheral vascular, and psychiatric systems. Let your patient lead you through the history.

If your patient is critical and your time is limited, use the abbreviated SAMPLE format to elicit the history.

Focused Physical Exam

Once you have obtained the history, begin a focused physical exam based on the information you elicited from your patient. Let the diagnostic impression you formed during the history guide your examination. For example, if you suspect a myocardial infarction, examine areas pertinent to a patient having a heart attack: cardiac and respiratory systems, chest, neck, and peripheral perfusion. It would be pointless and impractical to test deep tendon reflexes, extraocular movements, or the elbow's range of motion. Use the exam techniques presented in the chapter "Secondary Assessment" that pertain to your patient's special situation and clinical status.

Three common presentations among your responsive medical patients will be cardiac chest pain/respiratory distress, altered mental status, and acute abdomen. The following sections outline problem-oriented physical exams for those complaints. For each of these cases, the focused physical exam is different. As you gain clinical experience, you will be able to quickly assess your patient's pertinent areas according to your suspected field diagnosis. Likewise, clinical judgment and the seriousness of your patient's condition will determine which exam techniques you use on the scene and which you use en route to the hospital.

In the Field

Patient 1: *Chest Pain/Respiratory Distress*
For a patient complaining of chest pain or respiratory distress, assess the following:

HEENT (Head, Eyes, Ears, Nose, and Throat). Note the color of the lips. Lip cyanosis is an ominous sign of central circulatory hypoxia. Examine the oral mucosa for pallor suggesting decreased circulation, as in shock. Inspect any fluids in the mouth. Pink, frothy sputum (the result of plasma proteins mixing with air and red blood cells in the alveoli) is a classic sign of acute pulmonary edema. Aggressively suction any fluids from the oropharynx that may compromise the upper airway. Note any swelling, redness, or hives, suggesting an allergic reaction.

Neck. Observe the neck for accessory muscle use and retractions, signs of acute respiratory distress. Retractions in the supraclavicular (above the clavicles) and suprasternal (above the sternum) notches indicate that your patient is having difficulty inhaling. Palpate the carotid arteries (one at a time) for rate, quality, and equality; if you detect weak or unequal pulses, auscultate for bruits.

As with the trauma patient, examine the jugular veins for abnormal distention. Normally, in a patient lying supine without circulatory compromise, these veins should distend slightly. This is normal. If the jugular veins do not distend in the supine position, your patient may be hypovolemic. In the semi-Fowler's position (sitting up at 45 degrees), the veins should disappear. Distention beyond 45 degrees is significant because something is inhibiting blood return to the chest. In the medical patient, this may be the result of congestive heart failure, constrictive pericarditis, or cardiac tamponade.

Inspect and palpate the position of the trachea. It should lie midline and remain fixed during the breathing cycle. Tugging to one side during inspiration suggests a pneumothorax on that side. Displacement to one side may indicate a tension pneumothorax on the opposite side as the entire mediastinum is displaced.

Chest. Assess the respiratory rate and pattern again and administer oxygen or ventilation as needed. Note the length of the inspiratory and expiratory phases. A prolonged inspiratory phase suggests an upper airway obstruction. A prolonged expiratory phase suggests a lower airway obstruction such as in asthma and emphysema. Inspect and palpate the chest wall for symmetry of movement and intercostal retractions. A barrel chest suggests a history of emphysema. Look for the classic midline scar from open heart surgery or the typical bulge of an implanted pacemaker or defibrillator.

Auscultate all lung fields (anterior to posterior, apices to bases) and compare side to side. Report and record the sounds you hear (crackles, wheezes), where you hear them (in the bases, apices, diffuse), and when they occur during the respiratory cycle (inspiratory, expiratory). For example, if your patient has bilateral inspiratory crackles, you might suspect congestive heart failure or pulmonary edema. If he has diffuse expiratory wheezing, you might suspect the bronchospasm associated with asthma or chronic obstructive pulmonary disease. The presence of both would suggest acute pulmonary edema. A localized wheeze might indicate a pulmonary embolism, a foreign body aspiration, or an infection.

Patients with unilateral (one-sided) decreased breath sounds require further testing, such as tactile fremitus, bronchophony, egophony, or whispered pectoriloquy. Percuss the chest and back for hyperresonance (asthma, emphysema, pneumothorax) and dullness (pulmonary edema, pleural effusion, pneumonia).

Cardiovascular. Inspect for signs of arterial insufficiency or occlusion in your patient's trunk and extremities. Look for skin pallor and other signs of decreased perfusion. Inspect and palpate the chest for the point of maximum impulse (PMI) at the fifth intercostal space near the midclavicular line. Assess central and peripheral pulses for equality, rate, regularity, and quality. Auscultate for heart sounds, identifying S1, S2, and any additional sounds.

Abdomen. Look for exaggerated abdominal muscle use during exhalation, a sign of lower airway obstruction as seen in asthma and emphysema. Inspect and palpate the abdomen for distention caused by air or fluid. Ascites is an accumulation of fluid within the abdominal cavity caused by increased pressure in the systemic circulation as seen in patients with right heart failure. It is also common in patients with cirrhosis of the liver, where portal circulation (to and from the liver) is increased.

Inspect and palpate the flanks and presacral area for edema in bedridden patients suspected of having congestive heart failure. Check for unusual pulsation of the descending aorta, just left of the umbilicus. Palpate for liver enlargement or upper quadrant tenderness, suggesting ulcer disease, gallbladder disease, or pancreas problems, all of which can be confused as chest pain.

Extremities. Perform neurovascular checks on both hands and feet. These consist of checking for pulses, sensation, and

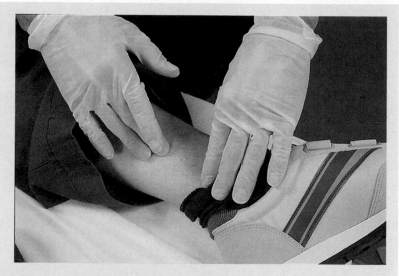

FIGURE 7-8 Check for peripheral edema.

the ability to move. Pay special attention to the equality of pulses in all extremities. Unequal pulses in the upper extremities suggest a thoracic aneurysm; unequal pulses in the lower extremities suggest an abdominal aneurysm. Assume vascular compromise if the pulse is absent, the limb is cool, or the skin is cyanotic or ashen.

In cardiac and respiratory emergencies, evaluate the lower extremities for pitting edema. Depress the skin on the tibial plateau (Figure 7-8). If the depression remains after you remove your finger, pitting edema exists. This is a sign of chronic fluid retention, as seen in heart and renal failure. Examine the fingernails for pitting. Check the wrists for MediAlert identification.[3]

In the Field

Patient 2: *Altered Mental Status*
For a patient with an altered mental status, assess the following:

Heent. Inspect and palpate the head to rule out any evidence of trauma. For example, your stroke patient may have suffered a skull fracture from falling on the floor. Palpate the fontanels of the infant for sunkenness (dehydration) and bulging (increasing intracranial pressure). Examine the face for symmetry. Unilateral facial drooping may indicate a stroke or inflammation of the facial nerve (Bell's palsy).

Examine the pupils for direct and consensual response to light. One pupil's getting larger or reacting more slowly to light could indicate a deteriorating brain pathology such as a stroke. A small portion of the population, however, has unequal pupils, a benign condition known as *anisocoria*. Bilaterally sluggish pupils usually suggest decreased blood flow to the brain and hypoxia. Fixed and dilated pupils indicate severe brain anoxia. Your patient's pupils also may dilate from sympathomimetic or anticholinergic drug use. Pinpoint pupils suggest a narcotic drug overdose or pontine hemorrhage (bleeding within the pons).

Next, test for near response and accommodation. Test the integrity of the extraocular muscles with the "II" test. Normally, your patient will move his eyes conjugately (together) to follow your finger. He may exhibit a nystagmus, a fine jerking of the eyes. At the far extremes of the test, nystagmus may be normal, but if you observe it during all extraocular movements, it suggests a pathology. Examine the conjunctiva for redness (irritation), pallor (hypoperfusion), or cyanosis (hypoxia). Inspect the sclera for jaundice.

Chest. Inspect, palpate, and auscultate the chest for any signs of cardiorespiratory involvement.

Abdomen. Look for evidence of trauma or internal bleeding. Listen for bowel sounds, which may be absent in anticholinergic drug ingestions.

Pelvis. Look for evidence of incontinence.

Extremities. Perform neurovascular checks on both hands and feet. These consist of checking for pulses, sensation, and the ability to move. Assume vascular compromise if the pulse is absent, the limb is cool, or the skin is cyanotic or ashen.

(continued)

Because the motor and sensory nerves run along different pathways in the spinal cord, you must check your patient's extremities both for mobility and for sensation of light touch and pain. As with trauma patients, the inability to feel and move both legs indicates complete spinal cord disruption. Diminished sensation or diminished motor ability indicates a partial disruption. Weakness or disability on only one side suggests brain dysfunction such as a stroke. Report and record all extremity function tests.

Posterior Body. Inspect the posterior body for deformities of the spine. Also check for evidence of incontinence or bleeding. In the supine patient, inspect the flanks for presacral edema.

Neurologic Assessment. Reassess your patient's level of consciousness and compare his response with your earlier findings. Note his speech pattern and any deficits in speech or language. Observe mood swings or behaviors that suggest anxiety or depression. Determine your patient's person, time, and place orientation. Does he know his name, the day of the week, and where he is?

Perform the one-minute cranial nerve exam outlined in Table 7-1. Inspect general body structure, muscle development, positioning, and coordination. Note any obvious asymmetries, deformities, or involuntary movements. Assess muscle tone by feeling the muscle's resistance to passive stretching in the extremities. Note the degree of resistance. Test for muscle strength by applying resistance during the range-of-motion

Table 7-1 One-Minute Cranial Nerve Exam

Cranial Nerve(s)	Test
I	Normally not done.
II, III	Direct response to light.
III, IV, VI	"H" test for extraocular movements.
V	Clench teeth; palpate masseter and temporal muscles. Test sensory response to touch of forehead, cheek, and chin.
VII	Show teeth.
IX, X	Say "aaaahhhh"; watch uvula movement. Test gag reflex.
XII	Stick out tongue.
VIII	Test balance (Romberg test) and hearing.
XI	Shrug shoulders, turn head.

evaluation. Check for pronator drift and watch for any drifting sideways or upward. Assess for coordination and cerebellar function, using rapid alternating movements and point-to-point testing. Note seizure activity tremors. Ask the primary caregivers whether your patient's presentation is normal for him or if this represents a change.

Assessment Pearls

Taking a Glucometer Reading for All Patients with Altered Mental Status. In a recent case, an unresponsive patient was transported to a community hospital by an ALS ambulance and then later transported by helicopter to a tertiary care facility. At the specialty care hospital, the first thing the ED staff did was check the patient's blood sugar. It was 40 mg/dL. The EMS crew and community hospital staff had overlooked this simple diagnostic test. The patient was given lunch and discharged within 1 hour of helicopter arrival.

Granted, this type of case is not a common occurrence; neither is it uncommon. *Always* check the blood glucose level in any patient with altered mental status—or any unexplained physical exam finding—because the condition might be the result of hypoglycemia. Many medical conditions, such as hemiparesis, headaches, delirium, abnormal behavior, coma, facial palsies, seizures, and many more, can be attributed to hypoglycemia. The test is easy to administer and the treatment easily provided. When in doubt about a patient's condition, always return first to the basics.

In the Field

Patient 3: *Acute Abdomen*
For a patient complaining of abdominal pain, assess the following:

Heent. Notice any unusual odors coming from your patient's mouth. The smell of alcohol does not rule out a serious medical condition. The sweet or fruity smell of ketones suggests diabetes. A fecal odor may indicate a lower bowel obstruction. The acidic smell of gastric contents means that your patient has vomited and may again. Inspect any fluids in the mouth. "Coffee-grounds" emesis (vomiting) results from blood mixing with stomach acids and suggests an upper gastrointestinal (GI) bleed. Fresh blood usually means recent hemorrhage from the upper GI tract.

Chest. Listen to breath sounds. Crackles may indicate pneumonia, a cause of upper abdomen pain.

Abdomen. Look for discoloration over the umbilicus (Cullen's sign), or over the flanks (Grey Turner's sign), suggesting intraabdominal bleeding. Check for any visible pulsation, peristalsis, or masses. If you notice a bounding or an exaggerated pulsation, suspect an aortic aneurysm. Visible peristalsis may indicate a bowel obstruction. Auscultate for bowel sounds and renal bruits. Percussing the abdomen produces different sounds based on the underlying tissues. Percuss the abdomen in the same sequence you used for auscultation. Note the distribution of tympany and dullness. Expect tympany in most of the abdomen; expect dullness over the solid abdominal organs, such as the liver and spleen.

Palpate the abdomen last to detect tenderness, muscular rigidity, and superficial organs and masses. The normal abdomen is soft and nontender. Abdominal pain on light palpation suggests peritoneal irritation or inflammation. If you feel rigidity or guarding while palpating, determine whether it is voluntary (patient anticipates the pain or is not relaxed) or involuntary (peritoneal inflammation). Then palpate the abdomen deeply to detect large masses or tenderness. If the peritoneum is inflamed, your patient will experience pain when you let go.

Posterior Body. Inspect the posterior body for evidence of rectal bleeding.[3]

The Unresponsive Medical Patient

Because he cannot tell you what is wrong, the unresponsive medical patient requires an entirely different approach than the responsive patient does. Assess the unresponsive medical patient much as you would a trauma patient. Begin with the primary assessment, conduct a rapid head-to-toe exam (the rapid secondary assessment), and finally take a brief history from family or friends. This approach to the unresponsive medical patient also will help you to detect whether trauma may be involved.

After conducting the primary assessment, position your patient so his airway is protected. If the cervical spine is not involved, place your patient in the recovery position—laterally recumbent. This will prevent secretions from obstructing his airway. Now begin the rapid secondary assessment. The rapid secondary assessment for medical patients is similar to the rapid secondary assessment for trauma patients, except that you will look for signs of illness, not injury.

Assess the head, neck, chest, abdomen, pelvis, extremities, and posterior aspect of the body. Perform the entire exam with the unresponsive patient. Then, assess baseline vital signs: pulse, blood pressure, respiration, pulse oximetry, and temperature. Finally, obtain a history from bystanders, family members, friends, or medical identification devices or services. If possible, this history should include the chief complaint, history of the present illness, past medical history, and current health status.

Evaluate your data and provide emergency medical care while performing additional tests, such as cardiac monitoring and blood glucose determination, as needed. Consider your unresponsive patient unstable and expedite transport to the hospital, performing a reassessment every 5 minutes en route. The following is an example of assessing an unresponsive medical patient.

In the Field

Unresponsive Medical Patient Case

The rapid secondary assessment is not a comprehensive history and physical exam, but a practical, systematic assessment aimed at quickly identifying the cause of your patient's unresponsive condition. Your care for a patient with a coma of unknown origin, for example, might go something like this.

You are dispatched to aid an "unresponsive person" in a residential neighborhood. Your patient is an elderly man who presents laterally recumbent on the floor of his bathroom. You conduct a primary assessment while your partner elicits information from the patient's wife.

General. Your patient appears pale and diaphoretic, moaning unintelligibly. You find no apparent signs of trauma, and he appears to have slumped to the floor from the toilet.

Mental Status. You establish your patient's mental status with the AVPU mnemonic. He responds to your voice but cannot answer your questions.

Airway. You open your patient's airway with a head-tilt/chin-lift maneuver and observe his breathing. His airway is clear. His breathing is rapid and shallow but not labored. You ask another rescuer to administer positive-pressure ventilation with supplemental oxygen while you continue with your assessment.

Circulation. You palpate the patient's radial pulse, and note its absence. His carotid pulse is slow, regular, and weak. His skin is pale, cool, and clammy, indicating poor peripheral perfusion.

You assign this patient a high priority because of his altered mental status, his rapid, shallow breathing, and his poor peripheral perfusion. You suspect shock and begin a rapid secondary assessment.

Heent. You note lip cyanosis, a sign of central hypoxia. You see no lip pursing, nasal flaring, or other signs of increased breathing effort, such as retractions or accessory muscle use. You smell no unusual odors or fluids from the mouth. The face is symmetrical; the pupils are equal and round but react to light sluggishly. The trachea is midline, there is no jugular venous distention (JVD).

Chest. You note symmetrical chest wall movement and an equal and adequate rise and fall of the chest with each ventilation. You note some crackles in the lung bases. Your patient has no surgical scars.

(continued)

Abdomen. You see no ascites or abdominal distention, no rigidity or guarding, no rebound tenderness, no renal or carotid bruits, no needle marks, no surgical scars or pulsating masses.

Pelvis. You see no evidence of bladder or bowel incontinence or of rectal bleeding.

Extremities. You notice no finger clubbing, no medical identification, no needle marks. Peripheral circulation is poor, with no radial or pedal pulses. You note no needle marks but some pitting edema in lower extremities.

Posterior. You note some edema in your patient's flanks.

Vital Signs. Heart rate, 46 and regular; blood pressure, 78/38 mmHg; respirations, 36 and shallow; pulse oximetry, 92 percent on room air, 99 percent with supplemental oxygen.

Additional. ECG monitor shows third-degree AV block; blood glucose, 110.

Your patient's wife reveals his long history of heart disease and a long list of cardiac medications. Your field diagnosis is cardiogenic shock resulting from the bradycardic rate of the third-degree block. While your partner initiates an IV, you set up for immediate external cardiac pacing.[6]

Reassessment

En route to the hospital, conduct an ongoing series of reassessments to detect trends, determine changes in your patient's condition, and assess the effectiveness of your interventions. Patient condition can change suddenly. You must steadfastly reassess mental status, airway patency, breathing adequacy, circulation, and any deterioration in areas that are already compromised (Procedure 7-4a). Conduct your reassessment every 15 minutes for stable patients, every 5 minutes for unstable patients. Compare your findings to the baseline findings and note any trends.

Mental Status

Recheck your patient's mental status by performing the AVPU exam frequently during transport. Any deterioration in mental status is cause for great concern. The brain demands a constant supply of oxygen and glucose and a constant elimination of waste products. When it is deprived of either, even briefly, expect rapid mental status changes. A falling level of response indicates either a direct or indirect brain pathology.

For example, following a head injury, your patient who was alert and oriented at the scene gradually becomes sleepy and eventually unarousable. You should suspect a life-threatening increase in intracranial pressure (pressure inside the enclosed skull) and expedite transport to the appropriate medical facility. Or, as another example, your patient with an intraabdominal hemorrhage becomes increasingly less arousable because of the decreased oxygenated blood flow to the brain (indirect pathology).

Sometimes patients improve following your interventions. After you administer 50 percent dextrose to your hypoglycemic diabetic patient, for instance, he becomes alert and begins talking.

CONTENT REVIEW

➤ Reassessment
- Detects trends
- Determines changes in patient's condition
- Assess effects of interventions

Airway Patency

The patency of your patient's airway can change instantly. Bleeding, vomiting, and even secretions can suddenly obstruct the upper airway. Be prepared to suction your patient quickly. Respiratory burns and anaphylaxis can cause life-threatening swelling in a matter of minutes. Croup and epiglottitis also can quickly deteriorate into total upper airway occlusion.

Endotracheal intubation is the best way to secure the airway in patients with no gag reflex. However, endotracheal tubes can become dislodged easily during transport. Recheck for tube placement frequently during transport and every time you move your patient onto a backboard, onto the stretcher, or onto the hospital gurney.

The price of proper airway management is eternal vigilance and a pessimistic outlook—anything that can go wrong will go wrong. Be prepared for the worst.

Breathing Rate and Quality

A change in respiratory rate or quality might indicate improvement or deterioration. A sudden increase in rate or respiratory effort suggests deterioration. For example, if your patient suddenly begins to gasp for air, has retractions, and uses his accessory neck muscles, he has a serious problem.

Sometimes the signs are not so obvious. Subtle increases in respiratory rate can suggest a developing problem. A decrease in rate and effort could mean that your treatments are effective and your patient is improving. For example, after you administer an albuterol treatment, your patient breathes easier and his lung sounds improve. In infants and young children, however, a decrease in rate and effort may mean that your patient is exhausted and requires aggressive intervention.

If, while assisting ventilation with a bag-valve mask, your partner suddenly complains that squeezing the bag is becoming more difficult, consider the possibility that a tension pneumothorax is developing or that bronchospasm or

Procedure 7-4 Reassessment

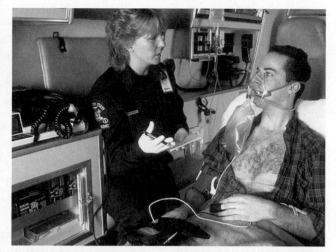

7-4a Reevaluate the ABCs.

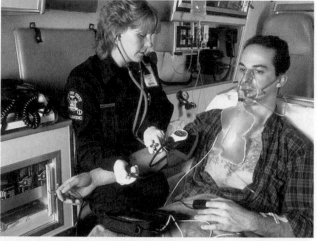

7-4b Take all vital signs again.

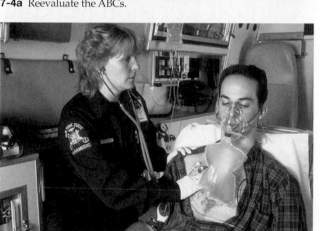

7-4c Perform your focused assessment again.

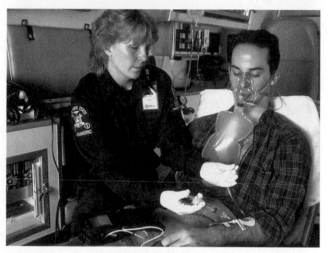

7-4d Evaluate your interventions' effects.

laryngospasm may be occurring. Airway and breathing management requires constant reevaluation.

Pulse Rate and Quality

Check central and peripheral pulses and compare the findings with earlier measurements. A rising pulse rate could indicate shock, hypoxia, or cardiac dysrhythmia. A falling rate could mean the terminal stage of shock or a rise in intracranial pressure. A sudden change in rate or regularity may suggest a cardiac dysrhythmia. The loss of peripheral pulses could mean decompensating shock.

Skin Condition

Similar to mental status, the skin quickly reflects the body's hemodynamic status. Reevaluate your patient's skin color, temperature, and condition. Cyanosis suggests decreased

oxygenation. Lip cyanosis indicates central hypoxia (overall oxygen status), whereas peripheral cyanosis indicates decreased oxygen to the tissues. Pallor and coolness suggest decreased circulation to the skin, as seen in shock.

If your patient suddenly develops hives after you administer a medication, suspect an allergic reaction. A localized redness and warmth could indicate bleeding under the skin or vasodilation. Cyanosis and coolness in a lower extremity suggest a peripheral vascular problem such as an arterial occlusion. A deep venous thrombosis will result in redness, swelling, and warmth in the lower leg.

Transport Priorities

Sometimes, stable patients suddenly deteriorate en route to the hospital. For example, the formerly conscious and alert head injury patient now responds only to pain. Or your stable cardiac patient suddenly develops a life-threatening arrhythmia. Or your patient suddenly cannot breathe because his simple pneumothorax has developed into a tension pneumothorax. In these cases, while you provide lifesaving treatments, change your transport decision to a higher priority. By the same token, if your unstable patient becomes stable, you may wish to downgrade your priority transport decision and decrease the danger and liability of driving with lights and siren on.

Vital Signs

Reassessing vital signs reveals trends clearly (Procedure 7-4b). A rising pulse rate combined with a falling blood pressure indicates shock. A decreasing pulse rate combined with a rising blood pressure, associated with an irregular respiratory pattern, suggests a rise in intracranial pressure. Any change in heart rate could indicate a cardiac dysrhythmia. A narrowing pulse pressure with a weakening pulse indicates cardiac tamponade, a tension pneumothorax, or hypovolemic shock.

Reevaluate your critical patient's vital signs every 5 minutes and look for changes, especially in his pulse oximetry.

Secondary Assessment

Elicit your patient's chief complaint again to determine whether the problem still exists or whether other problems have arisen. Often, following trauma, your patient will develop more complaints en route to the hospital as the excitement of the incident begins to wear off. Patients often focus on their major injuries and might not even be aware of other problems. Repeat your focused assessment as your patient's chief complaint dictates (Procedure 7-4c).

Effects of Interventions

Evaluate the effects of any interventions (Procedure 7-4d). Did the albuterol treatment help open the lower airways? Did the oxygen and nitroglycerin relieve the chest pain? What are the effects of the fluid challenge? Did your intervention help or harm your patient? Is he getting better or worse? Know the expected therapeutic benefits of your interventions, and then evaluate whether they worked. For example, you administer amiodarone to convert ventricular tachycardia. Following administration, observe your patient's electrocardiogram for changes while noting any harmful side effects, such as nausea, vomiting, or seizures.

Management Plans

Evaluate whether your care is working. If it is not, consider another management plan. Develop the courage to admit when your plan is not working and the flexibility to change your course of action. For example, your patient,

an elderly man with a history of congestive heart failure (CHF) and chronic obstructive pulmonary disease (COPD), presents with severe difficulty breathing and audible wheezing. You suspect he is having an exacerbation of his COPD and administer two nebulizer treatments and begin transporting. En route, however, he is not improving, and now you also can hear crackles bilaterally. At this point, you suspect he is in CHF and change your management to administering nitroglycerin and continuous positive airway pressure (CPAP).

Patients often present with multiple complaints, symptoms, and histories. Formulating a definitive diagnosis is difficult without the hospital's labs, X-rays, and other assessment tools. Your ability to reassess your patient, reevaluate your field diagnosis, and alter your management plan will optimize patient care.

Clinical Decision Making

Understanding the critical thinking process is essential for a paramedic. Your ability to analyze data effectively and devise a practical management plan optimizes patient care. You may be able to conduct the most comprehensive history and physical exam, but if you cannot analyze the data and devise the proper management plan, your efforts will be fruitless.

The critical thinking process has five steps: forming a concept, interpreting the data, applying the principles, evaluating the results, and reflecting on the incident. To explain the critical decision-making process, we will consider a 19-year-old female patient with a sudden onset of sharp pain to her right lower quadrant with some vaginal bleeding.

Form a Concept

The first step in critical decision making is to gather information and form a concept of your patient and the scene. You will get this information by assessing the general environment and the immediate surroundings. Note the mechanism of injury, if applicable. Then observe your patient's mental status, skin color, and positioning and note any deformities or asymmetry. In our sample case, your patient presents at home, sitting on a sofa. At first glance, she appears pale, diaphoretic, and anxious.

Next, you conduct a primary assessment, focusing on the MS-ABCs. Your initial goal is to identify and manage critical life threats. In this case, your general impression is of an alert and oriented but anxious young woman in moderate distress who presents with a clear airway; good air movement, as evidenced

CONTENT REVIEW
➤ Critical Thinking
 • Form a concept
 • Interpret the data
 • Apply principles
 • Evaluate results
 • Reflect on the incident

by her ability to converse in complete sentences; a strong, rapid, regular pulse; and cool, moist skin.

Ascertain your patient's chief complaint, history of present illness, past history, and current health status, while observing her affect (her general demeanor and attitude) and her degree of distress. You determine that her chief complaint is lower right quadrant pain that began suddenly 30 minutes ago. She also states she began bleeding at around the same time. She denies any nausea, vomiting, or diarrhea. You learn she has a past history of pelvic inflammatory disease and an active, unprotected sex life with multiple partners. Her last menstrual period was 6 weeks ago. She has had four pregnancies but no viable births. She appears in moderate distress.

Finally, you conduct a focused physical exam of the appropriate areas. This includes any diagnostic testing, such as an electrocardiogram, pulse oximetry, and blood glucose testing. You take a full set of vital signs, which can help you identify most life-threatening conditions. Remember that your patient's age, underlying physical and medical condition, and current medications can influence her vital signs. For example, the use of beta-blockers could cause a general decrease in her pulse and blood pressure.

Your patient has some deep palpation tenderness in the lower right quadrant but no rebound tenderness, and the rest of her abdomen is soft and nontender. She has minor bleeding at this time and has used only one sanitary pad since the bleeding began. Her vital signs are HR, 110 and regular; respirations 20, not labored; blood pressure 120/86 mmHg.

Interpret the Data

After you assess the patient, you will interpret all your data in light of your knowledge and experience. In this case, your knowledge base includes female reproductive anatomy, the physiology of a normal pregnancy, and the pathophysiology of pregnancy complications, along with their classic signs and symptoms. It also involves the anatomy, physiology, and pathophysiology of the cardiovascular system and the signs and symptoms of shock.

Your experience base includes every patient you have assessed and managed with a similar presentation. Your attitude toward managing patients with these symptoms also becomes a factor, because your experience may prejudice you.

Consider all the data and determine the most common and statistically probable conditions that fit your patient's initial presentation. This is your differential field diagnosis. Then, consider the most serious condition that fits your patient's situation. In our example, a field diagnosis of a ruptured ectopic pregnancy is obvious. When a clear medical diagnosis is elusive, base your treatment on the presenting signs and symptoms.

Apply the Principles

With your field diagnosis in mind, you devise a management plan that covers all contingencies. You will use written protocols, standing orders, and all the interventions at your disposal to manage your patient's particular problem.

Sometimes patients present with atypical signs and symptoms. For example, a patient who presents with a sore throat and cough may actually be having a heart attack and congestive heart failure. Other times, a protocol for your patient's problem simply may not exist. For example, your system may not have a protocol for facilitated intubation in head injuries. In these cases, consult with your medical direction physician for guidance in providing optimal care to your patient. The physician's emergency medical expertise and experience can be invaluable to you and your patient in unusual and difficult cases.

In our example, although your patient presents with relatively normal vital signs and is fully alert and oriented, you are very concerned. A basic principle of medicine is that all women of childbearing age with lower abdominal pain are pregnant until proven otherwise. You initiate advanced life support precautions en route to the hospital, including high-concentration oxygen if the patient becomes hypoxic, and two large-bore intravenous lines.

The patient's presentation has led you to expect the worst. If her fallopian tube ruptures and begins to hemorrhage, she will need rapid fluid resuscitation and general shock management. Your experience includes similar patients who suddenly suffered a life-threatening hemorrhage from a ruptured fallopian tube. Again, your attitude becomes a factor in that you will not allow her stable presentation to undermine your initial instinct—that she is potentially in serious trouble.

Evaluate the Results

During the reassessment, you reassess your patient's condition and the effects of your standing order/protocol interventions. In other words, you determine whether your treatment is improving your patient's condition and status. For example, has the albuterol helped your patient's breathing? Did the nitroglycerin and oxygen relieve the chest pain? Is the hemorrhage under control? Reflect on your actions and either continue your original plan, discontinue treatment, or take a completely different approach. You may alter your initial impression if your patient's condition worsens or if you discover new information. If time and circumstances allow a detailed exam, you may discover less obvious problems.

In our sample case, your patient remains in potentially unstable condition. Your reassessment shows that her vital signs are holding with the infusion of IV fluids. She is alert and not as anxious as before, and her skin is becoming warm and normal in color. You deliver her to the emergency department in stable, but guarded, condition.

Reflect on the Case

After the call, discuss your field diagnosis and care with the emergency physician. Compare your field diagnosis with his diagnosis. Conduct a run critique with your crew and discuss ways to improve your assessment and management of this case and future cases. Add these data to your information and experience base for future calls. Make every patient contact a learning experience. In this case, the emergency physician confirms your field diagnosis with lab tests and an ultrasound.

Clinical decision making is an essential paramedic skill that you will develop with time and experience. The prehospital environment is unlike any other medical care setting, and you will have to make decisions in less-than-optimal and sometimes dangerous conditions. Most times you will have the benefit of consulting with your medical direction physician in difficult and unusual situations; other times you may not.

Your ability to gather information, analyze it, and make a critical decision may someday make the difference between your patient's life and death. This is inevitable. How well you prepare for that challenge will determine your ultimate success. The process begins in your paramedic education program. You must develop a good working knowledge of anatomy, physiology, pathophysiology, and the principles of emergency medicine. In time, through repeated patient contacts, you will develop the clinical judgment you need to make effective patient care decisions.

The critical decision-making process involves a series of steps that experienced clinicians do almost unconsciously. First, you gather information (history and physical exam) to form an initial impression and then interpret it against your knowledge and experience to develop a working field diagnosis. You next apply the principles of emergency medicine to devise and implement a management plan and evaluate the effects of your treatments. Then you reevaluate and revise your plan as necessary. Finally, you compare your findings with the emergency physician's diagnosis and discuss alternate ways to manage similar patients. With every patient contact, your experience grows and your clinical judgment improves. This is the essence of paramedic practice.

Summary

Patient assessment is the key to providing effective prehospital emergency medical care. Its components include the primary assessment, the secondary assessment, vital signs, and reassessment. The primary assessment is designed to identify and treat life-threatening airway, breathing, and circulation problems. The secondary assessment is designed to identify the signs and symptoms surrounding your patient's chief complaint. It is a problem-oriented approach that is easily modified to match your patient's clinical situation. The reassessment is designed to reevaluate your patient for changes in status en route to the hospital.

The four general types of patients require distinctly different assessment approaches. The trauma patient with a significant mechanism of injury should receive a primary assessment, a rapid secondary assessment, and rapid transport. The patient with isolated, minor trauma, such as a cut finger or sprained ankle, should receive a physical exam focused on his particular problem or area. The responsive medical patient requires a primary assessment, a secondary assessment that focuses on his chief complaint, and vital signs. The unresponsive medical patient requires a primary assessment, followed by a rapid secondary assessment and rapid transport.

The patient assessment templates in this chapter are only guidelines. They do not dictate an exact procedure for assessing every patient. Instead, they provide general chronological guidelines to help you make critical transport and management decisions. As a paramedic, you will be expected to use clinical judgment when deciding which assessment tools to use for your particular patient and situation. With time and experience, you will become adept at assessing real patients in crisis. The more effective and efficient you become with this process, the better your patient care will be.

You Make the Call

You are dispatched to a motor vehicle collision on the highway that runs through your town. Law enforcement and fire resources are on scene already, however you are the first ambulance to arrive. As you approach the scene, a firefighter tells you "We have multiple patients, we are going to need another ambulance." Your partner contacts dispatch for additional resources while you continue to take report from the fire department first responder. He informs you that there are three patients.

The first patient was the restrained driver of a minivan who self-extricated and is standing near her vehicle. She is conscious, alert, and oriented and complains of isolated right wrist pain.

The second patient has also self-extricated, from the passenger seat of the minivan. She has a history of asthma and is complaining of shortness of breath following the accident. She is anxious, but denies any other pain or complaint, saying, "It's just the stress of the accident aggravating my asthma".

The final patient was the unrestrained driver of the other vehicle, a small sedan that hit the median at approximately 60 mph. He is unresponsive and shows signs of significant trauma.

1. Each of these patients will require a slightly different assessment approach. For each patient, outline the patient assessment format you would choose to use.

See Suggested Responses at the back of this book.

Review Questions

1. As you approach a scene, something just does not seem right. It is not anything you can put your finger on, just a sense that something is wrong or is about to happen. What should you do about it?
   a. Wait until law enforcement arrives before entering.
   b. Ignore your feelings and enter the scene.
   c. Enter the scene with something with which to protect yourself.
   d. Call out for the patient to come outside.

2. You are caring for a trauma patient whom you have categorized as a "priority patient" based on your primary assessment. In this situation, what type of physical exam will you perform during your secondary assessment?
   a. Detailed secondary assessment
   b. Focused secondary assessment
   c. Rapid secondary assessment
   d. No secondary assessment at all is performed on high-priority trauma patients.

3. Which of the following is a possible field diagnosis for a patient with inspiratory stridor?
   a. Epiglottitis   c. Asthma
   b. Bronchitis   d. Bronchiolitis

4. Your patient presents unconscious, without a gag reflex, and with a decreased minute volume. You should perform all of the following interventions *except* _____

   a. intubating the patient.
   b. bag-valve-mask ventilation.
   c. administering 100 percent oxygen.
   d. full immobilization of the patient.

5. Your patient presents with warm, pink skin, a radial pulse rate of 80/minute, and a capillary refill time of 2 seconds. From this information, what can you conclude about his circulatory condition?
   a. It is currently acceptable.
   b. It shows signs of spinal cord injury.
   c. It shows signs of diminished peripheral perfusion.
   d. The patient is in need of intravenous access and fluid therapy.

6. The rapid secondary assessment is designed to _____
   a. provide a detailed physical exam.
   b. identify the presence of any life-threatening injuries not found in the primary assessment.
   c. find and treat minor injuries.
   d. rule out the need for rapid transport.

7. Your patient presents with a major jugular vein laceration following a knife attack by an assailant. Your priority treatment for this injury is _____
   a. stopping the bleeding with a gauze pressure dressing.
   b. clamping the vessel with a hemostat.
   c. tying the vessel off with a surgical string.
   d. application of an occlusive dressing.

8. While assessing an unresponsive patient found in the park, you note that the patient's chest wall is not expanding normally, and, in fact, one section of the chest wall is moving in the opposite direction as the rest of the chest wall during breathing. This is a finding consistent with _____

    a. pneumothorax.

    b. diaphragmatic hernia.

    c. tracheobronchial tear.

    d. flail chest.

9. Your patient presents with jugular vein distention, absent breath sounds on the left side, diminished breath sounds on the right side, tachycardia, and profound hypotension. You should _____

    a. monitor and transport the patient to the trauma center.

    b. decompress the left chest immediately.

    c. place your patient on his right side.

    d. perform pericardiocentesis.

10. Which of the following is *not* a component of a SAMPLE history?

    a. Past medical history

    b. Medications

    c. Signs and symptoms

    d. Quality of pain experienced

11. Generally, when assessing a responsive medical patient, what part of your assessment often contributes the most significantly to your differential field diagnosis?

    a. Vital signs

    b. Medical interview findings

    c. Pulse oximetry and 12-lead ECG findings

    d. Physical assessment determinations

12. In a stable patient, which of the following findings is *least* contributory to arriving at a field diagnosis?

    a. Unilateral wheezing

    b. Tachycardia

    c. Blood glucose level of 368 mg/dL

    d. Abnormal capnogram

13. Your cardiac patient presents with jugular vein distention while sitting up. This finding is suggestive of _____

    a. right heart failure.

    b. left heart failure.

    c. simple pneumothorax.

    d. systemic hypertension.

14. A localized wheeze heard on auscultation could be the result of what pathology?

    a. Asthma

    b. Pneumonia

    c. Acute pulmonary edema

    d. COPD

15. In an unresponsive patient, the finding of pinpoint pupils could be part of a differential diagnosis of _____

    a. shock.

    b. anticholinergic poisoning.

    c. brain anoxia.

    d. narcotic overdose.

16. In a responsive patient with a complaint of abdominal pain, you should initiate your secondary assessment with _____

    a. assessment of the vital signs.

    b. determination of the SpO_2 and $ETCO_2$ values.

    c. obtaining the patient's medical history.

    d. establishing oxygen therapy, cardiac monitoring, and IV access.

17. The reassessment phase of patient assessment is designed to _____

    a. reevaluate the effectiveness of your interventions.

    b. detect trends in the patient's status.

    c. ascertain whether any new signs or symptoms have developed.

    d. all of the above.

18. You are transporting a patient with a chest injury following a motor vehicle crash. Your partner has intubated the patient and is performing bag-valve ventilation. He suddenly complains that the bag is becoming increasingly more difficult to squeeze. You reassess your patient and note pronounced JVD, tachycardia, and hypotension. The most likely cause for this sudden change in condition is _____

    a. pericardial tamponade.

    b. tension pneumothorax.

    c. massive hemothorax.

    d. diaphragmatic hernia.

19. What phase of assessment is performed in essentially the same manner for the stable or unstable patient suffering from either a trauma or a medical incident?

    a. Primary assessment

    b. Secondary assessment

    c. Obtaining vital signs

    d. Reassessment phase

See Answers to Review Questions at the back of this book.

References

1. Campbell, J. E. Alson, R. L. *International Trauma Life Support for Emergency Care Providers*, 8th ed. Upper Saddle River, NJ: Pearson/Prentice Hall, 2016.

2. Cordell, W. H., Hollingsworth, J. C, Olinger M. L., et al. "Pain and Tissue-Interface Pressures during Spine-Board Immobilization." *Ann Emerg Med* 1995;26(1): 31–36.

3. Luscombe, M. D., Williams J. L. "Comparison of a Long Spinal Board and Vacuum Mattress for Spinal Immobilisation." *Emerg Med J* 2003;20(5): 476–478.

4. Dalton, T. M., et al. *Advanced Medical Life Support*, 3rd ed. Upper Saddle River, NJ: Pearson/Prentice Hall, 2006.

5. Tintinalli, J. E., ed. *Tintinalli's Emergency Medicine: A Comprehensive Guide*, 7th ed. New York: McGraw-Hill, 2010.

6. Neumar, R. W., Shuster, M., Callaway, C. W., et al. Part 1: Executive Summary: 2015 American Heart Association Guidelines Update for Cardiopulmonary Resuscitation and Emergency Cardiovascular Care. *Circulation*. 2015;132:S315-S367.

Further Reading

Bledsoe, B. E. and R. W. Benner. *Critical Care Paramedic*. Upper Saddle River, NJ: Pearson/Prentice Hall, 2006.

Campbell, J. E. Alson, R. L. *International Trauma Life Support for Emergency Care Providers*, 8th ed. Upper Saddle River, NJ: Pearson/Prentice Hall, 2016.

Limmer, D., M. F. O'Keefe, et al. *Emergency Care*, 13th ed. Upper Saddle River, NJ: Pearson/Prentice Hall, 2015.

Mistovich, J., et al. *Prehospital Emergency Care,* 10th ed. Upper Saddle River, NJ: Pearson/Prentice Hall, 2013.

Prehospital Trauma Life Support, 7th ed. St. Louis: Mosby Lifeline, 2007.

Ralston, M., et al., eds. *Pediatric Advanced Life Support Provider Manual*. Dallas: American Heart Association, 2006.

Morrissey, J. Research Suggests Time for Change in Prehospital Spinal Immobilization. (Available at http://www.jems.com/articles/print/volume-38/issue-3/patient-care/research-suggests-time-change-prehospita.html, Accessed on August 13, 2015.)

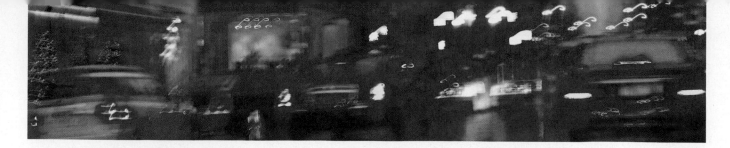

Precautions on Bloodborne Pathogens and Infectious Diseases

Prehospital emergency personnel, like all health care workers, are at risk for exposure to bloodborne pathogens and infectious diseases. In emergency situations it is often difficult to take or enforce proper infection control measures. However, as a paramedic, you must recognize your high-risk status. Study the following information on infection control carefully.

Infection control is designed to protect emergency personnel, their families, and their patients from unnecessary exposure to communicable diseases. Laws, regulations, and standards regarding infection control include:

- *Centers for Disease Control and Prevention (CDC) Guidelines.* The CDC has published extensive guidelines on infection control. Proper equipment and techniques that should be used by emergency response personnel to prevent or minimize risk of exposure are defined.

- *The Ryan White Act.* The Ryan White Act of 1990 allows emergency personnel to find out if they were exposed to an infectious disease while rendering patient care. Employers are required to name a "designated officer" to coordinate communications with the treating hospital.

- *Americans with Disabilities Act.* This act prohibits discrimination against individuals with disabilities, including those with contagious diseases. It guarantees equal employment opportunities and job protection if the infected individual can perform essential job functions and does not pose a threat to the safety and health of patients and coworkers.

- *Occupational Safety and Health Administration (OSHA) Regulations.* OSHA has enacted a regulation entitled Occupational Exposure to Bloodborne Pathogens that classifies emergency response personnel as being at the greatest risk of occupational exposure to communicable diseases. This regulation requires employers to provide hepatitis B (HBV) vaccinations free of charge, maintain a written exposure control plan, and provide personal protective equipment. These requirements primarily apply to private employers. Applicability to local and state governmental employees varies by locality. Many states have developed their own OSHA plans.

- *National Fire Protection Association (NFPA) Guidelines.* This is a national organization that has established specific guidelines and requirements regarding infection control for emergency response agencies, particularly fire departments and EMS services.

Standard Precautions and Personal Protective Equipment

Emergency response personnel should practice Standard Precautions by which ALL body substances are considered to be potentially infectious. To practice Standard Precautions, all emergency personnel should utilize personal protective equipment (PPE). Appropriate PPE should be available on every emergency vehicle. The minimum recommended PPE includes the following:

- *Gloves.* Disposable gloves should be donned by all emergency response personnel BEFORE initiating any emergency care. When an emergency incident involves more than one patient, you should attempt to change gloves between patients. When gloves have been contaminated, they should be removed as soon as possible. To properly remove contaminated gloves, grasp one glove approximately 1 inch from the wrist. Without touching the inside of the glove, pull the glove halfway off and stop. With that half-gloved hand, pull the glove on the opposite hand completely off. Place the removed glove in the palm of the other glove, with the inside of the removed glove exposed. Pull the second glove completely off with the ungloved hand, only touching the inside of the glove. Always wash hands after gloves are removed, even when the gloves appear intact.

- *Masks and Protective Eyewear.* Masks and protective eyewear should be present on all emergency vehicles and used in accordance with the level of exposure encountered. Masks and protective eyewear should be worn together whenever blood spatter is likely to occur, such as during arterial bleeding, childbirth, endotracheal intubation, invasive procedures, oral suctioning, and cleanup of equipment that requires heavy scrubbing or brushing. Both you and the patient should wear masks whenever the potential for airborne transmission of disease exists.

- *HEPA and N-95 Respirators.* Due to the resurgence of tuberculosis (TB), prehospital personnel should protect themselves from TB infection through use of an N-95 or a high-efficiency particulate air (HEPA) respirator, as approved by the National Institute of Occupational Safety and Health (NIOSH). It should fit snugly and be capable of filtering out the tuberculosis bacillus. An N-95 or HEPA respirator should be worn when caring for patients with confirmed or suspected TB. This is especially true when performing "high-hazard" procedures such as administration of nebulized medications, endotracheal intubation, or suctioning on such a patient.

- *Gowns.* Gowns protect clothing from blood splashes. If large splashes of blood are expected, such as with childbirth, wear impervious gowns.

- *Resuscitation Equipment.* Disposable resuscitation equipment should be the primary means of artificial ventilation in emergency care. Such items should be used once, then disposed of.

Remember, the proper use of personal protective equipment ensures effective infection control and minimizes risk. Use ALL protective equipment recommended for any particular situation to ensure maximum protection.

Consider ALL body substances potentially infectious and ALWAYS practice Standard Precautions.

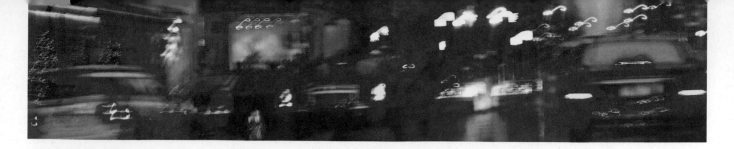

Suggested Responses to "You Make the Call"

The following are suggested responses to the "You Make the Call" scenarios presented in each chapter of Volume 2, Patient Assessment. Each represents an acceptable response to the scenario but should not be interpreted as the only correct response.

Chapter 1—Scene Size-Up

1. *Describe how you would size up this scene. Make sure you cover the following areas:*

   - *Vehicle placement*
   - *Initial radio report*
   - *Assuming incident command*
   - *Safety*
   - *Hazard control*
   - *Standard Precautions*
   - *Location and triaging of patients*
   - *Mechanism of injury*
   - *Resource determination*

Initially, it is appropriate to park the ambulance past the incident, if at all possible. Parking past the incident allows for easy egress from the scene when needed, and allows space for other resources as they arrive.

Next, you want to try to do a "windshield assessment" by looking at the scene to determine what, if any, additional resources you will need. Given the location of the vehicle, the presence of standing water, and the potential for multiple patients, it would be reasonable to request additional fire and EMS resources at this time. If an initial radio report describing the scene has not been given, it is appropriate to contact dispatch and briefly describe what you see so all incoming units are advised of the situation. At major scenes it is important to identify yourself as Incident Command and direct the scene until relieved by higher ranking personnel.

There are multiple safety considerations at this scene. First, the inclement weather and nighttime conditions make visibility a concern. All appropriate emergency lights should be utilized, and all personnel should wear reflective safety vests. The standing water is also a safety concern, as multiple objects or debris could be hidden under the water. Depending on the depth of the water, this situation may be considered a water rescue, requiring trained responders. The stability of the vehicle should also be established and maintained, as vehicle movement may pose a hazard to responders.

The location and triage of patients may prompt you to expand your requested resources, or cancel resources en-route if no further patients are found. By looking at the mechanism of injury, you can gain a high index of suspicion as to which patients should be higher priority. It may be necessary to establish an incident command structure, should this be determined a multiple casualty incident. Standard precautions should be taken by all responders, and special equipment, such as leather gloves, rain gear, or helmets may be required.

Chapter 2—Primary Assessment

1. *How would you describe this patient's respiratory status? What factors influence this determination? What immediate interventions, if any, would you provide at this time?*

This patient is in respiratory failure. Although his respiratory rate is technically within normal limits, he shows multiple other signs of impending respiratory arrest. The patient is obviously fatigued, evidenced by his head bobbing with each breath and accessory muscle use. You also have information from the patient's mother that the asthma attack has been ongoing for "several hours".

Immediate interventions for this patient include positive pressure ventilation, either via CPAP or a bag-valve-mask. Nebulized bronchodilators should be administered per local protocols. If respiratory arrest appears imminent, epinephrine should be considered and advanced airway management devices should be prepared.

Chapter 3—Therapeutic Communications

1. *Would you allow the patient's father to ride in the ambulance to the hospital? What communication techniques could you use when navigating the situation?*

The patient's body language combined with the father's anger and agitation indicate that it may be best to separate the patient from his father. It would be appropriate to suggest to the father that he follow in his own vehicle, or ride with another family member. Reassuring the father that the best possible care will be given may be helpful. It may also be helpful to calmly and firmly tell the father that there is not room for additional passengers in the ambulance. If it is necessary to take the father in the ambulance, it would likely benefit the patient to ensure that the father rides in the front passenger seat, rather than the patient compartment.

2. *List out your strategies for communicating with this patient, given that he is crying and not readily answering your questions.*

It will be important to be extremely patient and gentle in your questioning of this patient. Acknowledging the legitimacy of your patient's feeling may be helpful. Simply saying "I can see that you are upset and need to cry right now. If you feel up to answering some questions, it would be helpful, but I understand if you'd rather just be quiet."

Chapter 4—History Taking

1. *What potential challenges does this patient present with regards to history taking? List at least three, and describe your strategies for effectively overcoming these challenges.*

History taking challenges with this patient include:

- Residence in a skilled nursing facility. Although these facilities often have detailed medical records for their patients, this is not always the case. It is also possible that the staff member you interact with is not familiar with the patient's history or medications. It may be helpful to request to see the patient's actual paper file, or view the computer-based chart to see recent medications, vital signs, etc.

- Altered mental status. Obtaining a history from a patient who is confused may be difficult. The patient may not be an accurate historian, so other resources should be utilized. Facility staff may provide some information. It may also be helpful to obtain the phone number of a family member who you can call for additional information regarding the patient's health.

- Hearing impairment. It will be necessary to speak slowly and clearly, when questioning this patient. Checking to ensure that her hearing aides are turned on and not out of battery power may also be helpful.

Chapter 5—Secondary Assessment

1. *A thorough physical exam involves auscultation, inspection, palpation, and percussion. Beginning with the head, list specifically what you will assess for in each area of the body. Identify the exam technique you will use. For example, you may assess the chest for the presence of a flail segment by palpation.*

- Head
  - Palpate for pain, tenderness, crepitus, etc.
  - Inspect for bruising, bleeding, abrasions, lacerations, etc.

- Neck
  - Inspect for jugular venous distension, tracheal deviation, signs of trauma, etc.
  - Palpate for pain, tenderness, crepitus, etc.

- Chest (Anterior/posterior)
  - Palpate for pain, tenderness, crepitus, presence of a flail section, etc.
  - Inspect for punctures, penetrations, lacerations, etc.
  - Auscultate for lung sounds and heart tones
  - Percuss for possible hemo/pneumothorax.

- Abdomen
  - Palpate for pain, tenderness, rigidity, guarding, etc.
  - Inspect for bruising, abrasions, punctures, etc.
  - Auscultate for bowel sounds

- Pelvis
  - Palpate for pain, tenderness, crepitus, etc.
  - Inspect for incontinence, bleeding, bruising

- Extremities
  - Palpate for pain, tenderness, crepitus, etc.
  - Inspect for bruising, deformities, lacerations, swelling, etc.

Chapter 6—Patient Monitoring Technology

1. *What technological monitoring devices would you use for this patient?*

This patient is unresponsive and requires the full range of available diagnostic testing. Blood glucose determination, cardiac monitoring including a 12 lead EKG, end tidal capnography, pulse oximetry, and temperature should all be obtained with this young man.

Chapter 7—Patient Assessment in the Field

1. *Each of these patients will require a slightly different assessment approach. For each patient, outline the patient assessment format you would choose to use.*

Patient one has an isolated extremity injury. As such, she requires a primary assessment followed by a focused secondary exam centered on her area of injury. Patient two appears to be a conscious medical patient who may have associated trauma. This patient requires a primary assessment followed by a detailed secondary assessment to identify any further complaints. The final patient is an unresponsive trauma patient who requires a primary exam, rapid secondary exam, and rapid transport.

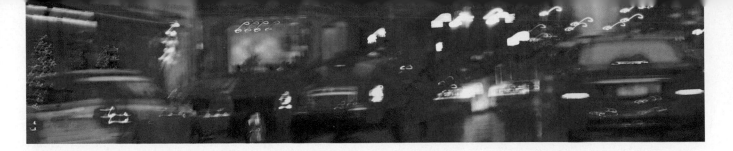

Answers to Review Questions

Below are the answers to the Review Questions presented in each chapter of Volume 2.

Chapter 1—Scene Size-Up

1. c
2. a
3. d
4. a
5. d
6. d
7. b
8. a
9. a
10. d

Chapter 2—Primary Assessment

1. d
2. c
3. a
4. c
5. a
6. d
7. c
8. d
9. d
10. c
11. b
12. d
13. b
14. d
15. b

Chapter 3—Therapeutic Communications

1. c
2. c
3. a
4. d
5. b
6. c
7. b
8. b
9. b
10. c

Chapter 4—History Taking

1. d
2. d
3. c
4. b
5. a
6. c
7. c

Matching

1. c
2. e
3. h
4. g
5. a
6. d
7. b
8. f

Chapter 5—Secondary Assessment

1. b
2. a
3. c
4. a
5. b
6. d
7. a
8. b
9. c
10. c
11. a
12. b
13. c
14. b
15. b
16. b
17. c
18. b
19. c
20. b

Chapter 6—Patient Monitoring Technology

1. b
2. d
3. b
4. c
5. d
6. a
7. d
8. b
9. b
10. d
11. a
12. c
13. a
14. b
15. b
16. c
17. c
18. a
19. b
20. a

Chapter 7—Patient Assessment in the Field

1. a
2. c
3. a
4. d
5. a

6. b
7. d
8. d
9. b
10. d
11. b
12. b

13. a
14. b
15. d
16. c
17. d
18. b
19. a

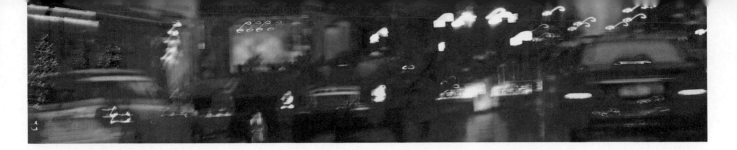

Glossary

advanced life support   life-support activities that go beyond basic procedures to include adjunctive equipment and invasive procedures.

afterload   resistance in the blood vessels that the heart must overcome to eject blood.

aphasia   defective language caused by neurologic damage to the brain.

arterial blood gas (ABG)   dissolved gases in the arterial circulation.

artifact   deflection on the ECG produced by factors other than the heart's electrical activity.

ascites   bulges in the flanks and across the abdomen, indicating edema caused by congestive heart failure.

augmented leads   another term for unipolar leads, reflecting the fact that the ground lead is disconnected, which increases the amplitude of deflection on the ECG tracing.

auscultation   listening with a stethoscope for sounds produced by the body.

Babinski's response   big toe dorsiflexes and the other toes fan out when the sole is stimulated.

bipolar leads   ECG leads applied to the arms and legs that contain one positive electrode and one negative electrode; leads I, II, and III.

blood pressure   force of blood against arteries' walls as the heart contracts and relaxes.

blood tube   glass container with color-coded, self-sealing rubber top.

B-natriuretic peptide   peptide found in the ventricles of the heart; increases when ventricular filling pressures are high; can be used to detect congestive heart failure.

borborygmi   loud, prolonged, gurgling bowel sounds, indicating hyperperistalsis.

bradycardia   pulse rate lower than 60.

bradypnea   slow breathing.

bronchophony   abnormal clarity of the patient's transmitted voice sounds.

Broselow tape   a measuring tape for infants that provides important information regarding airway equipment and medication doses based on the patient's length.

bruit   sound of turbulent blood flow around a partial obstruction.

carboxyhemoglobin   hemoglobin with carbon monoxide bound.

cardiac output   the amount of blood the heart ejects each minute, measured in milliliters.

chief complaint   the pain, discomfort, or dysfunction that caused the patient to request help.

circulation assessment   evaluation of the pulse and skin and control of hemorrhage.

closed questions   questions that ask for specific information and require only very short or yes-or-no answers; also called *direct questions*.

closed stance   a posture or body position that is tense and suggests negativity, discomfort, fear, disgust, or anger.

communication   the exchange of common symbols—written, spoken, or other kinds, such as signing and body language.

crackles   light crackling, popping, nonmusical sounds heard usually during inspiration; also called *rales*.

creatine kinase   isoenzyme important in energy utilization.

crepitus   crunching sounds of unlubricated parts in joints rubbing against each other.

Cullen's sign   discoloration around the umbilicus (occasionally the flanks) suggestive of intraabdominal hemorrhage.

cultural imposition   the imposition of one's beliefs, values, and patterns of behavior on people of another culture.

decerebrate   arms and legs extended.

decode   interpret a message.

decorticate   arms flexed, legs extended.

delirium   an acute alteration in mental functioning that is often reversible.

dementia   a deterioration of mental status that is usually associated with structural neurologic disease.

deoxyhemoglobina   hemoglobin with no oxygen bound.

depolarization   process in which electrolytes cross cell membranes and cause a shift in polarity.

depression a mood disorder characterized by hopelessness and malaise.

diastole phase of cardiac cycle when ventricles relax.

diastolic blood pressure force of blood against arteries when ventricles relax.

differential field diagnosis the list of possible causes for the patient's symptoms.

diuretic a medication that stimulates the kidneys to excrete water.

dysarthria defective speech caused by motor deficits.

dysmenorrhea difficult or painful menstruation.

dysphonia voice changes caused by vocal cord problems.

dyspnea the sensation of having difficulty breathing.

edema presence of an abnormal amount of fluid in the tissues.

egophony abnormal change in tone of the patient's transmitted voice sounds.

Einthoven's triangle the triangle around the heart formed by the bipolar leads.

electrodes adhesive pads, containing conductive gel, that stick to the patient's skin.

electrolyte substance that takes on a charge when dissolved in water.

empathy identification with and understanding of another's situation, feelings, and motives.

encode create a message.

ethnocentrism viewing one's own way of life as the most desirable, acceptable, or best, and acting in a superior manner to another culture's way of life.

feedback a response to a message.

focused history and physical exam problem-oriented assessment process based on initial assessment and chief complaint.

general impression the initial, intuitive evaluation of the patient.

glycogenolysis process in which glucagon is released into the bloodstream.

Grey Turner's sign discoloration over the flanks, suggesting intraabdominal bleeding.

hazardous materials substances that cause adverse health effects upon human exposure.

HEENT head, eyes, ears, nose, and throat.

hematemesis vomiting of blood.

hematuria blood in the urine.

heme iron-based structure where oxygen binds to hemoglobin.

hemoconcentration elevated numbers of red and white blood cells.

hemolysis the destruction of red blood cells.

hemoptysis coughing up of blood.

hypertension blood pressure higher than normal.

hyperthermia increase in the body's core temperature.

hypotension blood pressure lower than normal.

hypothermia decrease in the body's core temperature.

index of suspicion anticipation of possible injuries based on analysis of the event.

inspection the process of informed observation.

intermittent claudication intermittent calf pain while walking, which subsides with rest.

ischemia deprivation of oxygen to the myocardium.

Korotkoff sounds sounds of blood hitting arterial walls.

lactic dehydrogenase enzyme found in heart muscle, skeletal muscle, liver, erythrocytes, kidney, and some types of tumors.

leading questions questions framed to guide the direction of a patient's answers.

leads color-coded wires that connect to an ECG machine.

major trauma patient person who has suffered significant injury.

mechanism of injury combined strength, direction, and nature of forces that injured the patient.

methemoglobin hemoglobin that is oxidized.

multidraw needle long, exposed needle that screws into a vacutainer and is inserted directly into a vein.

myocardium the cardiac muscle tissue of the heart.

myoglobin heme protein found in striated muscle; contains iron, stores oxygen, gives muscle its red color.

nocturia excessive urination at night.

nonverbal communications gestures, mannerisms, and postures by which a person communicates with others; sometimes called *body language*.

open stance a posture or body position that is relaxed and suggests confidence, ease, warmth, and attentiveness.

open-ended questions questions that permit unguided, spontaneous answers.

ophthalmoscope handheld device used to examine the interior of the eye.

orthopnea difficulty breathing while lying supine.

otoscope handheld device used to examine the interior of the ears and nose.

oxyhemoglobin hemoglobin with oxygen bound.

palpation using one's sense of touch to gather information.

paroxysmal nocturnal dyspnea sudden onset of shortness of breath at night.

patient assessment problem-oriented evaluation of patient and establishment of priorities based on existing and potential threats to human life.

percussion the production of sound waves by striking one object against another.

perfusion passage of blood through an organ or tissue.

personal protective equipment (PPE) equipment designed to protect against infection. The minimum recommended PPE includes protective gloves, masks and protective eyewear, HEPA and N-95 respirators, gowns, and disposable resuscitation equipment.

pleural friction rub   the squeaking or grating sound of the pleural linings rubbing together.

polyuria   excessive urination.

precordial (chest) leads   ECG leads applied to the chest in a pattern that permits a view of the horizontal plane of the heart.

preload   amount of blood returned to the heart from the body; also known as *end-diastolic pressure*.

priapism   a painful and prolonged erection of the penis.

primary assessment   prehospital process designed to identify and correct life-threatening airway, breathing, and circulation problems.

primary problem   the underlying cause for the patient's symptoms.

pulse oximetry   a measurement of hemoglobin oxygen saturation in the peripheral tissues.

pulse pressure   difference between systolic and diastolic pressures.

pulse quality   strength of the pulse, which can be weak, thready, strong, or bounding.

pulse rate   number of pulses felt in 1 minute.

pulse rhythm   pattern and equality of intervals between beats.

quality of respiration   depth and pattern of breathing.

rapid secondary assessment   quick check for signs of serious injury.

referred pain   pain that is felt in a location away from its source.

respiration   exchange of oxygen and carbon dioxide in the lungs and at the cellular level.

respiratory effort   how hard the patient works to breathe.

respiratory rate   number of times the patient breathes in 1 minute.

rhonchi   continuous sounds with a lower pitch and a snoring quality.

scene safety   steps taken to ensure a safe environment at the site of an emergency.

semi-Fowler's position   sitting up at 45 degrees.

sphygmomanometer   blood pressure measuring device comprising a bulb, a cuff, and a manometer.

Standard Precautions   a strict form of infection control based on the assumption that all blood and other body fluids are infectious.

stethoscope   tool used to auscultate most sounds.

stridor   predominantly inspiratory wheeze associated with laryngeal obstruction.

stroke volume   the amount of blood the heart ejects in one beat.

subcutaneous emphysema   crackling sensation caused by air just underneath the skin.

systole   phase of cardiac cycle when ventricles contract.

systolic blood pressure   force of blood against arteries when ventricles contract.

tachycardia   pulse rate higher than 100.

tachypnea   rapid breathing.

tenderness   pain that is elicited through palpation.

thrill   vibration or humming felt when palpating the pulse.

tidal volume   amount of air one breath moves in and out of the lungs.

tinnitus   the sensation of ringing in the ears.

troponins   contractile proteins of the myofibril.

ultrasound   use of high frequency sound waves to produce images of internal body structures.

unipolar leads   ECG leads applied to the arms and legs, consisting of one polarized (positive) electrode and a nonpolarized reference point created by the ECG machine combining two additional electrodes; also called augmented leads; leads aVR, aVL, and aVF.

vacutainer   device that holds blood tubes.

visual acuity wall chart/card   wall chart or handheld card with lines of letters, used to test vision.

vital statistics   weight and height.

wheezes   continuous, high-pitched musical sounds similar to a whistle.

whispered pectoriloquy   abnormal clarity of the patient's transmitted whispers.

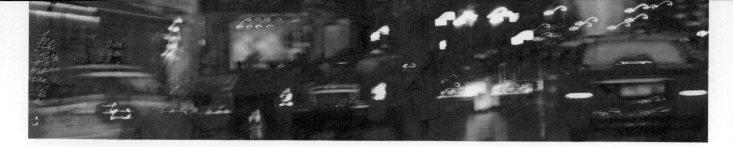

Index